REPRODUCTIVE GENETICS
AND THE LAW

Reproductive Genetics and the Law

SHERMAN ELIAS, M.D.
Director, Division of Reproductive Genetics
Professor of Obstetrics and Gynecology
College of Medicine
University of Tennessee, Memphis
Memphis, Tennessee

GEORGE J. ANNAS, J.D., M.P.H.
Edward Utley Professor of Health Law
Boston University School of Medicine
Chief, Health Law Section
Boston University School of Public Health
Boston, Massachusetts

YEAR BOOK MEDICAL PUBLISHERS, INC.
CHICAGO · LONDON · BOCA RATON

We dedicate this book, with love, to

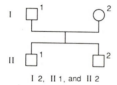

I 2, II 1, and II 2

and

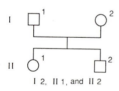

I 2, II 1, and II 2

1 2 3 4 5 6 7 8 9 0   91 90 89 88 87

Library of Congress Cataloging-in-Publication Data

Elias, Sherman.
  Reproductive genetics and the law.

  Bibliography: p.
  Includes index.
  1. Medical genetics—Law and legislation—United
States.   I. Annas, George J.   II. Title.
[DNLM: 1.   Genetics, Medical—legislation.
3.   Perinatology—legislation.   QZ 32.4. E42r]
KF3827.G4E44   1987   344.73'0419   86-28185
ISBN 0-8151-3062-7   347.304419

Sponsoring Editor: James D. Ryan, Jr.
Manager, Copyediting Services: Frances M. Perveiler
Production Manager, Text and Reference/Periodicals: Etta Worthington
Proofroom Supervisor: Shirley E. Taylor

FOREWORD

The title of Aldous Huxley's *Brave New World* is frequently invoked by those who are intrigued—or appalled—by the new genetics. The novel depicts a world in which humans are engineered in laboratories according to the formulae of mysterious and distant rulers. But Huxley took his title from Shakespeare's *The Tempest*. When Miranda, who has seen no humans other than her father, Prospero, and her beloved Ferdinand, beholds the retinue of noble gentlemen cast by the storm upon her remote island, she exclaims, "O, wonder! how many goodly creatures are there here! How beauteous mankind is! O brave new world, that has such people in't" (Act V, Scene 1). Since her infancy, she has dwelt with Caliban, Ariel and other creatures "engineered" by her father's magic art. She is now astonished, not at these strange and bizarre monsters with whom she has lived all her young life, but at quite normal, ordinarily proportioned, and modestly talented human beings.

When commentators on modern genetic science appropriate Miranda's exclamation, the meaning is reversed. The "creatures" of the brave new world are those shaped by the magic of genetic science. We wonder whether that magic is white or black, whether the creatures will be monstrous Calibans or enchanting Ariels. The commentators on genetic science ponder this question incessantly. Scientists will sometimes join them, but more often disclaim any intent or possibility of undoing the frame and structure of the human race in any malevolent way. The philosophers speculate about ambiguities latent in plans to "improve" and "cure;" the moralists raise the specter of eugenics. The debate is complex and often inconclusive. The original meaning of Miranda's words is lost. It may be helpful to recall that original meaning: a naive, innocent astonishment at normal, ordinary, imperfect, and sometimes ugly and evil, humans.

George Annas and Sherman Elias have written a book that, in my judgment, restores something of the original sense of Miranda's exclamation (even though they too invoke Huxley's title in its more ominous sense).

They describe the science of genetics and its diagnostic and therapeutic implications; they discuss the legal, ethical, and policy implications of the science. In their treatment of all this, there is a tone of calm normalcy, an appreciation of common sense. This is so because they place the admittedly extraordinary developments of genetics into the familiar world of medicine, attempting to cure obvious disease and relieve manifest pain and suffering. Chapters on genetic counseling and screening and on prenatal diagnosis focus on problems that are so obviously distressing and devastating that the specter of "eliminating the defective in order to create a perfect human race" fails to appear. Chapters on the more exotic forms of genetic manipulation, such as artificial reproduction and gene therapy, avoid the hysterical speculations about cloning and fabrication of subhumans and superhumans that often trouble their commentators. Similarly, the discussion of the legal and policy aspects of genetic developments remains within the realm of sound analysis of current law and realistic views of the capabilities of the persons and society. Throughout the book "the brave new world" is peopled with parents, infants, fetuses, and physicians striving to be "goodly creatures," that is, to struggle free of the ravages of disease and defect, and to live normally.

Still, all is not normal. Genetic science does reveal previously unimaginable facts and makes possible previously impossible modifications of nature. This is a science that, while presently dedicated to the removal of obvious abnormalities, can venture beyond the bounds of what we presently see as normal and natural. Even though Annas and Elias do not dwell on the challenge to common concepts of the normal, they are quite aware of it, and from time to time, allude to the issues that will have to be faced by ethics, law, and public policy. One of the difficulties that bedevils the debates over the new genetic science is the inability to recognize and appreciate the scope and range of normal human existence. Philosophers reveal the conceptual complexity of "norm," "normative," and "normal," as well as "nature," and "natural." They have taught us too well: acknowledging the complexity of the concept of normal, we abjure the concept as meaningless. Thus, when we find ourselves called upon to make judgments about previously inconceivable modes of human reproduction or modifications of human traits, we have no base; no solid ground from which our minds venture out.

One of the characters in *The Tempest*, Duke Alonso, says of the events related in the play, "this is as strange a maze as e'er men trod; and there is in this business more than nature was ever conduct of." But, he then goes on, "some oracle must rectify our knowledge" (Act V, Scene 1). It is obvious that we must rectify our knowledge about genetic science: the science will advance and the technological possibilities will grow. We must understand and direct these advances and possibilities. Policies must be devised, judgments rendered, laws enacted. We must do all this wisely and prudently, seeking to achieve benefits for persons and society and to avoid harms. How can the mind be rectified to enable it to perform so complex a task?

Shakespeare was inspired to write *The Tempest* by popular accounts of adventures in the new world. His magical island is "the still-vexed Bermoothes," or Bermuda, and his description of its indigenous creatures was modeled on reports about the "Indians." When European explorers first encountered the inhabitants of the lands that they "discovered," they were faced with a legal, ethical and policy problem of monumental proportions. They were quite uncertain what these creatures were, whose customs were so foreign and who had no knowledge of the Gospel. How were Christian men to deal with these natives? How did the concepts of rule, law and right pertain to them?

The problem was taken seriously. In 1539, the King of Spain commissioned one of the leading theologians of the time to prepare a *Report on the Indies* in which the dictates of "the law of nature and of mankind" were applied to the relationship between the Europeans and Americans. The author proceeded not by creating some grand theory, but by careful examination of the various situations or cases that might arise as Europeans and Americans encountered each other. This substantial treatise made a strong case in favor of the rights of the original inhabitants, and delineated the ethical principles that should govern dealings with them. The ethical argument was not as strong as the greed of the conquistadores, but the moral situation of those "discoverers" who faced a "brave new world" is similar to that of the scientific discoverers facing the new world of genetic science and technology.

The similarity lies in the absence of a known starting place from which to move into the new world. The Europeans were uncertain whether the native Americans should be considered "human," since, in their belief, the Gospel had been proclaimed to all members of the human race. Today we lack a sufficiently strong concept of the human to provide the basis for judgment about the departures from "normal" that genetic science makes possible. Yet, even lacking so fundamental a concept, the rectification of the mind about these issues can take place. It moves from cases and problems about the morality of which we are relatively satisfied, to cases which are more complex and perplexing. The creation of an ethics of genetics is, then, a kind of "casuistry." It eschews the building of a grand theory and inclines to the careful examination of cases: well-described examples of the sorts of information genetic science can provide, and of the effects genetic technology can produce.

Making no pretense to be the "oracle" that Duke Alonso desired, the book that George Annas and Sherman Elias have written is nonetheless a solid contribution to the rectification of mind that the Duke hoped for and that we need. While not primarily about the ethics of genetics, the authors refer to ethical problems again and again. The book is about science, the ways in which the accomplishments of the science of genetics affect the law and public policy, and the ways in which law and public policy can affect the human uses of the science of genetics. The authors thus feel no compulsion to elaborate a comprehensive theory of either law or ethics. This is a virtue, for they describe the science well, present realistic scenarios of the technological possibilities, and analyze and place in perspective already decided legal cases.

Proceeding in this fashion, they have initiated the casuistry that is required to build the law, ethics, and public policy of genetics. By careful description and analysis of scientific data and cases that have raised questions sufficiently grave to be brought to the court, a body of both fact and principle is collected. Several important principles, on which there is broad social consensus, are woven into these analyses: the principle of personal autonomy, realized in informed consent and in reproductive freedom, and the principle of pluralism of values in our society, together with the judiciously applied right of legitimate authority to protect society against serious threats to well-being. By staying close to the science and the cases, and by continually alluding to basic principle, rather than by moving at high levels of theory and generalization, Annas and Elias begin to collect the pieces that may eventually fit together into an oracular view of the human implications of the science and art of reproductive genetics.

ALBERT R. JONSEN, PH.D.
Professor of Ethics in Medicine
Chief, Division of Medical Ethics
University of California, San Francisco

PREFACE

Our increasing ability to control our reproduction and to determine prenatally the genetic endowment of our children changes both the practice of medicine and the concept of humanness. How should we as a society react to the new options and new dilemmas delivered by the "new genetics?" What information should couples have about their own genetic makeup and that of their fetuses and prospective children? Should laws require that all newborns, adults, and pregnant women be screened for genetic diseases? When should prenatal diagnosis be offered? Should limits be placed on reproductive liberty? What rights should handicapped newborns have? How can pregnant workers be protected from teratogens without discriminating against them? Should we encourage the development of new reproductive technologies that permit reproduction without sex? What should be the legal relevance of genetic connections between parents and offspring? Can we pursue fetal and gene therapy without compromising the rights of pregnant women?

These are just a few of the questions that both of us had dealt with individually before we met in 1980 and decided to write this book. There is considerable literature on the general subject of "Reproductive Genetics and the Law," but almost all of it suffers from extreme professional bias. Medical and scientific writers tend to ignore social policy issues, and lawyers and ethicists tend to misunderstand or ignore medical and scientific facts. Sound social policy (generally enunciated in law) must be based on an accurate and adequate understanding of relevant scientific facts. Developing social policy and law in the area of human reproduction requires an understanding of basic human genetics, and the medical principles and practices involved in screening, prenatal diagnosis, prenatal treatment, treatment of handicapped newborns, noncoital reproduction, and teratology.

Neither of us felt competent to attack this huge subject alone, and it would be presumptuous to contend that we have succeeded in conquering it. That was never a realistic goal. But we believe this collaboration of an obstetrician/geneticist and a health lawyer/medical ethicist has produced a unified and balanced summary of both the state of the art and the state of law, together with constructive suggestions that point in the general direction in which we should proceed as a society. It was our goal to present both sides of arguments where there are major disputes, but always to present our own views as well, together with the reasons for them. By working closely together, and by continuing our discussions until we ourselves reached agreement, we think we have been able to avoid the "Polyphemus syndrome:" the one-eyed view of the barbaric Cyclops who threatened to consume Ulysses and his entire crew for no reason other than that it pleased him. We believe that a subject as complex as social policy relating to human reproduction requires a "two-eyed" view, one that recognizes the problems faced by both law and medicine; one that takes pains to understand science and medical practice before making social policy regarding its use.

As "warm-up exercises" for this book, we wrote articles for the *Family Law Quarterly*, the *American Journal of Public Health*, the *American Journal of Obstetrics and Gynecology*, and the *Journal of the American Medical Association*. Almost none of the first article remains in this book, but much of the latter three can be found in updated and revised forms in Chapters 4, 9, and 10. We also developed two continuing education programs together (at Northwestern University School of Medicine), and worked together on presentations at international conferences in Dublin, Ireland, Rappallo, Italy, and Sydney, Australia, and national meetings in Boston, Chicago, San Francisco and Las Vegas. But the major project has always been this book. It is primarily directed to medical practitioners, genetic counselors, and their patients, as well as those interested in public policy and legal regulation. We believe that anyone contemplating having a child will also find this book valuable.

In keeping with our belief that a sound scientific basis is a prerequisite for sound social policy, the book begins with a chapter on the principles of human genetics. This chapter can, of course, be skipped by those familiar with this material. The next four chapters deal with the "nuts and bolts" of current social policy and medical practice: genetic counseling, genetic screening, and prenatal diagnosis. Two chapters then address the most controversial legal disputes in medicine: reproductive liberty and the treatment of handicapped newborns. The most recent U.S. Supreme Court decisions on abortion and the "Baby Doe" regulations are addressed in these chapters. The final three chapters deal with newer medical areas that are socially underdeveloped: teratology, noncoital reproduction, and fetal and gene therapy. Each of these chapters may be read independently, and all are cross-referenced where appropriate. Throughout the book we have attempted to interweave scientific fact with social policy discussion. Most chapters begin with a discussion of the current state of the art, and only thereafter entertain a discussion of social policy options.

Although we profess to take the "two-eyed view" of issues, we do have an overall perspective. We believe three general guidelines should inform policy development for reproductive genetics. The first is that the primary human value that should be protected is individual privacy, the "right to be left alone." Individuals should have the right to *refuse* any and all genetic interventions because of their interest in personal dignity and bodily integrity, and decisions to perform a medical or genetic intervention should always be *joint* decisions between the patient and the physician. The second guide is the principle of pluralism, which respects personal autonomy but recognizes the legitimacy of social rules to protect society's well-being. The third is that the "best interests" of the prospective child should be of paramount concern in policy formation. As will be seen, these guidelines do not answer every quandary addressed in this book, and at times even conflict with each other. They do, however, provide a principled framework from which to begin to develop a socially responsible reproductive genetics policy.

SHERMAN ELIAS, M.D.
GEORGE J. ANNAS, J.D., M.P.H.

ACKNOWLEDGMENTS

I would like to express my gratitude to the W.K. Kellogg Foundation for their encouragement and financial support which helped make this book a reality. I am especially indebted to Joe Leigh Simpson, M.D., my teacher, colleague, and friend who has inspired my career in academic medicine. I also wish to thank Carole Ober, Ph.D., for her excellent contribution on molecular genetics in prenatal diagnosis which appears in Chapter 5, as well as for her continuing research collaboration and friendship. I must also express my gratitude to my former teachers and colleagues: Albert B. Gerbie, M.D., Alice O. Martin, Ph.D., John W. Greene, M.D., Antonio Scommegna, M.D., John T. Queenan, M.D., and John J. Sciarra, M.D., Ph.D.

SHERMAN ELIAS, M.D.

I am deeply indebted to my two close friends and colleagues, Leonard H. Glantz, J.D., and Norman Scotch, Ph.D.: Leonard for his thoughtful and intelligent criticism and questioning that never fails to improve my arguments (even though they may still fail to convince him), and Norm for his generous and unfailing support of my work at the Boston University School of Public Health. Other colleagues who have contributed significantly to my thinking on these matters over the years are Seymour Lederberg, Ph.D., who team-taught a course on "Genetics and the Law" with me during the late 1970s and early 1980s, and John Robertson, J.D., a friend and legal scholar whose work is always solid and challenging. Research assistance by Doug Gleason and Priya Morganstern was invaluable.

GEORGE J. ANNAS, J.D., M.P.H.

xv

We are most grateful to James D. Ryan, Jr., our editor, and Year Book Medical Publishers for their insight and sensitivity in recognizing the importance and timeliness of this work. We wish to thank Shelley F. Elias and Mary F. Annas for their invaluable editorial assistance, and their literary skills that contributed to the clarity of this book. We also wish to gratefully thank Mary Lou Hannigan and Margaret Picariello for their careful typing, and Linda Seely and Shannon Jamison for their thorough proofreading.

SHERMAN ELIAS, M.D.
GEORGE J. ANNAS, J.D., M.P.H.

CONTENTS

Chapter 1 _____

Principles of Human Genetics

_____

The medical, legal, and social policy issues involved in reproductive genetics cannot be usefully discussed without a basic understanding of the science of genetics. Accordingly, we begin this book with a chapter devoted to the mechanisms of heredity: the determiners of inherited characteristics, and how they are transmitted.

MOLECULAR ASPECTS OF GENE EXPRESSION

DNA Structure and Replication

Hereditary information is transmitted from generation to generation by molecules of deoxyribonucleic acid (DNA). In 1953 Watson and Crick[1] described the structure of DNA as normally consisting of two long strands coiled around one another to form a double helix (Fig 1–1). Variability within the molecule is provided by four different bases: the *purines,* adenine (A) and guanine (G), and the *pyrimidines,* thymine (T) and cytosine (C). The stereochemical restrictions are such that G on one strand can only pair with C on the other, and A with T. The total number of pyrimidine bases always equals the total number of purine bases: that is, A + G = T + C.

The vertical support or backbone of each strand is a monotonous series of alternating deoxyribose sugar and phosphate groups, with the two transverse bases being like rungs on a ladder. During replication the two strands unwind and separate, and each acts as a template for the synthesis of a

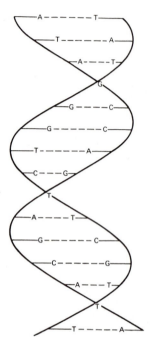

FIG 1–1.
The Watson-Crick double helix model of the stucture of deoxyribonucleic acid (DNA). A, T, G, and C represent adenine, thymine, guanine, and cytosine, respectively. (From Jackson L, Schimke RN: *Clinical Genetics. A Source Book for Physicians.* New York, John Wiley & Sons Inc, 1979, p 5. Used by permission.)

complementary strand (Fig 1–2). Each daughter cell contains a strand of DNA from the parent cell plus a newly synthesized complementary molecule. The DNA molecule of a single chromosome begins to replicate at hundreds or even thousands of sites. This requires an enzyme called DNA polymerase, which moves along the replicating strand and aids in the selec-

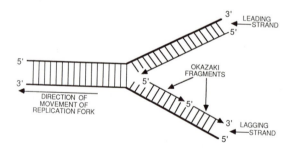

FIG 1–2.
DNA replication. The two strands of the duplex DNA molecule separate to form a *replication fork*. The enzyme DNA polymerase then adds complementary nucleotides at the 3' end. The strand that is continuously replicated is called the *leading strand*. The other strand that is replicated discontinuously in short pieces (Okazaki fragments) is called the *lagging strand*.

tion, placement, and bonding together of the correct complementary nucleotides.* The end product is two new double helixes, each a perfect copy of the original.

Gene Structure and Function

A major function of DNA is to direct the synthesis of polypeptides (linked amino acids) to form proteins. A gene represents the total sequence of bases in DNA that specify the amino acid sequence of a single polypeptide chain of a protein molecule. The genetic information is stored in the DNA by means of a triplet of bases that codes for a specific amino acid.

In Table 1–1, for example, the base triplet CAG codes for the amino acid glutamine. The sequence of such base triplets (called codons) determines the amino acid composition of the polypeptide. However, there are

TABLE 1–1.
The Genetic Code*

FIRST BASE	SECOND BASE†								THIRD BASE
	U		C		A		G		
U	UUU	phe	UCU	ser	UAU	tyr	UGU	cys	U
	UUC	phe	UCC	ser	UAC	tyr	UGC	cys	C
	UUA	leu	UCA	ser	UAA	stop‡	UGA	stop‡	A
	UUG	leu	UCG	ser	UAG	stop‡	UGG	tyr	G
C	CUU	leu	CCU	pro	CAU	his	CGU	arg	U
	CUC	leu	CCC	pro	CAC	his	CGC	arg	C
	CUA	leu	CCA	pro	CAA	gln	CGA	arg	A
	CUG	leu	CCG	pro	CAG	gln	CGG	arg	G
A	AUU	ile	ACU	thr	AAU	asn	AGU	ser	U
	AUC	ile	ACC	thr	AAC	asn	AGC	ser	C
	AUA	ile	ACA	thr	AAA	lys	AGA	arg	A
	AUG	met	ACG	thr	AAG	lys	AGG	arg	G
G	GUU	val	GCU	ala	GAU	asp	GGU	gly	U
	GUC	val	GCC	ala	GAC	asp	GGC	gly	C
	GUA	val	GCA	ala	GAA	glu	GGA	gly	A
	GUG	val	GCG	ala	GAG	glu	GGG	gly	G

*Codons are shown in terms of messenger RNA. The corresponding DNA codons are complementary to these. A = adenine; G = guanine; C = cytosine; U = uracil.
†Abbreviations for amino acids: ala = alanine; arg = arginine; asn = asparagine; asp = aspartic acid; cys = cysteine; gln = glutamine; glu = glutamic acid; gly = glycine; his = histidine; ile = isoleucine; leu = leucine; lys = lysine; met = methionine; phe = phenylalanine; pro = proline; ser = serine; thr = threonine; try = tryptophan; tyr = tyrosine; val = valine.
‡Stop = termination of a gene.

*A nucleotide is a purine or pyrimidine base attached to a 5-carbon sugar, deoxyribose or ribose, and a phosphate group.

more codon permutations, namely 4^3 or 64, than there are amino acids (only 20). Therefore, the code is said to be degenerate. More than one triplet may also code for a given amino acid (glutamine, for example, is determined by codons CAA and CAG). Some codons also initiate protein synthesis. Others, called nonsense codons, apparently code for nothing. With a few possible exceptions, the code is universal; the same amino acids are coded for by the same codons in all organisms from bacteria to humans.

Figure 1–3 is a schematic diagram of the genetic control of protein synthesis. The genetic information in the DNA is transferred or transcribed to a molecule of messenger ribonucleic acid (mRNA). The RNA differs from DNA in being single-stranded, with the sugar ribose instead of deoxyribose and the pyrimidine uracil (U) instead of thymine. Different regions of *either* DNA strand can serve as a template for coding for mRNA. However, with some exceptions, a given region of DNA usually uses only one of its strands for making mRNA from *that* particular region. The two strands of DNA dissociate, exposing the gene that is to be transcribed. The mRNA is then synthesized on the DNA strand by a synthetic sequence similar to DNA duplication (by the action of the enzyme RNA polymerase) with the same kind of complementary pairing as the two DNA strands. For example, a GTA triplet in the DNA would correspond to a CAU triplet in the RNA. The mRNA plays a key informational role during protein synthesis, having a sequence of bases determined by that of corresponding DNA strands. The length of the transcript varies with the length of the polypeptide. Since most polypeptides are at least 100 amino acids long, most mRNA molecules are at least 300 nucleotides long.

The DNA of many genes is composed of interspersed sequences. Coding for a particular protein *(exons)* is separated by "spacers" made up of sequences of DNA *(introns)* that do not code proteins.[2] The transcribed immature mRNA molecule is therefore a mosaic of exon and intron sequences. Prior to transport from the nucleus to the cytoplasm, the RNA transcript goes through an editing process in which the introns are excised and the exons are spliced together to form one continuous functional mRNA.

After the mature mRNA is transported into the cytoplasm, it becomes associated with *ribosomes*. Ribosomes consist of protein and a nonmessenger high molecular weight RNA (rRNA), and function as a "workbench" on which protein synthesis occurs. Amino acids from the chemical milieu of the cytoplasm are brought to their specific positions along the mRNA template by adaptor molecules called transfer RNA (tRNA). The tRNA has a double specificity: one end of the molecule is capable of binding only 1 of the 20 amino acids, and the other end contains a sequence of purine and pyrimidine bases complementary to the specific codon in the mRNA. Hence, the tRNA provides an interface between the free amino acids and the mRNA molecule. After bonds form between the amino acids, the polypeptide chain is completed and the protein is released from the ribosome. The synthesis of a polypeptide chain using mRNA to direct the amino acid sequence is called *translation*. This process involves a variety of cytoplasmic enzymes (initiation factors, elongation factors, and termination factors).

Regulation of Protein Synthesis

At any given time, relatively few of a cell's genes are being expressed through transcription into mRNA and translation into proteins. As a result of internal and environmental signals, an elaborate system of effectors, re-

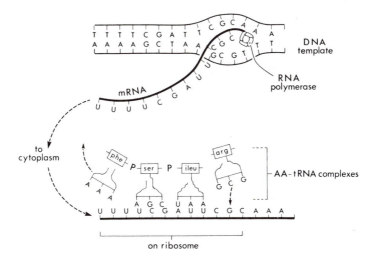

FIG 1–3.
An idealized representation of the synthesis of a protein with a specific amino acid sequence determined by the coding on the DNA molecule. One DNA strand, at a region of separation from the other, determines the synthesis of a complementary messenger RNA (mRNA) strand (with the T of DNA replaced by U in RNA). This process is catalyzed by the enzyme RNA polymerase. The mRNA leaves the nucleus and moves into the cytoplasm and associates with ribosomes. Transfer RNAs (tRNA) have a set of three bases at one end, whereas the corresponding amino acid is at the other. After activation, the amino—tRNA complexes move to the ribosomes, where they are lined up in the correct order by base-pairing between the codon of the mRNA and the complementary codon (or anti-codon) of the tRNA. The growing polypeptide chain is completed when a particular chain-termination codon is reached. *P* = polypeptide bond. (From Thompson JS, Thompson MW: *Genetics in Medicine*, ed 3. Philadelphia, WB Saunders Co, 1980, p 49. Used by permission.)

pressors, and promoters are combined into a regulatory circuit that enables cells to perform their designated functions. The factors that determine which genes will be expressed and in what amounts have not yet been well delineated. Such an understanding will be of great value because some genetic disorders may result from faulty gene regulation rather than from the production of abnormal proteins, and this suggests an approach to therapy. For example, most thalassemias are hereditary anemias characterized by diminished production of structurally normal hemoglobin.

Mutations

A *point mutation* is a permanent heritable change in the genetic makeup (genotype) as a result of a stable alteration in the DNA. Point mutations are of two general types: (1) *base substitutions,* and (2) *frameshift mutations.* In base substitutions there is a change in the DNA from one nucleotide to another that alters the genetic code of a single codon and, hence, may specify a new amino acid. This seemingly minor change may have profound implications. For example, a change in the sixth triplet of the gene for hemoglobin β-chains from CTT to CAT results in a coding for valine instead of glutamic acid in the sixth amino acid position. Such a single amino acid change is associated with sickle cell hemoglobin. A frameshift mutation is the result of a deletion or addition of a nucleotide, or any number of nucleotides other than three or multiples of three into or from DNA. This leads to an mRNA that is "misread" by the translation process (out-of-phase translation) from the point of the nucleotide addition or deletion. Thus, once a frameshift mutation occurs, all codons after the mutation are read out of phase. An example is hemoglobin Wayne, which is caused by a deletion of the third nucleotide of the 139th codon, resulting in an α-hemoglobin chain with an additional five amino acids. This abnormal hemoglobin is not associated with any known clinical problems.

THE CHROMOSOMAL BASIS FOR HEREDITY

Chromosomes (Greek: chromo = colored, -some = body) are discrete structures in the cell nucleus that store and transmit genetic information. The chromosomes of most organisms—both plants and animals, including humans—occur in pairs. The number of chromosomes is halved when the sex cells (gametes) are formed. Cells of the body (somatic cells) thus contain twice as many chromosomes as the nuclei of the gametes. In humans there are 46 chromosomes. Twenty-two of the pairs are similar in males and females and are called *autosomes* (Nos. 1–22). The remaining pair are called the *sex chromosomes*. In the female, the two sex chromosomes are called X chromosomes; in the male there is one X chromosome and a distinct Y chromosome.

During cell division, individual chromosomes can be identified by size, shape, and the color they exhibit under biologic stains. Since 1969, chromosome stains that produce patterns of dark and light horizontal bands, rather than uniform coloring, have been developed. Each stained chromosome reveals bands that define regions distinguishable by shade from adjacent segments. Various banding techniques are available. For example, certain chromosomal segments have an affinity for fluorescent dyes (such as quinacrine hydrochloride) that can be visualized by fluorescence microscopy. These methods are called Q-staining methods, and the resulting bands are Q bands. Another commonly employed technique utilizes Giemsa dye as the staining agent after treatment with a proteolytic enzyme (trypsin); it is called G-staining and the resulting bands, G bands. Other banding techniques are used to highlight different banding properties of the chromosomes. The recognition that these banding patterns are reproducible with a high degree of precision led to the adoption of a universally accepted nomenclature for the designation of chromosome numbers, regions, and alterations.[3]

Chromosomal analysis is usually performed on cells arrested at the metaphase of mitosis. The chromosomes of a human metaphase cell appear under the microscope as a *chromosome spread* (Fig 1–4). To analyze the spread, a photograph is taken and the pictures of the chromosomes are cut out and arrayed according to size and banding pattern. This display is called a *karyotype* (Fig 1–5).

Each metaphase chromosome consists of two *chromatids*, joined at a constriction site called a *centromere*. If a centromere is located in the middle of a chromosome, the chromosome is called *metacentric*; if it is located near one end, it is called *acrocentric*; and if it is off center, the chromosome is *submetacentric*. The short arm of a chromosome is designated by the letter "p," and the long arm by the letter "q."

Cell Division

Chromosomes are microscopically visible only for the relatively brief period of the cell cycle during mitosis and meiosis. The cell cycle is divided into four periods (Fig 1–6): gap 1 (G1), synthesis (S), gap 2 (G2), and division (D). During G1 the cell accumulates materials required for DNA

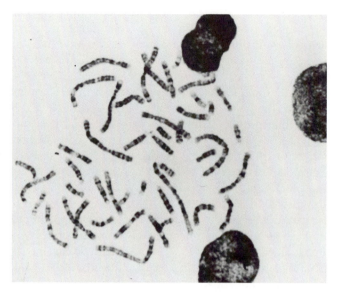

FIG 1–4.
A set of human chromosomes from a single nucleus as it appears on a microscope slide after preparation and staining.

replication (i.e., nucleotides, amino acids, proteins, etc.). Actual DNA synthesis occurs only in the S period, in which all the chromosomal DNA is replicated. Thus, at the end of the S period, the DNA content is doubled. After the S period, there is a resting period (G2) that lasts until the time of cell division (D).

Mitosis

Mitosis is the process by which cell division occurs. It results in the formation of two daughter cells, each with the identical chromosome complement as the parent cell (Fig 1–7). For descriptive purposes, mitosis is divided into four stages. However, the process is continuous and does not occur in discrete steps.

Prophase.—In the initial stage of mitosis, the chromosomes become shortened and thickened. They are then microscopically visible as result of condensation. The *centrioles* are two small bodies (organelles) that form the points of focus to which protein fibers (called spindle fibers) attach, and from which they migrate to opposite poles of the nucleus. The other ends of the spindle fibers are attached to the centromeres.

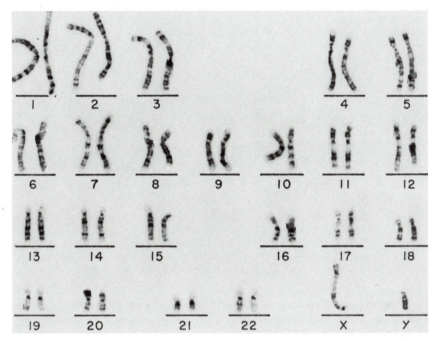

FIG 1–5.
A set of human chromosomes after they are photographed and cut out and the similar chromosomes (homologs) are arranged in pairs to give the 22 pairs of autosomes (numbered 1 to 22) and the pair of sex chromosomes (labeled X and Y).

Metaphase.—This stage begins with the disappearance of the nuclear membrane and the chromosomes lining up along the equator of the cell (the so-called equatorial plate). It is at this time that the chromosomes are best seen. Each chromosome resembles the letter "X" because the chromatids have divided longitudinally, being held together only at the centromere.

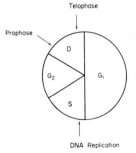

FIG 1–6.
Schematic representation of the cell cycle. S = synthetic period; G1 = first gap (resting) period; G2 = second gap period; D = Division (meiosis or mitosis). G1 is usually the longest. (From Simpson JL: *Disorders of Sexual Differentiation. Etiology and Clinical Delineation.* New York, Academic Press, 1976, p 10. Used by permission.)

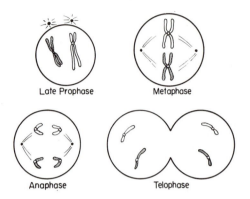

Late Prophase   Metaphase

Anaphase   Telophase

FIG 1–7.
Schematic representation of the stages of mitosis. Two pairs of chromosomes are represented. After DNA synthesis, each chromosome consists of two sister chromatids (late prophase and metaphase). After centromeric division (anaphase), these sister chromatids pass to different daughter cells (telophase). (From Simpson JL: *Disorders of Sexual Differentiation. Etiology and Clinical Delineation.* New York, Academic Press, 1976, p 10. Used by permission.)

Anaphase.—This stage begins with the separation of the two chromatids (now called chromosomes) from each other, each drawn toward opposite poles by the shortening of the spindle fibers.

Telophase.—When the chromosomes reach their respective poles, telophase begins. The spindle fibers disappear, and the two groups of daughter chromosomes become invested in a nuclear membrane. Following division of the cell membrane (cytokinesis), two complete cells are formed, each with a set of chromosomes identical to the original nucleus.

Meiosis

Meiosis is a special type of nuclear division that occurs when the gametes (ovum or sperm) are formed (Fig 1–8). During meiosis each gamete receives at random either of each pair of homologous chromosomes. Accordingly, each gamete contains a haploid set of chromosomes (i.e., only one member of each chromosome pair, $n = 23$). This is in contrast to mitosis, in which each daughter has an identical chromosomal makeup to that of the parental cell (i.e., a diploid number of chromosomes, $n = 46$). Meiosis also provides a mechanism, called *crossing-over,* for exchange of portions of chromosomes of homologous chromosomes. This generates variability, which plays an important biologic role in natural selection. When crossing-over occurs, daughter chromosomes have new combinations of genes different from either parent *(recombination).*

Meiosis consists of two stages, a reductional stage (meiosis I) and a divisional stage (meiosis II). In other words, there are two divisions of the nucleus, but only one of the chromosomes. As with mitosis a number of stages may be identified for meiosis I:

Prophase I.—The prophase of meiosis I is itself characterized by several stages. During *leptotene,* the chromosomes become visible as long slender strands that begin to coil, becoming shorter and thicker. Although each chromosome appears as a single unit, the DNA has already reduplicated with each chromosome actually consisting of two chromatids.

The next stage, *zygotene,* is signaled by the lengthwise pairing of homologous chromosomes, a process known as *synapsis.* An exception occurs in males, where the X and Y chromosomes show end-to-end pairing involving the short arm of each. This suggests some limited homology and, hence,

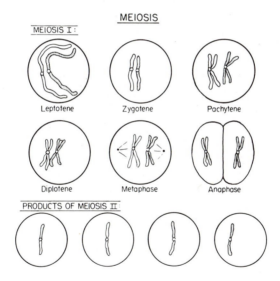

FIG 1–8.
Schematic representation of the stages of meiosis I and the gametic products that are present after meiosis II. The behavior of one pair of autosomes is shown. At zygotene, homologous chromosomes pair with each other along their longitudinal planes, a process known as synapsis. Synapsis occurs between segments of homologous chromosomes, presumably originating a homologous loci. At some sites different alleles at a single locus are exchanged between nonhomologous chromosomes. This can be recognized at diplotene. During metaphase chromosomes began to separate. If crossing-over occurs, no two of the four chromatids of a given chromosome pair are genetically identical, as illustrated by the four different products of meiosis II. (From Simpson JL: *Disorders of Sexual Differentiation, Etiology and Clinical Delineation.* New York, Academic Press, 1976, p 12. Used by permission.)

synapsis. At the completion of synapsis, the chromosomes enter *pachytene,* in which each chromosome is visible as a double strand consisting of two sister chromatids. Since there are two homologous chromosomes, each consisting of two chromatids, there is a total of four chromatids, called a tetrad.

At this time the homologous chromosomes pair and an exchange of homologous segments between non-sister chromatids occurs, i.e., crossing-over. The physical evidence of these exchanges is seen during the next stage, *diplotene.* The homologous chromosomes are drawn apart and held together only by X-shaped connections or bridges between non-sister chromatids, *chiasmata.** During the final stage of prophase, called *diakinesis,* the chromosomes become maximally contracted, and the chiasmata move towards the ends of the chromosome arms (terminalization), allowing normal disjunction to follow.

Metaphase I.—After terminalization of the chiasmata is completed, the homologues (each consisting of two chromatids) align on the equatorial plane. The homologues remain connected by the chiasmata, but usually only at the ends.

Anaphase I.—After terminalization of the chiasmata is completed, the homologues separate toward the appropriate poles. The bivalents assort themselves independently of one another. The chromosomes received originally as a maternal and paternal set are sorted into random combinations of paternal and maternal chromosomes, with one of each pair going to opposite poles. This gives rise to a very large number of possible combinations. In humans with 23 chromosomes, the number of possible combinations in one gamete is 2^{23} or 8,388,608. This potential variation is further increased by crossing over during the pairing of homologue chromosomes.

Telophase I.—This phase is comparable to that of mitosis, except that 23 bivalents migrate to the poles rather than 46 single-stranded chromosomes. This stage may or may not occur, depending on the species. Thus, the overall result of meiosis is the formation of four haploid cells from a single diploid cell.

In meiosis II, the second meiotic division occurs without a preceding DNA duplication. It resembles the corresponding stages of mitosis I—meta-

---

*In addition to being points of interchange of genetic material between "homologues" in the bivalent chromosome pair, chiasmata play an important role in the normal segregation (disjunction) of the homologue pair. Premature separation or suppression of chiasma formation could predispose to nondisjunction (i.e., failure of the sister chromatids to disjoin, leading to a numerical aberration of chromosome number in the gamete).

phase II, anaphase II, and telophase II. However, there is no prophase II stage during meiosis II; the chromosomes pass directly into metaphase II.

Formation of Gametes

In the male, spermatogenesis, the production of sperm, begins at puberty and continues throughout life. The early male stem cells in the testes, spermatogonia, undergo a series of transformational changes in the seminiferous tubules of the testes that incorporate meiosis I and II as previously described. During this process, virtually all the cytoplasm is lost and the sperm acquires its tail for motility. The entire process of differentiation from spermatogonia to mature sperm is about 64 days.[4] An average ejaculate contains about 200 million sperm. Many play a cooperative physiologic role, but only one will normally contribute its single set of chromosomes to pair with the set from the ovum in fertilization.

In oogenesis, human ova develop from the early female germ cells called oogoniae in the cortical tissue of the ovary. Meiosis begins before birth and proceeds as far as prophase I of meiosis I. These germ cells (called primary oocytes at this stage) remain suspended *(dictyotene)* until sexual maturity. Between puberty and menopause, usually only a single ovarian follicle progresses to maturity each month. Meiosis I is completed shortly prior to the ovum being released from the ovary. In contrast to the male, in females only one of the four meiotic products develops into an oocyte, the others being cast off as *polar bodies* that are not normally fertilized. This is an unequal division in which almost all of the cytoplasm remains with the ovum and very little is included in the polar body. The second meiotic division occurs only after the sperm enters the ovum. At this time meiosis II occurs, and the second polar body is formed.

Chromosomal Aberrations

Chromosomal aberrations may be manifested by changes in the number or structure of the chromosomes, or both. In humans the expected number of chromosomes in the haploid gamete is 23, and the diploid cell has 46 chromosomes. Any number of chromosomes that is an exact multiple of the haploid number is *euploid.* Euploid numbers are not always normal. For example, 3n (triploid) or 4n (tetraploid) chromosome numbers are found almost exclusively among abortuses. Any number that is not an exact multiple of n is said to be *aneuploid.* The addition of a single chromosome to a diploid cell is a *trisomy,* i.e., 47 rather than 46 chromosomes. If a single chromosome is missing from a diploid set, *monosomy* is the result. Trisomies and monosomies arise primarily through the process of *nondisjunction,* i.e., failure of paired chromosomes or sister chromatids to disjoin at anaphase, either in a mitotic division or in meiosis I or II. Nondisjunction during mitosis can result in more than one cell line, called *mosaicism.* Another source of monosomy is anaphase lag, a situation in which there is failure of a chromatid to move quickly enough during anaphase to become incorporated into the daughter nucleus. This results in a deficiency of the chromosome in one daughter cell.

With the advent of banding techniques, more structural chromosomal aberrations have been recognized. In general, any imbalance of chromosomal material, particularly a deficiency, is reflected in serious phenotypic consequences. This is to be expected because even the smallest imbalance visible through the light microscope likely involves many genes.

Loss of a portion of a single chromosome is called a *deletion;* it can either involve the end of the chromosome (terminal deletion) or can occur within an arm (interstitial deletion). Only banding can distinguish these. The genetic consequences of unequal crossing-over in meiosis are a deletion in one chromatid and a duplication (i.e., the presence of an extra piece of chromosome) in the other. In humans, duplications are usually associated with phenotypic abnormalities. A *ring chromosome* occurs when the end of each arm has been deleted and the broken arms have reunited in a ring formation. If two breaks occur in a chromosome, the intermediate segment may become inverted prior to repair of the breaks. Thus, a sequence of genes ABCDEFG might become ABCFEDGH. Such an *inversion* is termed *paracentric* if the centromere is not included in the inverted segment, and *pericentric* if the centromere is included. A chromosome with an inversion still has a full complement of genes, albeit in an abnormal sequence; hence, no adverse phenotypic effects would be expected. However, problems may arise during meiosis because inversions interfere with pairing between homologous chromosomes. In order for homologous regions to properly align where one chromosome of a pair contains inversions and the other chromosome of the pair does not, one of them must form a loop (Fig 1–9). If a chiasma does not form within a loop, the products of meiosis are balanced. However, if a chiasma forms within a loop, the gametes formed will have unbalanced chromosomal complements, hence leading to abnormal progeny.

A *translocation* is an exchange of segments between nonhomologous chromosomes. If this exchange is complete (i.e., no leftover segments), the translocation is reciprocal and said to be balanced. Such an individual, known as a translocation heterozygote, is phenotypically normal. During meiosis I there are several ways in which the two translocation chromosomes and two structurally normal homologues may segregate. Gametes are

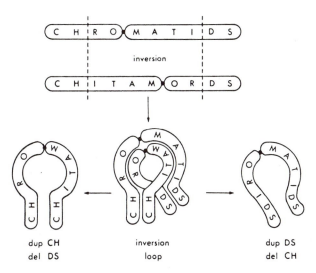

FIG 1–9.
Diagram of an inversion *(top two lines)* and how pairing is accomplished at meiosis formation of an inversion loop. Crossing-over within the inversion will result in unbalanced recombinants, with a duplication of one end and deletion of the other. (From Nora JJ, Fraser FC: *Medical Genetics: Principles and Practice,* ed 2. Philadelphia, Lea & Febiger, 1981, p 30. Used by permission.)

genetically balanced if both translocation chromosomes pass to one gamete, with the two normal chromosomes passing to the other gamete. However, if one of the translocation chromosomes and one of the normal chromosomes pass to the same gamete, the gamete will be genetically abnormal. Translocations are an important cause of repetitive spontaneous abortions and developmental abnormalities. The significance of a translocation can be illustrated by considering the most common translocation, which may lead to an offspring with Down syndrome, a translocation between chromosomes 14 and 21.*

Individuals whose cells do not all have the same chromosome constitution but in whom two, or even more, chromosomal complements are present in different cell lines are said to be *mosaics.* Mosaicism usually results

*The theoretical risk that a parent carrying a t(14q;21q) chromosome will have a child with Down syndrome is 33%. However, the empirical risk is considerably less. If the father carries the translocation, the risk is 2% to 3%; whereas if the mother carries the translocation, the risk is about 10%.[5] The deviation from the predicted 33% probably results from an increased likelihood of a Down syndrome fetus spontaneously aborting. Why the risk is less for a live-born infant with Down syndrome if the father carries the translocation as compared to the mother is uncertain, but presumably it is the result of unbalanced products being selected against at the gametic level. See discussion infra at page 9.

from mitotic nondisjunction or anaphase lag at an early cleavage division of the zygote rather than gametogenesis.

Chromosome Abnormalities

About 15% of all clinically recognized pregnancies terminate in spontaneous abortions.[6] Approximately 50% to 60% of all first trimester spontaneous abortions are associated with changes in the number or structure of the chromosomal complement.[7] The earlier the embryonic age, the more likely the chromosomal complement will be abnormal. By contrast, about 0.5% of live-born infants are chromosomally abnormal, suggesting that maternal selection may be an important factor in the elimination of abnormal embryos.[8]

A comprehensive review of the hundreds of syndromes associated with chromosomal abnormalities is far beyond the scope of this book, but brief discussions of the clinical features associated with some of the most common chromosome abnormalities among live-born infants are useful.[†]

Trisomy 21 (Down syndrome) is by far the most common and best known chromosomal disorder, with a frequency of about 1 of every 700 live births. One of the earliest comprehensive descriptions was provided in 1866 by Langdon Down, who referred to individuals with this condition as having "mongolian idiocy."[‡] LeJeune and associates were the first to demonstrate that individuals with Down syndrome had an additional small chromosome thought to be number 21.[11] Their work is a classic in human genetics, since it was the first time a chromosomal aberration was described in a human being.

The clinical diagnosis of Down syndrome is usually apparent at birth (Fig 1–10); however, no single physical finding is diagnostic, and virtually all the features may be observed in a normal individual as an isolated finding. The average birth weight of infants with Down syndrome is several hundred grams less than that of normal controls. Newborns are usually limp (hypotonic) and have decreased sucking and swallowing reflexes. There are characteristic craniofacial features, which include brachycephaly (disproportionately short head); mild microcephaly; epicanthal folds (a fold of skin extending from the root of the nose to the medial end of the eyebrow); upward and outward slant of the palpebral fissures (opening between the eyelids); broad and flattened nasal bridge; protruding tongue; high arched palate; speckling of the iris (called Brushfield spots); and small, rounded, low-set ears with overhanging, angular helixes. The hands and feet are

[†]The reader is referred to other texts for detailed information.[9, 10]

[‡]The term "Mongoloid" is obviously not acceptable because of its racial implications. Down syndrome should be used.

broad and stocky with short fingers and toes. The fifth finger is short and incurved (clinodactyly), and has a single flexion crease due to an abnormality in the middle phalanx. A single transverse palmar crease (simian line) is common (45% of cases), but it is also found in 5% of normal individuals. The feet usually show a wide gap between the first and second toes. Visceral

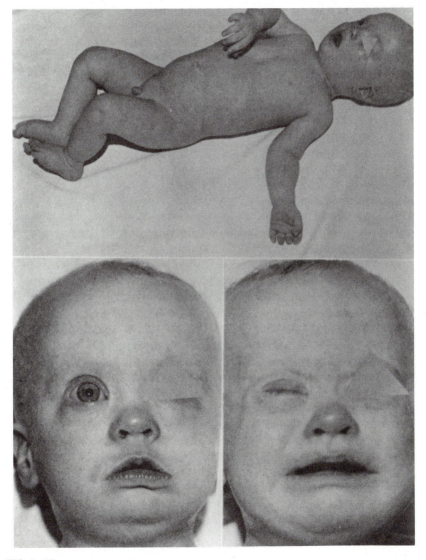

FIG 1–10.
Trisomy 21 (Down syndrome). (From Smith DW: Autosomal trisomies. *Am J Obstet Gynecol* 1964; 90:1055-1077. Used by permission.)

malformations are frequent; the most important are cardiac malformations (40% of cases), which include—in decreasing order of frequency—endocardial cushion defects, ventricular septal defects, patent ductus arteriosus, auricular septal defect, and aberrant subclavian artery. Other serious malformations that may be present include gastrointestinal atresias (most commonly duodenal atresia), tracheoesophageal fistula, annular pancreas, aganglionic megacolon (Hirschsprung disease), rectal prolapse, anal atresia, vertebral anomalies, and dysplastic pelvis. The risk of acute leukemia is about 1%, and thyroid abnormalities (goiter, hyperthyroidism) may also be present. Chronic upper respiratory tract infections, rhinitis, conjunctivitis, and periodontal disease are common.

Psychomotor development is the major area of concern. The IQ scores are generally in the range of 25 to 50, with an occasional individual score above 50. The parental IQ and intensive development enrichment programs are factors in achievement; however, development into the normal range cannot be expected. Some Down syndrome individuals have been said to have an IQ in the 70–80 range, but in such cases $46/47, +21$ mosaicism should be suspected.

The life expectancy of Down syndrome individuals is reduced, with about 30% dying within the first year of life, 50% before 5 years. Survival has increased greatly over recent decades because of advances in the treatment of cardiac defects, antibiotic therapy, and so forth, with 8% of patients surviving beyond 40 years.[10]

Trisomy 21 (i.e., 3 rather than the normal two number 21 chromosomes) is found in about 95% of individuals with Down syndrome, with the extra chromosome being of paternal origin in 20% to 25% of cases.[12] The risk of trisomy 21, as well as other chromosomal abnormalities, increases significantly with advancing maternal age. The likelihood of a 35-year-old woman having a child with Down syndrome is 1 in 384; at age 39 the risk is 1 in 140; at age 45 the risk is 1 in 30.* Although the relationship betwen aneuploidy and increased maternal age is better recognized and more established, Down syndrome may also be associated with advanced paternal age.[13–15] However, paternal age effect does not appear to occur until about the fifth decade, and then it may generally be considered to double the corresponding maternal age risk for having a child with Down syndrome. Some investigators have not confirmed a paternal age effect.[16]

Once a couple has had a child with Down syndrome, the risk that subsequent progeny will have a chromosomal abnormality (trisomy 21 or other) is in the range of 1% if the mother was aged 29 or younger when the index case was born (assuming the parental chromosome complements

*See Chapter 4.

are normal).[17] Beyond the age of 29, the risks are the same as the background maternal age risks.

In about 5% of individuals with Down syndrome, the extra chromosome 21 material is present not as a separate chromosome, but as a translocation. There is no evidence for any phenotypic difference between the translocation and trisomic cases of Down syndrome. Maternal age is not a factor in such cases because nondisjunction is not the cause. Among these cases of Down syndrome due to a translocation, about half occur sporadically *(de novo)*, and half are inherited from a balanced translocation carrier parent.†

Trisomy 18 (Edwards' syndrome) was first described in 1960.[19] It occurs with a frequency of about 1 in 8,000 live births, making it the second most common chromosomal multiple malformation syndrome.[20] There is a 4:1 preponderance of females to males. More than 130 different abnormalities have been reported to occur in patients with trisomy 18.[21] Distinctive features (Fig 1–11) include microcephaly; short palpebral fissures; prominent occiput (back part of the skull); receding jaw; low-set malformed ears; short sternum; clenched hands with a tendency of the index and fifth fingers to overlap the third and fourth fingers; "rocker-bottom" shaped feet with protruding heels; heart malformations; renal anomalies; inguinal or umbilical hernias; undescended testes in males. Postnatal survival is poor, with a mean survival of two to three months for males and ten months for females, although some individuals may live for years. Survivors are all severely mentally retarded.

Following the birth of a child with trisomy 18, the recurrence risk for either trisomy 18 or for a different chromosomal abnormality is in the range of 1% to 2%.[22] Cases involving translocations are usually sporadic and, unless a familial chromosomal aberration coexists, the recurrence risk is no greater for such a couple having a chromosomally abnormal child than the population risk at the corresponding parental ages.

Trisomy 13 (Patau syndrome) was first described in 1960.[23] It occurs with a frequency of between 1 per 4,000 and 1 per 10,000 live births.[20] Distinctive features (Fig 1–12) include: cleft lip and palate; eye abnormalities, which range from coloboma (a cleft of the iris, ciliary body, or choroid) through microphthalmia, to complete absence of the eyes; incomplete

†If inherited, the recurrence risk depends upon the chromosomes involved in the translocation. For example, if the father carries a translocation between chromosome 14 and 21, the recurrence risk is 2% to 3%; if the mother carries such a translocation, the recurrence risk is about 10%. By contrast, if *either* parent carries a translocation between two number 21 chromosomes, t(21q; 21q), the risk of either a child with Down syndrome or a spontaneous abortion is 100%.[18] If a *de novo* translocation occurs (i.e., neither parent carries the translocation), the recurrence risk for having another child with Down syndrome is no greater than the population risk at the corresponding parental ages.

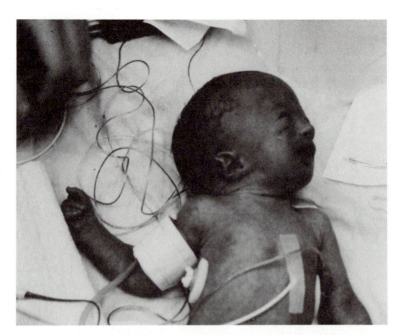

FIG 1–11.
Trisomy 18.

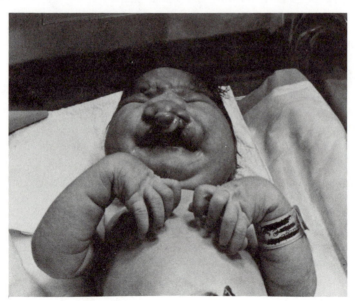

FIG 1–12.
Trisomy 13.

development of the forebrain; microcephaly with a sloping forehead; low-set and malformed ears; heart malformations; extra fingers or toes; skin defects of the scalp; single umbilical artery; urogenital abnormalities. Most infants die within the first three months of life; however, 18% survive the first year.[21] Mental retardation is severe in survivors.

As with trisomy 18, after the delivery of a child with a trisomy 13, the recurrence risk to a couple of having a future child with a chromosomal abnormality is 1% to 2%.[22] Also, most cases involving translocations are sporadic and, unless a familial translocation coexists, the recurrence risk for a child with a chromosomal abnormality is that of the corresponding parental ages only.

46,XY,del(5)(p13) ("cri-du-chat" or cat cry syndrome), associated with an absence of the distal portion of the short arm (p) of a number 5 chromosome, was first delineated in 1963.[24] The physical features of this syndrome are not as diagnostic as those of the aforementioned conditions. However, a striking clinical feature is a distinctive cat-like cry in the newborn period ascribed to abnormal laryngeal development. In addition, the face is often round with widely spaced eyes, and there is a paradoxically alert appearance. About 20% of these children have congenital heart defects. All these children are microcephalic and are severely mentally retarded (mean IQ, 20). With age the mewing cry diminishes, making the clinical diagnosis difficult. Many of these individuals attain adult age, and it has been estimated that this syndrome accounts for about 1% of institutionalized individuals with IQs below 35.[25]

About 90% of these cases are sporadic, conferring no additional recurrence risks for a subsequent child with a chromosomal abnormality beyond those of the corresponding parental age risks. However, in about 10% of cases, there is a balanced parental chromosomal rearrangement, most commonly a maternal translocation.[10] In these families, recurrence risks must be based on their specific chromosomal rearrangement.

45,X (Turner stigmata) was first described in 1938.[26] Seven girls were studied who exhibited sexual infantilism, short stature, webbed neck, primary amenorrhea, and certain skeletal anomalies, which Turner believed were due to pituitary dysfunction.[26] In 1959 it was reported that the complement 45,X (i.e., only a single sex chromosome, that being an X) was associated with gonadal dysgenesis and "Turner stigmata."[27] The frequency of 45,X among live-born infants is about 1 in 2,500. Although no single physical finding is diagnostic nor always present, characteristic features (Fig 1–13) include short stature; primary amenorrhea; sterility; sexual infantilism; peripheral lymphedema; webbed neck; cubitus valgus (lateral deviation of the forearms at the elbows); low hairline at the back of the neck; "shield"-shaped chest; cardiovascular anomalies; hypertension; retruded

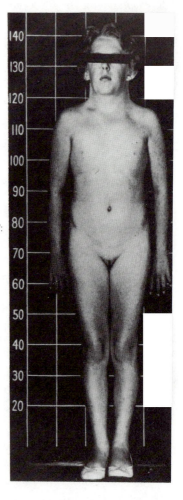

FIG 1–13.
45,X (Turner stigmata). (From Jones HW Jr, Scott WW: *Hermaphroditism, Genital Anomalies and Related Endocrine Disorders,* ed 2. Baltimore, Williams & Wilkins Co, 1971, p 78. Used by permission.)

jaw; urinary tract anomalies; hypoplastic or hyperconvex nails; multiple-pigmented nevi; high arched palate; auditory defects (sensorineural or secondary to middle ear infections).[28] Most 45,X patients have normal intelligence, but any given 45,X patient probably has a slightly higher probability of being retarded than a normal (46,XX) individual. The performance IQ is lower than the verbal IQ.[29] In particular, 45,X individuals have an unusual cognitive defect, characterized by an inability to appreciate the comparative shape of objects (space-form blindness).

In most 45,X adults the normal gonad is replaced by a white fibrous streak devoid of oocytes. Rarely, 45,X patients may have oocytes that persist from embryonic development and a few such patients have been fertile.[30] From a practical standpoint, however, 45,X patients should be counseled to anticipate primary amenorrhea and sterility.

In contrast to trisomies, the risk of having a child with 45,X is not correlated with advancing maternal age.[31] After a couple has had a 45,X child, the recurrence risk is no greater for the same or any other chromosomally abnormal child as compared to the general population risk at the corresponding parental ages. Among the rare 45,X women who themselves become pregnant, there are at least theoretical reasons to suspect an increased risk of producing a chromosomally abnormal offspring; however, suitable empirical risk figures are not available.[32] Finally, in addition to 45,X, a variety of other chromosomal abnormalities may be associated with gonadal dysgenesis with or without the Turner stigmata, including various forms of mosaicism and structural abnormalities of the X chromosome.[28]

47,XXY (Klinefelter syndrome) is defined as the spectrum of phenotypic abnormalities resulting from a chromosomal complement with at least one Y chromosome and at least two X chromosomes. It occurs with a frequency of about 1 per 1,000 live-born males and accounts for 10% to 20% of males attending infertility clinics. This syndrome, first described in 1942 by Klinefelter and coworkers, is characterized in adult males by the following: small firm testes; azoospermia (absence of sperm in the semen, hence infertility); gynecomastia (abnormally large breasts); scant facial and pubic hair; small penis; decreased testosterone levels; abnormal skeletal proportions, with relatively long legs and a decreased upper/lower segment ratio.[33] Newborns with 47,XXY chromosomal complements are phenotypically normal.[34] Although 47,XXY individuals are more likely to be retarded or socially maladjusted than normal (46,XY) males, the exact risk is uncertain.[35, 36] Klinefelter individuals frequently exhibit certain behavioral peculiarities such as poor self-motivation, passivity, and absence of anxiety.

About 15% of patients with Klinefelter syndrome have been found to have two or more chromosomally distinct cell populations, the most common being 46,XY/47,XXY. The clinical expression of these mosaic individuals is variable, ranging from near-normal male phenotype to a moderate form of Klinefelter syndrome. Other rare chromosomal variations include 48,XXXY; 49,XXXXY; 48,XXYY; and 49,XXXYY. In addition to manifesting the Klinefelter syndrome phenotype, these individuals are severely mentally retarded. There are currently no data available regarding the recurrence risks for 47,XXY or other chromosomal variants of Klinefelter syndrome, but there is an association with advanced maternal age.

47,XYY was first described in 1961.[37] For several years thereafter, relatively few cases were reported. But in 1965 and 1966, several investigators reported that among mentally retarded criminals the prevalence of 47,XYY was higher than that expected by chance, creating a resurgence of interest in this disorder.[38, 39] Approximately 1 per 1,000 live-born males has a 47,XYY chromosomal complement. There are no discernible phenotypic abnormalities in 47,XYY newborns.[40] The phenotype of adult 47,XYY males does not vary appreciably from normal (46,XY) males.[41] The 47,XYY males are sometimes quite tall (mean height, 71.3 in.), frequently have severe acne, and their deciduous teeth have been found to be larger than those of controls, suggesting that the Y chromosome regulates the quantitative variation of dental growth.[42, 32] Dermatoglyphic analysis has shown decreased total digital ridge counts consistent with the general observation of an inverse relationship between sex chromosome polysomy and total ridge count.[44, 45] Additional findings that have been implicated include electrocardiographic and electroencephalographic abnormalities.*[46–48]

Most offspring of 47,XYY males are chromosomally normal, in contrast to theoretical predictions that half would be 47,XXY or 47,XYY. Some 47,XYY men have purportedly had offspring with trisomy 21, which raises the possibility that the abnormal sex chromosome constitution affects segregation of autosomal chromosomes as well.[54] Further investigations are needed to understand gametogenesis in 47,XYY individuals.

47,XXX was first reported in 1959, and is estimated to occur in about 1 per 1,000 female births. Several studies have suggested that there is an increased likelihood that 47,XXX individuals will be retarded or mentally ill. The magnitude of the increased risk is difficult to estimate because most 47,XXX patients have been ascertained in surveys of the mentally retarded. However, the prevalence of 47,XXX is higher among the mentally retarded than among consecutively born neonates; these observations support the apparent relationship between mental retardation and 47,XXX. Prospective studies of the relatively few 47,XXX patients ascertained without bias at

---

*The first psychologic studies of 47,XYY males were studies of inmates at a Scottish maximum security prison.[49, 50] As compared to normal (46,XY) male inmates, it was found that 47,XYY inmates (1) incurred their first conviction at a younger age; (2) less often had a sibling who had received a conviction; and (3) committed crimes against property more often than against persons. These observations suggested that 47,XYY inmates are incarcerated for different reasons than other inmates. Probably the most objective study was from Denmark in which a 42% (5/12) rate of criminality was found among 47,XYY males, compared with 9.3% in 4,096 46,XY controls.[51] The difference is about 4.5-fold and is considered statistically significant. Hook suggested that despite the observation that IQs of 47,XYY males are lower than 46,XY controls in exclusively penal settings, it is not the lower intelligence per se that is solely responsible for the higher frequency of incarceration, but rather the increase in risk of social maldevelopment associated with the 47,XYY phenotype.[52] Other investigators object to these conclusions regarding the increased frequency of social maldevelopment and predisposition to "criminality."[53] The difficulties of assessing the clinical significance of the 47,XYY chromosomal complement have been extensively explored, and there are insufficient data to make any definitive conclusions regarding any increased frequency of psychosociopathic problems in these individuals. See discussion of XYY as a criminal defense, pp. 78–79.

birth indicate IQs 16 points below those of sibs.[55] One third show at least some mental or behavioral problems;[56] at least 5% of 47,XXX females are retarded, with an IQ between 45 and 70.

With the exception of dermatoglyphic abnormalities (decreased mean digital ridge count), it is difficult to determine whether other somatic anomalies are associated with 47,XXX complement more often than expected by chance. About 20% of 47,XXX women may experience delayed menarche, premature ovarian failure, and underdevelopment of secondary sexual characteristics.[57]

Most offspring of 47,XXX women have been chromosomally normal, despite theoretical expectations that 50% would be abnormal, i.e., 47,XXX or 47,XXY. Although controversial, there is also a suggestion that maternal trisomy X may affect the disjunction of the autosomes as well. At least two 47,XXX women have had trisomy 21 offspring.[58, 59] However, biases of ascertainment and reporting make the significance of the above findings uncertain. Nonetheless, it still seems prudent to offer prenatal diagnosis to 47,XXX women.

MENDELIAN INHERITANCE

Disorders resulting from the transmission of a mutant gene show one of three simple (or Mendelian) patterns of inheritance: (1) autosomal dominant; (2) autosomal recessive; or (3) sex-linked. Genes are situated on chromosomes at given locations in a definite linear relation to other genes. Each gene has an *allele* (an alternate form of a gene) that occupies the same locus on the other member of a chromosome pair. If a pair of alleles at a given locus are identical, the individual is *homozygous*. If the alleles are dissimilar, the individual is *heterozygous*. If the effects of the gene are evident in a single dose, i.e., the abnormal gene has been transmitted from only one parent and the individual is heterozygous for the particular trait, then the gene is said to be *dominant*. If on the other hand, the disorder is only expressed when the mutant gene has been inherited in double dose, i.e., from both parents and the individual is homozygous for the trait, then the mutant gene is said to be *recessive*. In addition to these considerations, the mutant gene may be located on the autosomal chromosomes or on the sex chromosomes; the inheritance of the disorder is then described as autosomal or sex-linked, respectively.

Diseases produced by single mutant genes, whether transmitted in dominant or recessive fashion, on an autosome or a sex chromosome, are uncommon disorders. Many Mendelian disorders occur only once per 10,000 to 50,000 births. However, although individually rare, mutant

PATTERNS OF TRANSMISSION OF SINGLE-GENE TRAITS

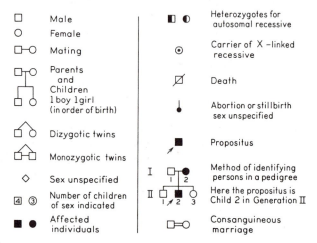

FIG 1–14.
Symbols commonly used in pedigree charts. (From Thompson JS, Thompson MW: *Genetics in Medicine,* ed 3. Philadelphia, WB Saunders Co, 1980, p 55. Used by permission.)

genes in aggregate cause abnormalities in about 1% of live-born infants, and the risk in certain families for an affected offspring is 25% or 50%, depending on the particular mode of inheritance.

Genetic information can be summarized in a family tree or *pedigree chart,* which is a useful shorthand method of organizing data for easy reference. The symbols used to construct such a pedigree chart are shown in Figure 1–14.

Autosomal Dominant Inheritance

An individual carrying a mutant autosomal dominant gene (allele) has a 50% risk of passing that allele to any given offspring, male or female. Thus, a dominant gene is considered to be one that produces an effect even if the other allele is normal (sometimes called a "wild type" allele). *Penetrance* is a term particularly relevant to autosomal dominant inheritance referring to the ability of a gene to be expressed if present, i.e., an all-or-none phenomenon. For example, consider a family in which a woman's father, brother, and two children all have polydactyly (extra digits), yet the woman has no manifestations of this condition; nonexpression of the gene indicates *incomplete penetrance.* If all individuals carrying a mutant autosomal dominant gene show its manifestations, there is *complete penetrance.* The term *variable expressivity* refers to the extent (mild to severe) to which a mutant gene is expressed.

At least 934 human genes are recognized as inherited in autosomal dominant fashion, and there are undoubtedly more.[60] In general, dominant traits are less severe than recessive ones. This is probably because when a gene mutation gives rise to a serious disorder it militates against reproduction and hence tends to die out quickly. Figure 1–15 shows a typical pedigree of a family with an autosomal dominant trait. Table 1–2 lists some common autosomal dominant disorders.

Autosomal Recessive Inheritance

An autosomal recessive trait is expressed only if an individual is homozygous for the appropriate allele. Affected individuals receive one mutant allele from each parent who is heterozygous for that same mutation. Usually the parents are clinically normal, although rarely a carrier of the mutant gene in single dose may show a mild manifestation. Each child (male or female) of parents who are both heterozygous (carriers) for a mutant gene has a 25% chance of being homozygous and thereby being affected with the disorder. Moreover, on a statistical basis, 50% of the offspring will be heterozygotes (like the parents) and 25% will be genetically as well as phenotypically normal. It is characteristic of autosomal recessive disorders that only siblings and no other relatives are affected with a disorder.

The chances of two parents carrying the same autosomal recessive trait

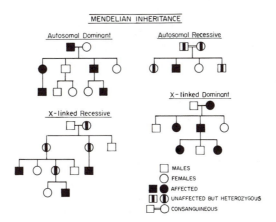

FIG 1–15.
Patterns of familial transmission expected of autosomal dominant, autosomal recessive, X-linked recessive, and X-linked dominant traits. (From Simpson JL: *Disorders of Sexual Differentiation. Etiology and Clinical Delineation.* New York, Academic Press, 1976, p 34. Used by permission.)

TABLE 1–2.

Selected Common Autosomal Dominant Disorders

Huntington chorea
Marfan syndrome
Neurofibromatosis
Achondroplasia
Familial hypercholesterolemia
Hereditary spherocytosis
Cleft lip with lip pits
Acute intermittent porphyria
Von Willebrand disease
Adult-type polycystic kidney disease
Tuberous sclerosis
Myotonic dystrophy
Craniofacial dysostosis (Crouzon disease)
Hyperbilirubinemia I (Gilbert disease)
Noonan syndrome
Idiopathic hypertrophic subaortic stenosis (IHSS)
Mandibulofacial dysostosis (Treacher Collins syndrome)
Peroneal muscular dystrophy (Charcot-Marie-Tooth disease)
Polyposis of the colon (Intestinal polyposis I)
Waardenburg syndrome

are increased if they are consanguineous (inbred). The rarer the mutant gene in the population, the more often will the parents be related. Inbreeding does not increase the frequency of the gene in the population, but it does increase the frequency of the homozygote and thus the number of clinically affected individuals. The increased likelihood of homozygous recessives is the biologic basis for prohibiting cousin marriages in many societies.

At least 588 autosomal recessive traits are recognized and there are undoubtedly more.[60] Figure 1–15 shows a typical pedigree of a family with an autosomal recessive trait. Table 1–3 lists some common autosomal recessive disorders.

X-Linked Recessive Inheritance

Since females have two X chromosomes and males only one, genes that are recessive in females are expressed in males (i.e., males are *hemizygous*). An X-linked recessive gene is transmitted through phenotypically normal yet heterozygous females. Thus, each son of a carrier female has a 50% chance of being affected, and each daughter of a carrier female has a 50% chance of being a carrier. In families with X-linked recessive disorders the proband (affected individual) might characteristically have affected male siblings, maternal uncles, maternal nephews, maternal male first cousins, and perhaps other maternal male relatives. Affected males never transmit the gene to their sons (who receive the Y chromosome), but they transmit it to all their daughters, who will be carriers. Unaffected males never transmit the gene to their offspring. Rarely, an affected homozygous female can occur as a result of an affected father having a child by a carrier mother. In families in which only a single male is affected with an X-linked recessive disorder, there is a one in three chance that the gene was not transmitted from a carrier mother, but resulted from a new mutation.*

There are currently at least 115 genetic disorders recognized to be inherited in X-linked recessive fashion and there are undoubtedly more.[60] Figure 1–15 shows a typical pedigree of a family with an X-linked recessive trait. Table 1–4 lists some common X-linked recessive disorders.

X-linked Dominant Inheritance

The rules for X-linked dominant inheritance are similar to those for X-linked recessive inheritance, except for the fact that the heterozygous fe-

TABLE 1–3.
Selected Common Autosomal Recessive Disorders

Cystic fibrosis
Sickle-cell disease
Tay-Sachs disease
Phenylketonuria
β-thalassemia
Albinism (various forms)
Adrenogenital syndrome (various forms)
Familial Mediterranean fever
α_1-antitrypsin deficiency
Homocystinuria
Friedreich ataxia
Total color blindness
Deafness (various forms)
Dysautonomia (Riley-Day syndrome)
Galactosemia
Glycogen storage disease (various forms)
Hepatolenticular degeneration (Wilson disease)
Laurence-Moon-Biedl syndrome
Methemoglobinemia
Meckel syndrome

---

*Under such circumstances geneticists may apply Bayesian analysis, a type of analysis that takes into account information such as the number of males in the pedigree who would be at risk under a heritable model hypothesis but who had no clinical disease.[61]

TABLE 1–4.
Selected Common X-Linked Recessive Disorders

Hemophilia A (factor VIII deficiency)
Hemophilia B (factor IX deficiency)
Duchenne muscular dystrophy
Glucose-6-phosphate dehydrogenase deficiency
Agammaglobulinemia (Bruton disease)
Testicular feminization syndrome
Diffuse angiokeratoma (Fabry disease)
Anhidrotic ectodermal dysplasia
X-linked hydrocephalus (aqueductal stenosis)
Chronic granulomatous disease
Lesch-Nyhan syndrome
Menkes kinky hair syndrome
Hunter syndrome
Wiskott-Aldrich syndrome
Cutis hyperelastosis
Color blindness
Ocular albinism
Diabetes insipidus (X-linked forms)
Hypospadias-dysphagia syndrome (G syndrome)
Fragile X syndrome

males express the condition. Thus, a male carrying an X-linked dominant allele transmits the allele to all his daughters but to none of his sons. The probability that a female with an X-linked dominant allele will pass the allele to any offspring (male or female) is 50%. Since females have twice as many X chromosomes as males, they are twice as commonly affected as males, although sometimes less severely.

There are relatively few conditions inherited in X-linked fashion. The best example is vitamin D-resistant rickets. Affected males show short stature, bowed legs, and striking roentgenographic skeletal changes. Females have a spectrum of disorders, ranging from a phenotype as severe as affected males to no apparent clinical findings, yet they can be identified as carriers by the demonstration of increased excretion of phosphate in the urine. Figure 1–15 shows a typical pedigree of a family with an X-linked dominant trait.

POLYGENIC/MULTIFACTORIAL INHERITANCE

In many heritable conditions the proportion of affected relatives cannot be explained on the basis of Mendelian inheritance, and there is no evidence for a chromosomal abnormality. The most common model suggested to explain such family patterns is that of polygenic/multifactorial inheritance.

One explanation for a trait whose recurrence risk is 2% to 5% is that the trait is influenced by multiple genes and so is *polygenic*. When environmental factors are also considered influential, the term multifactorial is often applied. The concept of polygenic inheritance assumes that there are a large number of nonallelic genes, each having a small individual effect, which cumulatively determine the phenotype of an individual with regard to a specific trait. The presence of several genes contributing to a phenotype produces a continuous frequency distribution curve in the population, both with regard to the distribution of genes and to the degree of phenotypic expression. The usual model is to assume that this continuous variation results in a normal distribution in the population (the so-called bell-shaped curve or gaussian distribution). These genes of presumably minor individual effect appear to govern ordinarily inherited traits including intelligence, stature, skin color, blood pressure, and certain components of ocular refraction. In disease states, patients can be graded according to the severity of clinical findings; however, it is not possible to grade patients according to their degree of "normality."

If one assumes that there is some underlying graded attribute (or *liability*) that is related to the causation of a disorder, then one can explain the heritable nature of most common birth defects not associated with a unifactorial etiology (i.e., single gene or chromosomal abnormality). The expression of a trait is manifest only when the total liability, genetic and environmental, exceeds a *threshold* (Fig 1–16). Thus, we can separate the population into two discrete groups—one affected and one unaffected with a particular defect, a discontinuous variation. For example, either an individual has a cleft palate or not; there is relatively little variability in the

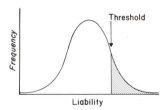

Liability

FIG 1–16.
Schematic representation of one model for polygenic or multifactorial inheritance, assuming an underlying continuous distribution with a threshold beyond which liability is so great that an abnormality is manifested. Parents of affected individuals presumably have a greater liability (i.e., they are closer to the threshold) than most other individuals in the population. (From Simpson JL: *Disorders of Sexual Differentiation. Etiology and Clinical Delineation.* New York, Academic Press, 1976, p 43. Used by permission.)

TABLE 1–5.

Some Common Abnormalities Considered To Be
Inherited in Polygenic/Multifactorial Fashion

Cleft lip and/or palate
Neural tube defects
Congenital hip dislocation
Congenital aganglionic megacolon
  (Hirschsprung disease)
Pyloric stenosis
Peptic ulcer disease
Congenital heart defects (most forms)
Hypertension
Talipes equinovarus (clubfoot)
Scoliosis
Epilepsy (most forms)
Hydrocephalus (most forms)
Asthma
Aseptic necrosis of the capital femoral epiphysis
  (Legg-Perthes disease)

degree of clefting, although some variation exists in all traits. The latest time in development when the palatal shelves can reach the horizontal plane and fuse can be considered the threshold.

Among the important implications of the polygenic/multifactorial model are: (1) the recurrence risk increases as the number of affected first-degree relatives increases; (2) when a sex difference in the population incidence of a disorder exists, the relatives of the less frequently affected sex will be more frequently affected; (3) the more severe a malformation, the higher the recurrence risk; and (4) the recurrence risk in a first-degree relative of an affected individual may be approximated by the square root of the population frequency.[62] Examples of some common abnormalities considered to be inherited in polygenic/multifactorial fashion are listed in Table 1–5.

Chapter 2 —————————————

Genetic Counseling

"Hereditary counseling" was one of the earliest applications of human genetics. Its primary scope was to provide information about a specific genetic disorder, including severity and prognosis; any effective treatment; the genetic mechanism that caused it; and the risks of its occurring in relatives. Counseling was usually provided by nonmedical geneticists whose interest centered on their research or teaching activities. Unfortunately, inaccurate information was often provided because of failure to correct for ascertainment biases, inappropriate attempts to fit data into simple Mendelian patterns, and lack of appreciation for the complexities involved in applying general principles of genetics to specific family situations.[1]

In the 1950s, a number of developments began to make genetics clinically important to physicians. Nongenetic diseases (i.e., those primarily due to environmental factors such as infections or nutritional deficiencies) were brought under control. This made it possible to identify genetic diseases as responsible for a greater proportion of human illnesses. The number of diseases recognized as inherited in Mendelian fashion rapidly increased. Empirical recurrence risks became available for some common familial (but not Mendelian) diseases.[2] Advances in cytogenetic and biochemical technologies and their applications in the diagnosis of many birth defects and intersex states brought human genetics into the mainstream of clinical medical practice. Changes in law and social attitudes toward contraception and abortion accompanied these advances in medical technology. Finally, in the late 1960s, the introduction of prenatal diagnosis, specifically genetic amniocentesis,* established medical genetics as an integral part of modern comprehensive obstetric care.[3] In this chapter, we review the definitions, goals, processes, responses, and social policy implications of genetic counseling.

DEFINITIONS AND GOALS

In 1974, The American Society of Human Genetics defined genetic counseling as:

> . . . a communication process which deals with the human problems associated with the occurrence, or risk of occurrence, of a genetic disorder in a family. This process involves an attempt by one or more appropriately trained persons to help the individual or the family to (1) comprehend the medical facts, including the diagnosis, the probable course of the disorder and the available management; (2) appreciate the way heredity contributes to the disorder and the risk of recurrence in specified relatives; (3) understand the options for dealing with the risk of recurrence; (4) choose the course of action which seems appropriate to them in view of their risk and their family goals and act in accordance with that decision; and (5) make the best possible adjustment to the disorder in an affected family member and/or to the risk of recurrence of that disorder.[4]

Stated more concisely: "Genetic counseling is the process whereby an individual or family obtains information about a real or possible genetic problem."[5]

These definitions have several important implications. First, persons providing genetic counseling must have accurate genetic and medical knowledge. Second, genetic counseling is a dynamic communicative process that includes making the diagnosis (i.e., taking the medical and family histories, performing the clinical examinations, and performing relevant laboratory investigations); providing information regarding risks of recurrence, explanations of genetic and medical implications of the disorder, prevention, and family planning; and the actual medical management of the condition. Third, genetic counseling is directly concerned with human behavior, so it must be based on an understanding of interpersonal psychodynamics, as well as an understanding of the psychological meanings of health and illness, procreation, and parenthood.[6] Finally, the responsibility of the modern professional genetic counselor must include helping clients adjust psychologically and socially to their genetic condition. Achievement of these goals requires an understanding of the genetic counseling process.

*See Chapter 5.

Who Should Provide Genetic Counseling?

Genetic counseling cannot and should not be exclusively provided by a single specialist, but is an interdisciplinary responsibility. There is also a growing recognition of the need to ensure that those providing genetic counseling are competent. In the clearest situations, such as advanced maternal age, the primary care physician can usually provide necessary counseling.[7] In many cases the primary care physician is also the most appropriate person to provide the counseling because the physician knows the family, their personal attitudes, and socioeconomic background better than a consultant.[8] However, in more complex situations, the primary care physician may lack the specific knowledge, time commitment, availability of specific diagnostic tests, or skills required for genetic counseling. In these cases patients are appropriately referred to a center with a medical genetics team. An effective medical genetics team should include individuals with expertise in medical diagnosis and genetic analysis, and skills in objective and subjective data collection, information presentation, and family support.[5] Such a team would generally include a physician, a medical geneticist who may be the immediate genetic counselor, a Ph.D. medical geneticist, genetic counselors, a social worker, a psychologist or psychiatrist, a child development specialist or vocational rehabilitation specialist, and a chaplain.

Consultation services must be available from other specialists with expertise that cannot be fully provided by the genetics team. A major advantage of the genetics center approach is that it promotes better quality control. Some areas have developed satellite counseling clinics, which appropriate members of a medical genetics team visit regularly. This helps ensure the widest availability of quality counseling services.[9] Finally, no single center can offer all genetic services. Under certain circumstances the special expertise of other centers must be called on for a secondary consultation or referral.

All who hold themselves out to the public as engaging in genetic counseling services must possess sufficient knowledge, training, and skill to provide these services in a reasonable manner. Practitioners must respect the limits of their individual competence, and avoid acting beyond the scope of their ability. The use of a genetics team approach has been endorsed as consistent with the notions of competence and appropriately shared responsibilities, as well as "consistent with the general shift in our society away from an exclusively physician-centered health care delivery system to one that allows properly trained nonphysicians a major role in the health care process."[10]

There are no state or federal licensing schemes for genetic counselors. There is, however, a detailed private certification process. In 1980, at the request of the American Society of Human Genetics, the American Board of Medical Genetics was incorporated to provide accreditation of training programs and to prepare and administer examinations that certify individuals providing services in medical genetics.[11] To be eligible for certification by the American Board of Medical Genetics, an individual must meet the criteria in the area of desired certification, provide the supporting credentials required, and pass the appropriate examination. The areas in which certification is offered are:

1. *Clinical Geneticist*—An individual who holds an M.D., D.D.S., D.M.D., or D.O. degree and can demonstrate competence to provide comprehensive diagnostic, management, and counseling services. Competence in this area implies that the clinical geneticist:

   a. has diagnostic and therapeutic skills in a wide range of genetic disorders;

   b. has an appreciation of their heterogeneity, variability, and natural history;

   c. is able to elicit and interpret individual and family histories;

   d. is able to integrate clinical and genetic information and appreciate the limitations, interpretation, and significance of specialized laboratory and clinical procedures;

   e. has expertise in genetic and mathematic principles to perform complex risk assessments;

   f. has the skills in interviewing and counseling techniques required: (1) to elicit from the patient or family the information necessary to reach an appropriate conclusion; (2) to anticipate areas of difficulty and conflict; (3) to help families and individuals recognize and cope with their emotional and psychological needs; (4) to recognize those situations requiring psychiatric referral; and (5) to transmit pertinent information effectively, i.e., in a way that is meaningful to the individual or family;

   g. has knowledge of available health care resources for appropriate referral.

2. *Ph.D. Medical Geneticist*—An individual with a Ph.D. degree may work in association with a medical specialist, be affiliated with a clinical genetics program, serve as a consultant to medical and dental specialists, and/or serve in a supervisory capacity in a clinical genetics program. Competence in this area implies that the individual:

   a. is able to elicit and interpret individual and family histories;

   b. has appreciation of the heterogeneity, variability, and natural history of the medical disorders in question;

   c. is able to integrate clinical and genetic information in order to appreciate the limitations, interpretation, and significance of specialized laboratory and clinical procedures;

d. has expertise in genetic and mathematic principles to perform complex risk assessments;

e. has the skills in interviewing and counseling techniques required: (1) to elicit from the patient or family the information necessary to reach an appropriate conclusion; (2) to anticipate areas of difficulty and conflict; (3) to help families and individuals recognize and cope with their emotional and psychological needs; (4) to recognize those situations requiring psychiatric referral; and (5) to transmit pertinent information effectively, i.e., in a way that is meaningful to the individuals or family.

3. *Clinical Laboratory Geneticist*—An individual with a doctoral degree (M.D., Ph.D., D.D.S., etc.) who works in a clinical laboratory performing diagnostic services, and as a consultant concerning the management of patients with disorders in his or her field. Two specialists are currently certified:

   Clinical Cytogeneticist has advanced knowledge of cytogenetics and its clinical application, including prenatal diagnosis, and technical proficiency in the techniques of cell culture and chromosomal analysis.

   Clinical Biochemical Geneticist has advanced knowledge of biochemical procedures currently used in diagnosis, screening, heterozygote detection, and prenatal diagnosis of genetic diseases.

4. *Genetic Counselor*—An individual who holds a post-baccalaureate degree, including the doctoral degree, who is qualified to participate and assist as a counselor and coordinator of services and resources in the care of persons with genetically caused and predisposed disorders. A genetic counselor without a clinical doctoral degree must work in association with a clinical genetics team, under the supervision of a clinical geneticist or Ph.D. medical geneticist. Competence in this area implies that the genetic counselor:

a. is able to elicit and interpret individual and family histories;

b. has sufficient appreciation of medical aspects of the problems;

c. has sufficient knowledge of genetic and mathematic principles to understand the limitations, interpretation, and significance of specialized laboratory and clinical procedures;

d. has the skills in interviewing and counseling techniques required to (1) elicit from the patient or family the information necessary to reach an appropriate conclusion; (2) anticipate areas of difficulty and conflict; (3) help the families and individuals recognize and cope with their emotional and psychological needs; (4) recognize those

situations requiring referral; (5) transmit pertinent information effectively, i.e., in a way that is meaningful to the individual or family;
e. has knowledge of available health care resources for appropriate referral.

ESSENTIALS OF THE PROCESS

Pedigree Analysis

Taking a family history involves construction of a pedigree. It includes inquiries about the health status of the couple, their first-degree relatives (siblings, parents, and offspring), second-degree relatives (uncles, aunts, nephews, nieces, and grandparents), and third-degree relatives (first cousins). It is especially important to check whether there is consanguinity in the family. It may be necessary to obtain medical records to confirm directly the diagnosis of a relevant disorder in family members. Untoward reproductive outcomes should be noted, including spontaneous abortions, stillborns, and anomalous infants, and details should be sought (e.g., gestational age, complications of pregnancy, autopsy reports, etc.). Exposure to drugs (including prescription, nonprescription, and "street" drugs) and toxic chemicals (e.g., in the workplace) in the patient or her spouse—either prior to conception or during the current pregnancy—should be determined. The amount of alcohol intake and cigarette smoking during pregnancy should also be evaluated.* Parental ages should be recorded. Prenatal diagnosis counseling is mandatory if the maternal age at the anticipated date of delivery is 35 years or older. Paternal age greater than 55 years confers an increased risk for new dominant mutations and, although controversial, may also increase the risk for aneuploid offspring.

Ethnic origin should be ascertained. All couples of Jewish ancestry should be offered screening to determine whether they are carriers for Tay-Sachs disease, since this could indicate the necessity for antenatal testing. Preferably, screening should be performed prior to pregnancy, since serum levels of hexosaminidase A may result in a false-positive carrier status during gestation; however, this can usually be resolved utilizing a leukocyte assay for the enzyme activity. Screening should also be done for β-thalassemia in Italians and Greeks, α-thalassemia in Orientals, and sickle cell anemia in blacks.†

A questionnaire that has been found useful for identifying those people

---

*See Chapter 8.

†Consult Chapters 4 and 5 for detailed discussion of the indications and methods for the prenatal diagnosis of genetic disorders, and Chapter 3 for discussion of genetic screening.

who could benefit from formal genetic counseling is presented in Table 2–1.[12] This questionnaire was designed to be simple enough for completion by patients with input by a physician or a nurse.

Medical Diagnosis

Good genetic advice requires certainty of diagnosis; even the best counseling cannot compensate for an inaccurate diagnosis. In addition to the pedigree analysis, the proband (if living) should be carefully examined, as should any other family members at risk. If the proband is no longer living, the appropriate medical records should be sought and inspected. Laboratory work often includes cytogenetic studies or biochemical analysis of blood, urine, or cultured cells. Nongenetic factors may mimic the action of genetic factors in the production of disease (so called phenocopies); a good history and various clinical and laboratory studies may be helpful in differentiation. Familial recurrence is unlikely with phenocopies. A new mutation of a dominant disorder may also be confused with a sporadic case. The possibility of nonpaternity must also be considered.[7]

Sometimes, however, despite the most intensive efforts, a precise diagnosis cannot be established. Some families will receive a measure of satisfac-

TABLE 2–1.
Information Requested on Genetic Questionnaire Utilized by Prentice Women's Hospital and Maternity Center*

1. Do you have any congenital abnormalities (birth defects) or serious illnesses? If so, what? Examples of birth defects include heart disease, clubfoot, cleft (hare) lip.
2. Do any of your relatives (especially your children, parents, brothers, or sisters) have a birth defect or mental retardation?
3. Do any of your relatives have health problems other than diabetes, heart attack, gallbladder disease, appendicitis, hernia repair, or surgery related to accidents? Examples include muscular dystrophy or sickle cell anemia.
4. Does the child's father or any of his relatives (especially his children, parents, brothers, or sisters) have a birth defect or mental retardation?
5. Do the relatives of the child's father have health problems other than diabetes, heart attack, gallbladder disease, appendicitis, hernia repair, or surgery related to accidents? Examples include muscular dystrophy or sickle cell anemia.
6. Have you or any of your relatives had more than one miscarriage in the first 3 months of pregnancy? If so, list the relationship and number of miscarriages.
7. Have you been exposed to any infectious diseases (such as measles) during this pregnancy?
8. Have you taken any drugs other than iron or vitamins during pregnancy? If so, list the drug(s).

*Age, last menstrual period, ethnic background, and race are requested along with patient identification.

tion and relief from the knowledge that all reasonable steps have been taken to try to answer their questions. For others, the answer "we do not know" leads to understandable dissatisfaction with the counseling experience.[5]

Estimating and Interpreting the Recurrence Risks

The counselor may predict the risks for family members by identifying the etiologic factor, which will fall into one of four categories: (1) single mutant gene; (2) chromosomal aberration; (3) polygenic; or (4) environmental. For diseases caused by single mutant genes, the risks may generally be calculated in straightforward fashion using Mendelian laws.‡ Among the latter three catagories, however, counseling must be based on *empirical* risk figures.

The next step is interpreting the risks to the family in meaningful and understandable terms. Evidence from many follow-up studies indicates that individuals generally remember the level of risks they were told at counseling; not always in numerical form, but whether it was a high or low recurrence risk.[13, 14] However, how different people *perceive* their genetic risks varies widely, from overly cautious to reckless. Perception is difficult to measure objectively either in a laboratory or in real life,[15] and the counselor must recognize that risk perception of a genetic disorder is a complex phenomenon.[16] First, the family must understand the consequences of the genetic problem. Factual information must be conveyed concerning its significance and natural history. The explanation should be developed in small, discrete steps, with frequent pauses so the counselees can ask questions. A realistic understanding of such information may require several counseling sessions.

Second, perception of risks is highly dependent upon the individual's subjective experiences and expectations. For example, a cleft lip may be perceived as a major tragedy by some parents. On the other hand, some couples may readily accept a child with Down syndrome. Third, the way the counselor presents risk figures has an important influence on how they are interpreted.[16] For example, a "1 in 4 risk of an abnormality" might be interpreted differently than a "3 to 1 likelihood of a normal child." Although most counselors claim to use a nondirective approach, few deny that an element of counselor bias always exists. Risk figures might usefully be presented in several alternative ways.

Interpretation of a risk is also subject to shift, i.e., odds previously regarded as high may subsequently assume more or less threatening proportions.[16] Discussion of a risk situation with the nuclear or extended family, friend, clergy, or other consultants may lead clients to "shift" their percep-

‡See Chapter 1.

tions of the significance of the risks. As noted by geneticist Margery Shaw, "Perhaps the most important factor in the counselee's interpretation of risks depends on the nature of the outcome if the gamble is lost. Thus the burden in question (medical, social, psychological and economic) may influence the decision more than the mathematical odds. Since rational decision making is more difficult when only one or a few gambles are taken (as in small families), risk taking may be quite unrelated to probabilities."[15]

Another writer has put the case more graphically, noting that most of us accept a 1 in a 100 chance of winning a prize at a carnival, but reject the 1 in 6 chance of losing our lives by playing Russian roulette. In one case what we stand to lose is a dollar; in the other, our life. The notion is that odds themselves are relevant only when one knows the consequences that follow from the event occurring or not occurring. In the genetic counseling situation this implies that "parents can assess specific genetic risks only if they are informed of the sequelae and all their implications. . . ."[17] For example, parents may be willing to take the risk of a genetic disease if the affected child is likely to be stillborn or die in early infancy, but would be less likely to take the risk of having a handicapped child who would require a lifetime of constant care.[17]

All of this, of course, implies that the more accurate information the couple has, the more likely they are to make a final decision that is consistent with their own values. As a policy matter, this conclusion underlines the role of the legal doctrine of informed consent in genetic counseling and its purpose: the promotion of self-determination and rational decision making in decisions that critically affect one's own life.

Options

A discussion of the available options makes the counseling process more relevant and comprehensive. Such discussions will vary according to the circumstances. Helping an individual or a family adjust to the realities of a genetic disorder is more accurately termed "disease counseling," rather than genetic counseling. This entails providing information about the condition, its prospects, treatment possibilities, and available support services, such as training and education.[5] With respect to reproductive options, the following may be relevant:
1. Adoption
2. Prenatal diagnosis
3. Artificial insemination by donor
4. Artificial insemination by husband's sperm and a surrogate mother
5. In vitro fertilization with sperm from the husband and ovum from a donor
6. Surrogate embryo transfer

7. Acceptance of risks and choosing to take the risk
8. Use of contraception in hopes that prenatal diagnosis or treatment will become available
9. Sterilization

Counselors must be careful not to misrepresent the availability of some of these technologies, many of which are still considered experimental or investigational.*

Follow-up

To avoid confusion, the relevant medical and genetic information should be reinforced with a letter to the couple and the referring physician. The number of follow-up sessions will vary, depending on the specific genetic disorder and the couple's needs. The couple should be informed that counseling services may be made available to their family members who may unknowingly be at risk. However, the couple must understand that such extended family counseling must be initiated by them and that confidentiality will be strictly respected. Finally, the couple should be encouraged to call or return at any time they wish to discuss any additional questions or concerns.

ATTITUDINAL STRATEGIES

All forms of counseling have the potential of modifying behavior. Indeed, an argument may be made that without behavior modification, genetic counseling cannot be considered effective. Nonetheless, counseling can be justified on the sole basis of making reproduction decisions more informed. Genetic counseling may take one of several attitudinal forms or strategies, and individual counselors may vary their approach from patient to patient. There are no rigid protocols for how genetic counseling should be offered, since it must be done in a comfortable way for the presenter as well as the recipient.[5]

Directive Genetic Counseling

In directive genetic counseling, the counselor seeks to direct the counselees' choice through a preconceived limitation on the options from which they may choose, resulting in their focusing on only one option and not realizing other alternatives.[18] In the most blatant form of directiveness, the

---

*See Chapter 9 for detailed discussion of noncoital methods of reproduction.

counselor may simply tell the counselees what they ought to do. This form of counseling has traditionally been employed by physicians in other areas where giving advice or "guidance" based on knowledge and experience is more expected.

The goal of imposing the beliefs of the counselor on the client is perhaps nowhere so openly stated as in a 1971 article by a group of Tennessee physicians on counseling young women with sickle cell anemia. Their conclusion, from a finding of a 6% maternal mortality rate and a 20% infant mortality rate, was that permitting a woman with sickle cell disease to undergo pregnancy could not be justified. In their words, "We advocate primary sterilization, abortion if conception occurs, and sterilization for those that have completed pregnancies. Patients with sickle cell disease should be unhesitatingly thus counseled."[19] While the authors might argue that such "counseling" is for the patient's own good, what really seems to be at stake is an attempt by a group of physicians to impose their own specific beliefs on a racially defined population. This is propaganda, not counseling; and today few, if any, geneticists ascribe to such a directive or "coercive" counseling approach.

Nondirective Genetic Counseling

The most widely used and promoted method is called nondirective genetic counseling. The counselor makes clear from the onset that the process is educational, and no decisions will be made for the counselees. The counselor tries to remain impartial and objective in providing information that will allow the counselees to make their own rational decisions. The assumption is that such decisions will reflect the values and needs of the family and not necessarily those of the counselor or those of society. The need to give emotional support to families who are receiving stressful information is recognized, and efforts are deliberately made to provide it.[20] A slight variation on this theme is that some counselors will not comment on the decisions families suggest, whereas others will support any decisions families make.[18] On the surface, nondirective counseling seems to border on passive or indifferent communication. However, counselors will not be able to keep from interjecting their own biases by either verbal or nonverbal messages. For example, a simple gesture (nonverbal body language) such as shifting in one's chair or the raising of eyebrows may be interpreted as approval or disapproval of a decision. Sometimes, despite conscious efforts to provide nondirective counseling, counselors may unknowingly be giving directive signals. Repetition of certain points or presenting them in a louder voice may influence the way counselees weigh the information. Even silence at certain crucial times in a discussion may be persuasive. As difficult as it is, the endeavor is to avoid letting the counselor's value system impinge on the right of the family to self-determination.

Until the day we are willing to forbid by legislation all reproduction by carriers of certain genetic defects, all women over 35, all women with sickle cell disease, or any other category of individuals (and we trust this day will never come), counselors should expend all of their efforts toward getting information across in an understandable and useful manner, and none of their efforts toward attempting to impose their own values and preferences on families.[21]

The entire purpose of the doctrine of informed consent is to permit individuals to decide for themselves on a course of action, and to give the individual the objective, material information needed to make a decision in a reasonable manner. No matter how irrational the decision of a woman or couple to have a child may seem to the counselor, it must be remembered that it is the individual's or couple's child, not the counselor's, and the individual's or couple's decision. As two leading legal commentators have put it:

> The very foundation of the doctrine of informed consent is every man's right to forego treatment or even cure if it entails what *for him* are intolerable consequences or risks, however warped or perverted his sense of values may be in the eyes of the medical profession, or even of the community, so long as any distortion falls short of what the law regards as incompetency. *Individual freedom here is guaranteed only if people are given the right to make choices which would generally be regarded as foolish* [emphasis added].[22]

The World Health Organization Expert Committee on Genetic Counseling[23] has endorsed the nondirective approach and we also ascribe to this method.[24] We recognize, however, that completely nondirective counseling does not exist. Merely offering prenatal diagnostic services implies approval of the process. Nonetheless, the primary objective must be to present information in as accurate, comprehensive, and objective a fashion as possible, making sure that all alternatives are presented. The final use of this information must remain the decision of the counselees and will be dictated by their private values, concerns, and desires.

Genetic counseling can also be seen as a psychotherapeutic modality in which families are assumed to be under stress with inner conflicts requiring resolution. Accordingly, genetic counseling would take the form of probing and working through their stressful situation. Such counseling must be provided by individuals qualified in psychotherapy and generally requires a long-term involvement. It is really a subset of psychotherapy, rather than a form of genetic counseling.[20]

PSYCHOLOGICAL AND SOCIAL CONSIDERATIONS

Timing

The time to initiate genetic counseling depends on the genetic problem. Following the birth of an abnormal child, the parents may be shocked, bewildered, grieved, frustrated, frightened, or angry. Counseling at this point is best directed toward explaining the nature of the infant's disorder and the prognosis, providing answers to questions, and offering emotional support. This information should be given by the primary physician, who knows the couple, along with the pediatrician and medical geneticist. The counselor should be prepared to accept emotional outbursts with empathy and sympathy, while maintaining professional objectivity. This initial stage is usually not the time to go into details concerning recurrence risks for future offspring or the possible availability of prenatal diagnosis. The couple should, however, be made aware that such information is available later. After the initial crisis is over, and the parents become aware of the significance of their child's abnormality, more detailed genetic counseling is required. Timing for subsequent genetic counseling will vary, depending on the psychological readiness of the couple. Sensitive intervention may help a person resolve inner defenses and conflicts, and the timing of each phase of the genetic counseling process can be a critical factor in determining whether genetic information will be accepted or rejected.[5]

Genetic counseling for reproductive considerations should not be delayed, because it could significantly alter the couple's reproductive options. For example, a Jewish couple in which both partners are carriers for Tay-Sachs disease must be informed of their risks and the availability of prenatal diagnosis. If counseling is provided early in a pregnancy, prenatal diagnosis is an option; if counseling is delayed until late in pregnancy, this option is lost.*

Psychological Defenses

Psychological defenses underlie all genetic counseling sessions and, if not appreciated, can impede the entire counseling process. A wide variety of defenses may be employed. Some, such as repression, denial, or isolation of affect, can usually be recognized by a perceptive counselor, whereas others are difficult to identify except in extended evaluation or in a psychotherapeutic relationship.[25]

It is useful to distinguish between two general contexts in which cou-

*See Chapter 5.

ples seek counseling. Some couples seek genetic counseling because an abnormality is present in a distant relative or because exposure to potentially teratogenic agents has occurred. Such couples are naturally concerned but have no intimate knowledge of the burden of anomalous offspring. Their anxiety is usually not so high as to impede the communication of genetic information. By contrast, other couples may have experienced an untoward event of immediate concern, such as a stillborn, an anomalous offspring, or multiple spontaneous abortions. Understandably, their anxiety level will usually be high, and retention may be impeded unless psychological receptiveness is carefully considered.

The Coping Process

Couples having experienced an abnormal pregnancy outcome, or other major life stress, may be expected to manifest clearly identifiable sequential coping responses in order to attain psychological homeostasis.[26, 27]

The first response is shock and disbelief. This denial is a psychological mechanism whereby the individual attempts to maintain the integrity of the personality simply by denying the stressful situation. The individual may insist that a mistake has been made, not comprehend what has been said, and so on. The counselor must be alert to this coping response because frequently such individuals appear to be "very mature in handling the situation." This stage may vary considerably in duration. If prolonged, it can be self-defeating and interfere with an understanding and acceptance of the genetic problem. The counselor must recognize that during this denial phase the counselee is usually unable to absorb new information.

During the second stage, the individual begins to comprehend the reality of the situation and attempts to deal with it at the intellectual level. Anxiety may manifest itself by nervousness, irritability, hyperactivity, fatigue, insomnia, loss of appetite, or somatic complaints such as headaches or indigestion. The individual may experience fear and become panic stricken. The stressful event has been recognized at the intellectual level, but there has not yet been a change in psychological equilibrium at the emotional level. In this phase the counselee may also be resistant to new information, although a "low-key" presentation of the threatening information may be effective.

As intellectual attempts at disregarding the new information fail, the individual may become frustrated and angry. Fault may be assigned to others (e.g., spouse, the affected child, the physician, the counselor) without a rational basis. Alternatively, the anger may be directed inward and be manifested by guilt. Such feelings may be intensified if the individual already suffers neurotic tendencies.

The next stage of the coping reaction, depression, results from the repeated frustrating attempts to resolve the problem. The symptoms of depression include feelings of worthlessness, uselessness, despair, and helplessness. Physical symptoms may include anorexia, weight loss, fatigue, constipation, headaches, photophobia, crying spells, and poor sleep. A common symptom pattern is early morning wakening when all depressive symptoms are at their worst. The counselor must recognize severe depression because of the high risk of suicide, and any counselee who mentions suicide or has made a suicidal gesture should be seen by a psychiatrist immediately.

A turning point is reached when the individual begins to abandon old modes of behavior and thought, and reaches psychological homeostasis. The person becomes active in trying adaptive changes. As new behavioral patterns are learned, repeated, and found successful, they will become established as normal response reactions to the problem.[28] This is a most critical time in the genetic counseling process because the individual is most receptive to new ideas. During this stage the role of the counselor should be supportive. The counselor should prevent the individual from simply incorporating his or her point of view without evaluation. Rather, the individual should be encouraged to evaluate self-generated alternative courses of action with regard to decision making and outcome.[27]

Appreciation of these psychological defenses helps explain the seeming failure of some intelligent couples to comprehend genetic information. For this reason, some geneticists routinely schedule multiple sessions. In our opinion, this is usually not necessary. Genetic counseling should not be equated with psychotherapy, even though an occasional individual exhibits such denial or distortion that psychotherapy is indicated.

Stigmatization

Stigmatization should be considered both from the perspective of the family and the affected individual. Genetic disorders are often viewed with disdain in a sociocultural sense because parents transmit them to their children.[9] Aside from the issue of loss of privacy, disclosure may engender feelings of unworthiness and inadequacy and burden the establishment or maintenance of social relationships because it defines the individual as less capable of fulfilling expected fertility roles.[29] A genetic disorder is characteristically a family problem; whenever heredity is implicated, family members are automatically identified as high risk.

The individual affected by a genetic disorder may also stigmatize himself or herself as inadequate or unworthy because the effect of the condition is extrapolated to the whole person. This may, in part at least, result from maternal rejection with delayed or defective bonding and permanent impairment of mother-child relationships.[30] As the child grows older, there is a recognition that peers are physically or intellectually superior. This may lead to attempts at overcompensation, withdrawal and depression, or anger. Later, increasing dependence—at a time when the child should be gaining independence—precludes an easy transition through adolescence.[30] Thus, the realization of a genetic disorder poses a threat to the integrity and self-esteem of the person and brings the psychological coping mechanisms previously discussed into operation.

Confidentiality

In addition to stigmatization, other hazards include loss of or inability to obtain employment and insurance. Because genetic information has these potential implications, genetic counselors have a high responsibility to maintain it in strict confidence. But do counselors ever have an obligation to inform potentially affected relatives of the genetic finding? For example, if the mother is diagnosed as a carrier of Lesch-Nyhan syndrome through an affected son, can the counselor inform the mother's sisters? The mother could, of course, be urged to notify her sisters herself, but assuming she adamantly refuses, what should the counselor do?

This extremely difficult question has no entirely satisfactory answer. There is, for example, a long line of legal cases that *permits* physicians to disclose otherwise confidential medical information to public authorities in certain circumstances (e.g., child abuse, gunshot wounds, certain diseases) to protect the health and safety of society's members.[31, 32] In such cases the physician has an affirmative duty to disclose what would otherwise be confidential information.

In the courts, the most analogous case involved a psychologist who failed to warn a woman that his patient, a disturbed graduate student from India who wanted to marry her, had threatened to kill her. The woman was subsequently murdered by the patient, and her parents sued for failure to warn her (or them) of the danger. The court enunciated the following rule: "Where a doctor. . .in the exercise of his professional skill and knowledge, determines, or should determine, that a warning is essential to avert danger arising from the medical or psychological condition of his patient, he incurs a legal obligation to give that warning."[33] The basis for this broadly worded and arguably unprecedented decision was the court's view that we live in an "interdependent" and "risk-infested" society, and that society cannot tolerate additional risks that physicians could eliminate by a simple act of communication. It would, of course, be stretching this decision considerably to use it to find a duty on the part of a genetic counselor to warn other family members that their *offspring* might be in danger because of a genetic condition the family member *might* be carrying. However, in view of the public policy enunciated by the courts, a strong argument can be made that such a disclosure, assuming it was carefully made to potentially affected individuals only, would be *legally permissible* even though not required.[32]

Given this type of uncertainty in the law and the fact that this situation can be easily anticipated, each genetic counseling group should have a clear, written policy defining the circumstances, if any, under which it will disclose information learned in the counseling program. This policy should be spelled out *before* the counseling and medical diagnosis process begins, so that the individual or couple can opt out immediately if the policy is not accepted. Our own bias is toward a policy of strict nondisclosure without counselee consent. We think this policy fosters client self-determination and confidence in the integrity of the counseling process. On the other hand, we recognize the serious implications of many genetic disorders and understand why a counselor might want to breach confidentiality in certain instances.

EFFECTIVENESS

To assess the effectiveness of genetic counseling, various aspects may be evaluated. Margery Shaw extensively reviewed the literature to determine the aims of genetic counseling; the methods by which knowledge is transmitted; the degree to which genetic disease information is comprehended and retained; the attitudes, beliefs, and value systems of the counselors and counselees; and the changes in reproductive behavior, if any, after counseling.[15] After reviewing over 200 articles on genetic counseling, she observed that many authors did not address these questions but, instead, gave narrative accounts of their experiences as counselors and their opinions about the value of genetic counseling. Other authors gave data addressing only specific questions, with widely varying results. Most were retrospective studies with little or no record of what transpired during the counseling sessions.

Nonetheless, Shaw's literature review provides evidence of certain trends in the evaluation of the genetic counseling process. First, the objectives of genetic counseling can be separated into two broad categories: (1) to promote societal goals by encouraging rational decision making, and (2) to protect individual autonomy by encouraging clients to make their own decisions, whether rational or not. Table 2–2 lists some of the stated objectives of counselors from the studies surveyed. Second, the methodology of counseling is highly variable. In some centers, counseling is a team effort including physicians, geneticists, and social workers. In other units, physicians are the only counselors. Third, in reviewing studies addressing the reception and retention of information by counselees, some investigators

TABLE 2–2.

Genetic Counseling Objectives*

Directed at the affected individual
  Decrease the pain and suffering of the disease
  Advise if treatment is possible
  Quote risk figures for offspring and other relatives
  Reduce anxiety and guilt
  Help patient to cope with affliction
Directed at the parents
  Help couples make rational decisions about their reproduction
  Give family planning options to at-risk matings
  Reduce anxiety and guilt in the parents
  Educate the parents about the disease in question
  Encourage couples to make their own decisions
  Discourage high-risk couples from reproducing
Societal goals
  Eliminate genetic disease
  Prevent genetic disease
  Reduce the incidence of genetic disease
  Reduce the burden of genetic disease
  Decrease the frequency of deleterious genes
  Upgrade awareness of genetics in the public
  Influence mate selection

---

*From Shaw MW: Review of published studies of genetic counseling: A critique, in Lubs HA, de la Cruz F (eds): *Genetic Counseling.* New York, Raven Press, 1977, pp 35–52. Used by permission.

have attempted to determine preknowledge (i.e., before counseling); others tested counselees immediately after, shortly after, or a long while after counseling. Although study designs varied considerably, the level of retention was generally reported as encouraging. Fourth, the issue of attitudes and beliefs was difficult to evaluate because it is subjective, and most comments concern statements that couples make in their decisions to reproduce or curtail reproduction. The most objective data come from follow-up studies of actual reproductive behavior. The study concludes that to evaluate genetic counseling, one must clearly state the objectives sought by the counselor.[15] The assessments should not, of course, be made by the counselors themselves, since self-assessors have a tendency to "draw the bull's-eye around the arrow," wherever it may have landed.

Other reviewers also note that centers that have attempted to evaluate their own effectiveness have often fallen into the trap of measuring their success by whether or not a family decision seemed rational to the counselor.[20] Instead, evaluation of the nondirective counseling process should be based on (1) whether a patient or family comprehended the counseling facts and used them in their decision making, and (2) whether the family felt that the counseling was supportive.[20]

A review of published follow-up studies to assess the impact of genetic counseling concluded that many parents of children with a genetic disorder inadequately understand the genetic implications of the disease, even after one or more genetic counseling sessions.[34] The authors of the review also criticized the design of most studies, noting that it was impossible to correlate this lack of genetic knowledge with insufficient transmission of information during the counseling session. On the other hand, their review also led them to conclude that, "Genetic counseling, if adequately available to families at risk, allows them to plan in reasonable freedom, and can thus be a powerful tool in the fight against the burden genetic diseases impose on individuals and society."[34]

One of the main goals of genetic counseling is to provide information that clients can use in making decisions about whether or not to have children.[35] Presumably counseling would facilitate more informed reproductive decision making among these clients and reduce the number of clients who are "reproductively uncertain." However, there is often a gap between the counselor's expectations and the consequences of counseling.[36] For example, in a two-year follow-up study of 200 consecutive couples seen in a genetic counseling clinic, investigators found that over a third of those who were told they were at high risk of having a child with a serious genetic disease were undeterred and actually planned further pregnancies.[37] In the past, such behavior was often regarded as "irresponsible," a failure on the part of the counselor, and an indictment of counseling in general. But when the couples in this study were carefully questioned, their reasons for planning further children were often considered very understandable.[37]

These findings were further substantiated in a prospective longitudinal self-administered questionnaire study of 836 clients undergoing genetic counseling.[36] The investigators found that genetic counseling did *not* eliminate reproductive uncertainty in a significant number of cases. They found that reproductive uncertainty after counseling was significantly associated with (1) uncertainty before counseling; (2) uncertainty about the client's perception of "ideal" family size; (3) concern about the effects of an affected child on the client's social life; (4) perceived serious problems caring for a child with a defect now living at home; and (5) new concerns raised in counseling. The investigators suggest that (despite their findings) counseling should not necessarily be regarded as a failure even if it does not reduce the reproductive uncertainty of most clients. There are other important goals of counseling, including the reduction of guilt and anxiety, helping families to adjust to the presence of a genetic disorder, and providing information regarding possible treatment or prenatal diagnosis.[38]

Medical sociologist James Sorenson has examined 39 studies of genetic counseling.[39] Cautioning that these studies varied widely in design and methodology and that what constitutes "genetic counseling" also varies from center to center, he concluded that the available evidence suggests, among other things, that the following statements are more *false* than true:

1. The majority of individuals coming to genetic counseling know little about their medical/genetic problem.

2. The majority of counselees have uncertain reproductive plans before counseling.

3. Before counseling, there is little, if any, concordance between patients' recurrence risk and their reproductive plans.

4. The majority of individuals report that genetic counseling influences their reproductive plans.

5. When actually given direct reproductive advice by a counselor, couples find it useful and follow it.

6. Genetic counseling reduces substantially disagreements between spouses about reproductive plans and the problems associated with raising a child with a birth defect.[39]

These conclusions are surprising to many because they seem to indicate that genetic counseling is not effective. This, however, is not the proper conclusion. Individuals make reproductive decisions for a wide variety of reasons. The possibility of having a handicapped child is only one of them, and probably not the major one, for most couples. Therefore, the proper test for effective genetic counseling is not, "Did it convince the couple to have (or not to have) another child?" The proper test is, "Did it increase the couple's awareness of their genetic status and the risks of having a handicapped child, such that their decision to reproduce was a "genetically informed one?" This test places genetic counseling where it belongs in health care delivery: a method of enhancing individual reproductive liberty.

Chapter 3 —————————————

Genetic Screening

Unlike traditional medicine, which responds to illness and injury presented to physicians, screening is a public health endeavor that actively seeks out asymptomatic people, many of whom are not otherwise receiving medical care. Screening tests have become pervasive and accepted in our society, even though they raise serious questions of autonomy, stigmatization, confidentiality, informed consent, and efficacy. In the realm of genetics, the past two decades have witnessed three waves of newborn genetic screening laws that have covered most of the states in the country. Phenylketonuria screening programs were mandated by 43 states between 1963 and 1968; from 1971 to 1974, 17 states passed laws to promote screening for sickle cell anemia; and by 1986,[1] 48 states and the District of Columbia had statutes (usually based on their original PKU enactment) governing newborn screening.[2] Genetic screening can also be performed on potential carriers, the fetus, and genetic donors. Screening of all but genetic donors will be discussed in this chapter,* but the emphasis will be on neonatal genetic screening, the most pervasive form of screening currently practiced.

Genetic screening is a "search in a population for persons possessing certain genotypes that (1) are already associated with disease or predisposed to disease, (2) may lead to disease in their descendants, or (3) may produce other variations not known to be associated with disease."[3] Persons in the first category are identified for treatment. The second group is identified so that individuals in it can receive counseling about their reproductive options

---

*For a discussion of genetic and gestational donors, see Chapter 9.

and risks. Both of these categories are also counted for epidemiologic studies establishing incidence or prevalence figures. The third group is identified for research purposes, specifically to help determine the genetic constitutions of populations. Thus, genetic screening has different meanings and contexts and may be of almost any order of magnitude, ranging from testing only selected individuals to testing all individuals regardless of age or clinical state.

Technological advances in the detection and treatment of diseases have spawned pressure for their use from the public (particularly from those who have experienced a disabling disease for which new technologies promise amelioration), from scientists who have made the discoveries, and from commercial firms eager to market them.[4] Increasing demand for genetic screening and limited resources are forcing decisions about who should be screened and how the choice should be made. Important factors include: (1) frequency and severity of the condition; (2) availability of a therapy of documented efficacy; (3) extent to which detection by screening improves the outcome; (4) validity and safety of the screening tests; (5) adequacy of resources to assure effective screening and follow-up; (6) costs; and (7) acceptance of the screening program by the community, including both consumers and practicing physicians.[5] The optimal genetic program would only be initiated after adequate public education, with community support and involvement in the program; those screened would be informed of the purpose of the screening and give consent; confidentiality would be maintained; results would be conveyed through nondirective counseling; screening tests would be inexpensive, simple, and accurate; there would be sufficient qualified personnel and laboratory facilities for required follow-up; and the program would provide means of self-assessment.

In this chapter we review genetic screening, carrier screening, and maternal serum α-fetoprotein screening; we will also discuss some future prospects in screening. Prenatal diagnosis of genetic disorders may also properly be considered as screening and is dealt with in detail in Chapters 4 and 5.

NEWBORN GENETIC SCREENING

Table 3–1 provides a list of disorders for which newborn screening tests are currently available.

Phenylketonuria

The genetic disorder that best illustrates the potential value of mass screening is phenylketonuria (PKU). This disease, first described by Folling

TABLE 3–1.
Disorders for Which Newborn Screening
Tests Are Available

Phenylketonuria
Congenital hypothyroidism
Maple syrup urine disease
Galactosemia
Cystinuria
α-1-antitrypsin deficiency
Histidinemia
Iminoglycinuria
Hartnup disease
Hyperprolinemia
Adenosine deaminase deficiency
Homocystinuria
Tyrosinemia
Valinemia
Arginosuccinic aciduria
Orotic aciduria
Angioneurotic edema (absence of inhibitor
    of C-1 esterase)
Sickle cell anemia
β-thalassemia
Familial hyperlipidemia
Biotinidase deficiency

in 1934, is estimated to occur in 1 in 15,000 to 1 in 20,000 live births.[6, 7] In its classic form, children appear normal at birth and during the perinatal period. An increased frequency of vomiting in early infancy has been described, and some infants have even had surgery for suspected pyloric stenosis.[8] If untreated, these children develop neurologic deterioration, seizures, and mental retardation. Such children lose approximately 50 IQ points during the first year of life and 98% will have an IQ below 70.[9, 10] Other clinical manifestations include reduced pigmentation (blond hair, blue eyes), eczema, delayed psychomotor development, failure to walk or talk, hyperactivity, agitation, aggressive behavior, hypertonicity tremor, microcephaly, enamel hypoplasia of the teeth, prominent jaw with widened spaces between the teeth, decalcification of the long bones, and decreased rate of growth. The urine of such untreated children has a characteristic "mousy" odor.

The metabolic error in PKU results from a defect in the enzyme phenylalanine hydroxylase, and the inheritance pattern is autosomal recessive.[10, 11] Early postnatal treatment with diets low in phenylalanine content can restore nearly normal homeostasis to phenylalanine metabolism and may prevent impaired brain development.[12, 13] An ongoing controversy is when to end the low phenylalanine diet. Some studies indicate that it is safe to terminate the diet at about age five.[14, 15] However, other studies indicate that longer treatment would be beneficial, at least for some patients.[16–18] Until the issue is resolved, it is prudent to maintain dietary treatment as long as familial and social factors permit, and then employ a relaxed but still restricted low-phenylalanine diet.[19, 20]

Phenylketonuria was the first condition for which newborn screening was widely adopted.[1, 19, 20] The routine hospital screening of newborns became practical only in the early 1960s with the development of the Guthrie test.[21] In this test, the growth of a laboratory culture bacteria is inhibited *unless* phenylalanine is added to the medium. Several drops of capillary blood are obtained from the newborn's heel directly onto a filter paper. Small discs of the dried blood (cut from the filter paper) collected from numerous newborns, along with control discs containing known concentrations of phenylalanine, are spaced on a large nutrient surface inoculated with bacteria. The amount of bacterial growth is directly proportional to the amount of phenylalanine in the blood; a halo around a disc indicates a high level of phenylalanine in the dried blood and is usually diagnostic of PKU. Confirmatory tests using more refined techniques are then performed to rule out false-positive tests. Alternatively, some laboratories now utilize the McCaman-Robins fluorometric test for screening newborns.[22] Early newborn discharge and home deliveries make achieving 100% testing impossible, but about 90% of all US infants are screened for PKU. When an infant is discharged under the age of 24 hours, a predischarge specimen must be taken, followed by a collection of a second specimen between the fourth and tenth day of life.*[23]

The PKU screening may be judged on several criteria. From a public health standpoint, screening and initiation of a low phenylalanine diet in the first few weeks of life prevent marked mental retardation in affected children. Since screening has become widespread in the United States, the admission of children with PKU to institutions for the mentally retarded has virtually ceased.[24] Cost-effectiveness analysis indicates that the cost of PKU screening programs, including treatment, is more than offset by the savings in health care, usually institutionalization, required without screening.[11, 25, 26]

---

*At least seven other conditions may exhibit elevated serum and urine phenylalanine levels. In addition to classic PKU, there is a transient hyperphenylalanemia due to delayed development of enzymes in some newborns.[9] This abnormality disappears within the first few weeks of life and requires no treatment. Of great concern are variants of PKU that involve the cofactor system rather than phenylalanine hydroxylase per se (i.e., either a deficiency of dihydropteridine reductase or a defect in dihydrobiopterin synthesis).[10] These disorders require special procedures for diagnosis. Unfortunately, mental retardation is not prevented by phenylalanine restriction alone, and no therapy is currently available.[19, 20]

There are now thousands of children and adolescents with PKU who have received dietary restriction therapy and who are of normal intelligence. Since PKU is an autosomal recessive condition, half of all affected individuals are female and are potentially subject to the maternal PKU syndrome. In 1957, attention was first directed to maternal PKU in a report of three nonphenylketonuric mentally retarded offspring of a mother with PKU.[27] Most infants born to untreated PKU mothers have, in fact, shown mental retardation and other anomalies, even though the infant did not have PKU. An analysis of 524 pregnancies in 155 women having PKU or other forms of hyperphenylalanemia found a higher frequency of spontaneous abortion, and among the 423 live-born offspring, there was a marked increase in the frequencies of mental retardation, microcephaly, and congenital heart defects.[28] Although beginning treatment with a low phenylalanine diet prior to conception would appear the most reasonable approach to preventing the adverse sequelae, it is uncertain at present what constitutes appropriate prenatal dietary therapy and if therapy is effective in preventing fetal damage.[29]

Galactosemia

The term "galactosemia" describes several autosomal recessive disorders of galactose metabolism. The most frequent form is expressed as a cellular deficiency of galactose-1-phosphate uridyl transferase, an important enzyme that catalyzes the reaction by which galactose is converted to glucose.[30] This disorder occurs with a frequency of about 1 in 75,000.[31] Affected infants frequently develop vomiting, lethargy, jaundice, diarrhea, hepatomegaly (enlarged liver), edema, and failure to thrive during the first days or weeks following ingestion of milk.[32–34] If untreated, the disease may be rapidly fatal or may develop into a chronic phase characterized by cirrhosis, cataracts, and mental retardation.[34, 35]

A diet free of galactose is effective in reducing the biochemical and clinical severity of the disease. In those children with manifestations of the toxicity syndrome, the galactose-free diet will cause striking regression of symptoms and signs.[30] Complete elimination of the sugar from the diet is the desired goal, but this is usually difficult to accomplish. As the children grow, it is important to be aware of sources of galactose in addition to milk, and a list of permitted foods should be given to the parents.[36] Unlike PKU, severe mental retardation is not inevitable, even in those patients whose dietary therapy is started late in the first year.[37, 38] However, impairment of mental function is least if the galactose-free diet is begun early, and the best results are in cases in which intrauterine exposure to galactose was prevented by restricting galactose intake during pregnancy.[39]

The presumptive diagnosis of galactosemia may be made by the identification of galactose in the urine and blood, but the definitive diagnosis
depends upon assay of transferase activity in red blood cells.*[30, 39]

Newborn screening for disorders of galactose metabolism came as a by-
product of PKU screening.[33] Several screening tests have been designed to
use blood collected and dried on filter paper, and, therefore, galactosemia
screening is usually done in connection with PKU screening. As with PKU,
it is optimal to obtain the blood sample after the third day of life. The
overall birth incidence for complete transferase deficiency is approximately
1:60,000.[40] There is limited information about the cost-effectiveness for
newborn screening for galactosemia.[33]

Maple Syrup Urine Disease (Branched-Chain Ketoaciduria)

Maple syrup urine disease (MSUD), also known as branched-chain ketoaciduria, was first described in 1954.[41] This autosomal recessive disorder
has a frequency of about 1:175,000 newborns, and at least five different
clinical forms are recognized.[6] In the classic type, the infant is apparently
healthy at birth, but by the end of the first week of life, the infant fails to
thrive, feeds poorly, and vomits frequently. This is followed by lethargy,
muscular hypertonicity, seizures, coma, and death. Untreated or improperly
treated infants who survive will generally have severe mental and motor
retardation.[42] Infections often hasten death. A distinctive odor, described as
that of maple syrup, is often noted, particularly in the urine. Maple syrup
urine disease results from defective decarboxylation of all of the keto deriv-
atives of the branched-chain amino acids, and the diagnosis is made by finding elevated concentrations of the branched-chain amino acids (valine, leucine, and isoleucine) in plasma and urine with an amino acid analyzer.[42]

---

*Several variant forms of transferase deficiency have been described: the Duarte variant,
with 50% normal red blood cell transferase in the homozygote; the Rennes variant, with 7%
residual activity; the Indiana variant, with 0% to 45% residual activity; the Chicago variant,
with 27% activity; and the Los Angeles variant, with the red blood cell transferase activity
actually increased to 140% of normal. In the Negro variant, red blood cell transferase activity
is undetectable, but liver and intestinal activity is in the range of 10%. Heterozygotes for the
Negro variant have normal activity, in contrast to heterozygotes for the classic type, in which
activity is 50% of normal. The clinical course in each of these variants depends upon the level
of enzymatic activity; the more the activity, the fewer the symptoms.[30] In addition to a galac-
tose-1-phosphate uridyl transferase, other more rare causes of galactosemia are galactokinase
deficiency and uridine diphosphate galactose-4-epimerase deficiency. The former enzyme deficiency leads to cataract formation in untreated patients without other evidence of galactose
toxicity, whereas the latter enzyme deficiency appears to be without clinical significance. As
with the transferase form, treatment of patients with the galactokinase deficiency is directed
toward exclusion of galactose from the diet, and, if initiated early, appears to be effective in
preventing most or all of the adverse sequelae.[30]

Arrest of neurologic damage has been achieved by dietary treatment with restriction of valine, leucine, and isoleucine.[43] Dietary formulas are now commercially available. Unfortunately, dietary treatment of patients with MSUD is difficult because of its acute neonatal course, and the involvement of three essential amino acids.[42] Accordingly, dietary management is best provided through centers with the appropriate experience and resources.

Routine neonatal screening for MSUD has been carried out since 1964, and over 12.5 million newborns have been tested around the world. It is difficult to justify screening for MSUD alone simply on a cost-effectiveness or cost-benefit basis; however, as part of a more comprehensive program including screening for other diseases (e.g., PKU, galactosemia, congenital hypothyroidism), MSUD can be justified on medical, economic, and humanitarian grounds.

Biotinidase Deficiency

Biotinidase deficiency is an autosomal recessive disorder that causes a deficiency in multiple carboxylase enzymes, which in turn leads to an inability to recycle the vitamin biotin.[44, 45] Affected infants appear normal at birth, but if untreated, become biotin deficient and develop seizures, skin rash, alopecia, ataxia, hearing loss, developmental delay, and metabolic decompensation that can terminate in coma and death. Infants with this disorder may be successfully treated with pharmacologic doses of biotin. In some cases, biotin supplementation has been lifesaving; if appropriate treatment is delayed, irreversible brain damage may develop. Biotinidase activity can be determined by a semiquantitative colorimetric method on filter papers impregnated with dried blood; this can serve as a simple, reliable, and inexpensive assay that is applicable to the mass screening of entire populations of newborns. The incidence of the disease is approximately 1:20,000,[46] and it has been recommended that neonatal screening for biotinidase deficiency be incorporated into the various state programs of neonatal screening for metabolic diseases.[47]

Congenital Hypothyroidism

A deficiency of thyroid hormone during critical periods of development causes irreversible brain damage and mental retardation.[48] The most common cause of congenital hypothyroidism is a developmental defect in thyroid embryogenesis (i.e., aplasia or arrested development and descent); the condition is often referred to as athyrotic cretinism or thyroid dysgenesis. Most cases are sporadic; however, on occasion, congenital hypothyroidism may result from an autosomal recessive or X-linked recessive disorder.[48] The incidence of congenital hypothyroidism is in the range of 1 in 5,000 births.[49] The early detection and treatment of hypothyroidism before 3 months of age greatly reduces the risk of mental retardation.[50–52] Owing to the difficulty of establishing an early clinical diagnosis, laboratory screening programs to detect neonatal hypothyroidism have been advocated.[23, 53]

Currently, the recommended approach is measurement of blood thyroxine (T_4) and the follow-up estimation of blood thyroid-stimulating hormone (TSH) on all samples with low (lowest 5% to 10%) T_4 values.[54] These hormones may be measured on the same dried blood spotted on filter paper as used for PKU screening. The sample should be collected before the infant is discharged from the hospital, but at least 72 hours after birth to be certain that the elevated TSH values due to the normal neonatal TSH surge have passed. In cases of early discharge, the infant should return for screening in one week. Every infant with pathologic values must have confirmatory testing.

Newborn screening for hypothyroidism is at least as justifiable as screening for PKU.[55, 56] The frequency of congenital hypothyroidism may be more than twice that of PKU and the benefit-cost ratio of screening may be 6 or greater, as compared to a ratio of about 2 for newborn screening limited to PKU and related inborn errors of metabolism.*

CARRIER SCREENING

From a clinical standpoint, the term "carrier screening" generally implies identification of heterozygotes (i.e., carriers) for an autosomal recessive

---

*Pooled data from five of the oldest newborn screening programs in North America (Quebec, Pittsburgh, Toronto, Oregon Regional, and New England Regional) indicated the results of 1,046,362 infants that had been screened for congenital hypothyroidism.[57] A total of 277 cases of congenital hypothyroidism were detected and 7 were missed, resulting in a total of 284 affected infants in the screened population, for an overall incidence of one in 3,684 live births. The cost of screening varied from $0.70 to $1.60 per infant, depending on which costs were included in the estimate. Results of preliminary developmental testing of 20 infants, 18 months of age, in whom treatment was begun at a mean of 6 weeks in the Quebec program, showed normal psychologic and neuromuscular development. Growth and bone maturation were also normal in these infants.

In the New England Hypothyroid Collaborative Study, 336,000 newborns were screened. Among 63 hypothyroid infants treated before recognizable clinical manifestations appeared and for whom Stanford-Binet scores were available (administration at ages 3 and 4 years), the mean IQ score was 106 ± 16, with a normal distribution. The only factor apparently influencing the IQ results was adequacy of treatment in the first year of life. These data gave strong evidence that children with infantile hypothyroidism, treated adequately before clinically diagnostic signs and symptoms appear, are protected against the mental retardation seen in hypothyroid infants treated only after a clinical diagnosis can be made.[58]

or X-linked recessive disease. The considerations that should be weighed in establishing carrier screening programs are:

> First, the disease in question should be serious. Second, the test to be performed on the population at risk should be simple, relatively inexpensive, and sensitive enough not to miss positive individuals. Third, the individual identified as positive should have some options. For example, married couples identified as being at risk for a recessive disease for which there is no prenatal diagnosis might choose to take the risk, undergo artificial insemination, or adopt a child and forego pregnancy . . . Fourth, the costs avoided should exceed the costs incurred. A major determination of the cost is the frequency of the disorder in the population screened.[59]

The most common purpose for carrier screening is to provide prospective parents with reproductive alternatives. In this regard, parental screening is not unique to genetic disorders, as premarital detection of incompatibilities in blood groups, venereal diseases, or prenatal detection of microbial infections are analogous situations. Individuals' knowledge of their carrier status may have important therapeutic or preventive health care implications for them.[60] For example, heterozygotes for type II hypercholesterolemia may develop coronary heart disease as early as the third and fourth decade of life. It is believed that diet, weight control, and specific medications may obviate substantially the increased risk for early myocardial infarction in carriers of this autosomal dominant disorder. Individuals with sickle cell trait may be at risk for life-threatening complications under conditions of lowered oxygen tension, e.g., flying in unpressurized aircraft, or inadvertent hypoxia while under general anesthesia. Carriers for α-l-antitrypsin deficiency are clearly predisposed to chronic obstructive pulmonary disease. Smoking is considered an important exacerbating factor to the development of chronic bronchitis and emphysema. Accordingly, carriers should be counseled to avoid smoking and other noxious inhalants.

Screening all individuals for carrier status, regardless of family history or ethnic background, would be impossible. How, then, does one decide who should be screened? This decision is generally based on several relatively simple criteria, including the availability of an accurate test for a genetic disorder and an ethnic, racial, or geographic heritage associated with an increased risk for that specific genetic trait. These criteria should provide some direction for determining which carrier screening tests are warranted. For relatively "common" autosomal recessive disorders occurring in defined ethnic groups, there is usually no known prior history of the disorder in either side of the family.[61] Table 3–2 provides a selected list of genetic traits and diseases associated with ethnic, racial, and religious groups.

In the United States, carrier screening programs have been implemented for Tay-Sachs disease, sickle cell anemia, and the thalassemias, largely because of the availability of laboratory tests, definition of select groups to screen, and adequate education of these groups about their risks for the diseases.

Tay-Sachs Disease (GM$_2$ Gangliosidosis)

Tay-Sachs disease was the first disorder for which large-scale carrier screening was done in the United States. It occurs primarily in infants of Ashkenazi Jewish parents. Approximately 1 in 3,600 Jewish children born

TABLE 3–2.
Genetic Traits and Diseases Associated With Ethnic, Racial, and Religious Groups*

GROUP	DISORDERS FOUND WITH INCREASED FREQUENCY
Ashkenazi Jews	Tay-Sachs disease
	Stub thumbs
	Abetalipoproteinemia
	Dystonia musculorum deformans (recessive form)
	Spongy degeneration of brain
	Bloom syndrome
	Familial dysautonomia
	Factor XI (plasma thromboplastin antecedent) deficiency
	Gaucher disease (adult form)
	Iminoglycinuria
	Pentosuria
	Niemann-Pick disease
	Meckel syndrome
Mediterranean peoples (Italians, Greeks, Sephardic Jews)	β-thalassemia
	Glucose-6-phosphate dehydrogenase deficiency (Mediterranean type)
	Familial Mediterranean fever
	Glycogen storage disease (type III)
Blacks	Hemoglobinopathies (especially hemoglobin S, hemoglobin C, α-thalassemia, β-thalassemia, persistent fetal hemoglobin)
	Glucose-6-phosphate dehydrogenase deficiency
	Adult lactase deficiency (African type)
French Canadians	Tyrosinemia
	Morquio syndrome
	Agenesis of corpus callosum
South Africans	Variegate prophyria
Japanese/Koreans	Acatalasia
	Oguchi disease
	Dyschromatopsia universalis hereditaria

Chinese	α-thalassemia
	Glucose-6-phosphate deficiency
	Adult lactase deficiency
Nova Scotia-Acadians	Niemann-Pick disease (Type D)
Armenians	Familial Mediterranean fever
Finns	Congenital nephrosis
	Lysinuric protein intolerance
	Aspartylglycosaminuria
	Neuronal ceroid lipofuscinosis (infantile type)
	Cornea plana
	Gyrate atrophy with hyperornithenemia
Norwegians	Cholestasis-lymphedema
Irish-English	Neural tube defects
Lebanese	Dyggve-Melchior-Clausen syndrome
	Juvenile Tay-Sachs disease
Eskimos	Pseudocholinesterase deficiency, 21-hydroxylase deficiency

*Adapted from the following: McCormack MK: Medical genetics and family practice. *Am Fam Physician* 1979; 20:154. Damon A: Race, ethnic group and disease. *Soc Biol* 1969; 16:69. McKusick VA: The ethnic distribution of disease in the United States. *J Chronic Dis* 1967; 20:115. McKusick VA: Ethnic distribution of disease in non-Jews. *Israel J Med Sci* 1973; 9:1375.

is affected with this condition as compared with 1 in 360,000 non-Jewish births.[62] Calculations based on these data show that about 1 in 30 Ashkenazi Jews in the United States are carriers of Tay-Sachs disease as compared with 1 in 300 non-Jewish individuals.[63]

Tay-Sachs disease (GM_2 gangliosidosis) is an autosomal recessive disorder caused by a generalized deficiency of an enzyme, hexosaminidase A, that is involved in the metabolism of a class of nervous system lipids called gangliosides. In the absence of the enzyme, one of the gangliosides, GM_2, accumulates in neurons of the brain. The clinical picture is characterized by motor weakness, usually beginning between 3 and 6 months of age. There is a persistent exaggerated response to sounds. Psychomotor retardation is evident from 4 to 6 months of age when the child fails to develop normal milestones. Deafness, blindness, convulsions, and generalized spasticity are usually in evidence by 18 months of age. "Cherry-red" spots in the macular region of the eye are present in over 95% of patients. As the disease progresses, the child develops a state of decerebrate rigidity, with death usually resulting from bronchopneumonia by 3 years of age.[64] No specific therapy for Tay-Sachs disease is available.

Tay-Sachs disease meets the major criteria for screening because (1) the disease occurs predominantly in a defined population, Ashkenazi Jews; (2) the carrier state can be simply, accurately, and relatively inexpensively determined with readily available biological material, which can be automated for mass screening; and (3) the prenatal diagnosis of the condition is possible so that selective abortion of affected fetuses is a viable alternative.[64, 65] Detection of Tay-Sachs carriers is accomplished by assay of hexosaminidase A in white blood cells or by measurement of resistance of serum hexosaminidase A to heat inactivation.[64, 65]

Worldwide, Tay-Sachs screening has been carried out in 73 cities and 13 countries, with 312,214 individuals screened from 1969 through 1980.[65] These programs identified 12,763 carriers and 268 at-risk couples with no family history of the condition. Among these couples, 252 pregnancies occurred with 39 Tay-Sachs fetuses identified prenatally; 212 unaffected offspring have been born.[66] Recent data indicate that these efforts have contributed to a 60% to 85% decrease in the incidence of this disorder in Jewish infants in North America.[61] When program costs are compared with the medical care costs that ensue from those Tay-Sachs patients who are born if the screening program is not carried out, the program costs are about one third to one fifth of the care costs.[67, 68]

Sickle Cell Anemia

Sickle cell anemia occurs almost exclusively in African blacks and their descendants. Among American blacks, the overall frequency is about 1 in 600. This disease is a severe hemolytic anemia, occurring in persons homozygous for the sickle gene. It is characterized by a tendency for the red blood cells to become distorted, "sickle-shaped," under conditions of low oxygen tension, resulting in increased blood viscosity, which produces capillary stasis, vascular occlusion, and infarction in various tissues such as the bones, spleen and lungs. Infection, dehydration, or other physical stresses often instigate the above cycle, which is referred to as a "crisis" and is associated with severe pain. The diagnosis is made by demonstration of the sickling phenomenon on a peripheral blood smear and confirmed by hemoglobin electrophoresis, which reveals hemoglobin S. There is no successful treatment at present. Management consists of avoiding low oxygen tension situations and promptly treating infections. Crises are treated symptomatically with analgesics and hydration. If the hemoglobin level drops to low levels, blood transfusion may be required; however, patients usually tolerate hemoglobin levels of 5 to 6 gm/100 ml blood very well (normal, around 12 gm/100 ml blood). About 10% of sickle cell anemia patients born in the United States die by the age of 10 years.[69]

Heterozygous occurrence of the sickle gene (sickle cell trait) is associated with a benign clinical course under most circumstances. Persons who are heterozygous, A/S (A is the normal allele for the β-chain, S is the abnormal allele for the sickle gene), enjoy an immunity to malaria, a common infectious disease to which normal homozygotes (A/A) are not immune.[70] As a consequence, in regions of the world in which malaria is still a problem, the sickle cell allele is maintained by selection at relatively high frequencies.

Recently sickle cell screening has taken on a new dimension, namely the advent of reliable and readily available methods for prenatal diagnosis through direct analysis of genes in DNA extracted from fetal cells obtained either by amniocentesis or chorionic villus sampling.*

β-Thalassemia

The β-thalassemias constitute one of the most serious worldwide health problems, accounting for 100,000 childhood deaths annually.[71] The thalassemias are a heterogeneous group of hereditary anemias in which the common feature is diminished synthesis of hemoglobin.[72, 73] As with sickle-cell trait, the high frequency of various thalassemia alleles is probably due to the protection it offers from malaria.[74.]

Recently developed techniques in molecular biology have helped define the precise molecular defects in several thalassemias. The β-thalassemias may be broadly classified into several groups. The most common form is further subdivided into two groups, one in which no β-globin is synthesized from the affected locus (β^-) and another where some, albeit a reduced amount, is produced (β^+).[74]

Since individuals inherit only one β-chain gene from each parent, affected individuals are either heterozygotes, homozygotes, or double heterozygotes. Statistically, one quarter of the offspring of two heterozygotes (β-thalassemia trait) will have the homozygous state (i.e., β-thalassemia major or Cooley's anemia). Moreover, an individual may inherit a β-thalassemia gene from one parent and a β-chain structural variant from the other parent. Sickle β-thalassemia is a commonly encountered example of such a double heterozygous state.

The β-thalassemias are distributed widely in populations in Mediterranean countries, the Middle East, parts of India and Pakistan, and throughout Southeast Asia. The incidence of heterozygous β-thalassemia in Italy ranges between 2% and 20%.[75-77] Similar frequencies have been reported in Greece. It should be remembered, however, that β-thalassemia occurs sporadically in all racial groups, so a patient's racial background does not necessarily preclude the diagnosis.

The heterozygous (carrier) state for β-thalassemia (thalassemia minor) is not usually associated with any clinical disability except in periods of

*See Chapter 4 for a discussion of DNA analysis.

stress, such as pregnancy or during severe infection. Hemoglobin levels range from normal to slightly decreased; in the adult, they seldom drop below 10 gm/100 ml of blood. The red blood cell indices are particularly useful in screening for carriers in population surveys. The red blood cells appear small and poorly hemoglobinized (mean corpuscular hemoglobin values of 20 to 22 pg and mean corpuscular volume values of 50 to 70 fentoliters). Demonstration of an elevated proportion of hemoglobin A_2 (3% to 7%), which requires a chromatographic or an elution procedure, is generally confirmatory.[74, 78]

Of the various thalassemia syndromes, homozygous β-thalassemia (thalassemia major) has the most pronounced medical, social, and economic impact throughout the world. The clinical picture was first described by Thomas Cooley in 1925. Affected infants usually appear healthy at birth because the normal presence of high levels of fetal hemoglobin mask the lack of β-chain production. Gradually within the first six months of life, the infants fail to thrive and develop feeding problems, listlessness, pallor, and diarrhea. The abdomen becomes distended due to liver and spleen enlargement. Unless maintained on an adequate transfusion program, the child develops characteristic facial features with bossing of the skull and overgrowth of the maxillary region. Growth is stunted and sexual development is retarded. These children are particularly prone to infection, skeletal fractures, bleeding tendencies, diabetes mellitus, adrenal insufficiency, and complications of repeated blood transfusions. Although in the past such individuals have succumbed to their disease by early adulthood, modern medical management with hypertransfusion and iron chelation has significantly improved the outlook.[74, 78]

Recently, efforts directed at the prevention of β-thalassemia through carrier screening and prenatal diagnosis have been initiated in several European countries and certain areas of North America.* This has been made possible by the advent of simple, inexpensive, and effective screening tests for this disorder.[79, 80]

---

*In one such study reported from Sardinia, 27,202 individuals were screened for β-thalassemia and 5,418 carriers detected.[81] This represented a voluntary participation of about 22% of the total population of subjects of childbearing age of the two Sardinian provinces screened. Of 613 couples determined to be at risk as a result of this screening program, 55 pregnancies have occurred; 475 (86%) couples elected to have antenatal testing; 50 (9%) decided against it and continued the pregnancy; and 30 (5.4%) spontaneously aborted. In 132 (27%) of the 475 pregnancies tested, antenatal testing showed the fetus to be affected with thalassemia major; in all but 3 instances elective abortion followed. Similar successful experiences have been reported from other screening programs. The number of newborns with thalassemia major has decreased by about 80% in the Cypriot and 40% in the Asian communities in the United Kingdom, by 50% in Greece, by 70% in Cyprus, and by 90% in the Italian province of Ferrara.[82]

SCREENING PREGNANT WOMEN

Although prenatal diagnosis should properly be considered as screening, such screening is generally targeted toward specific high-risk pregnancies.† In this section, we consider forms of screening that have been proposed for the *entire* pregnant population.

Routine Diagnostic Ultrasound Imaging During Pregancy

Ultrasonography during pregnancy has become a highly developed technology capable of detecting many fetal structural and functional abnormalities.† A 1984 National Institutes of Health Consensus Conference reviewed available data to assess the value of *routine* ultrasonographic examinations for all pregnancies.

> The information presented in the material reviewed by the panel, including the studies of Bennett, Eik-Nes, Bakketeig, Grennert, and others, allowed no consensus that routine ultrasound examinations for all pregnancies improved perinatal outcome or decreased morbidity or mortality. There was, however, evidence that there was a higher rate of detection of twins and congenital malformations, as well as more accurate dating of pregnancy, but without significant evidence of improved outcome. The evidence with respect to the number of antepartum days of hospitalization and induction rates was contradictory among trials. The data on perinatal outcome were inconclusive. The panel recognized the inadequacy of the clinical trials on which these conclusions are drawn. Furthermore, it is acutely aware of the difficulty associated with conducting ideally controlled clinical trials and the large numbers of patients that must be included to uncover differences between control and experimental groups, where a morbid event occurs infrequently and spontaneously in the control population.
>
> The panel concludes that diagnostic ultrasonography for pregnant women improves patient treatment and pregnancy outcome when there is an accepted medical indication. Randomized, controlled clinical trials would be the best way to determine the efficacy of routine screening of all pregnancies.[83]

The panel cited numerous epidemiologic studies that have tended to support the safety of diagnostic ultrasound exposure in humans. In particular, in the three randomized clinical trials in which half of the women were exposed routinely to ultrasound, there was no association of routine ultrasound exposure with birth weight. They also cited two studies that showed no association of ultrasound exposure to hearing loss. The panel concluded, however, that many of the studies reporting on the safety of diagnostic

†See Chapter 5.

ultrasonography were inadequate to address many other important issues because of technical problems in conducting such research.[83]

To help answer the questions about the safety of ultrasound in pregnancy, the panel recommended conducting animal studies designed to detect the long-term effects of exposure. From these studies reasonable estimates of the risk from diagnostic ultrasound could be made. They also recommended further studies on the fundamental mechanisms leading to bioeffects and studies of the interactions between ultrasound and developmentally significant agents such as drugs, ionizing irradiation, nutrition, hyperthermia, and hypoxia. A long-term follow-up on infants in a randomized clinical trial would help clarify questions about the effect of ultrasound on human development. The panel found that there are no data on the dose to either mother or fetus in the clinical setting. Documentation of "dwell time" and type of machine and transducer would begin to address this problem. They recommend that this information, at least, be recorded at each examination, either with imaging or Doppler devices.[83]

Taking into account the available bioeffects literature and data on clinical efficiency, as well as concern for psychosocial, economic, legal, and ethical issues, the panel came to the following conclusions:

1. Ultrasound examination during pregnancy should be performed for a specific medical indication. Routine screening is not recommended at this time.

2. Ultrasound examinations for "social" purposes (e.g., to satisfy the family's desire to know the fetal sex, to view the fetus, or to obtain a picture of the fetus) should be discouraged. Also, visualization of the fetus solely for educational or commercial demonstrations without medical benefit to the patient should not be performed.

3. Prior to an ultrasound examination, patients should be informed of the clinical indications for ultrasonography, specific benefit, potential risk, and alternatives, if any. In addition, the patient should be supplied with information about the exposure time and intensity, if requested.

4. There should be training requirements and uniform credentialing for all physicians and sonographers performing ultrasound examinations.

5. All health care providers performing ultrasound examinations should demonstrate adequate knowledge of the basic physical principles of ultrasonography, equipment, record-keeping requirements, indications, and safety.[83]

Genetic Screening Using Fetal Cells in Maternal Blood

The low but significant risks of amniocentesis and chorionic villus sampling restrict their use to pregnancies in which the risk of fetal defects is relatively high.* It has been known for many years that fetal cells normally

*See Chapter 5.

enter into the maternal circulation during pregnancy.[84–86] Accordingly, if a reliable method of isolating and analyzing fetal cells from maternal blood were available, a screening approach similar to that utilized for neural tube defects could be envisioned. Blood could be obtained from all pregnant patients. Those whose blood samples showed a fetal abnormality would then be offered chorionic villus sampling or amniocentesis for confirmatory studies. Indeed, considerable research has been directed toward these ends using fetal lymphocytes or trophoblast cells separated from maternal blood cells by a fluorescein-activated cell sorter.[87, 88] Although promising, this approach to prenatal screening has not yet been proved successful. If universal screening were implemented, however, the demands for cytogenetic evaluation would be so great that automated methods for chromosomal analysis would be required. At present, automated methods are not practical, but work in this area has also been encouraging.

Maternal Serum α-Fetoprotein Screening

Neural tube defects (NTDs) are disorders of polygenic/multifactorial inheritance that occur with an overall incidence of 1 to 2 in every 1,000 live births in the United States.[89] The two major types of NTDs are anencephaly and spina bifida. In anencephaly, the cranial vault fails to develop; affected infants who are not stillborn die shortly after birth. In spina bifida there is incomplete closure of the spinal cord and surrounding structures that may result in paralysis of the lower limbs, sensory loss, lack of bladder and bowel control, scoliosis (curvature of the spine), hydrocephalus, and mental retardation.[90] Couples who are delivered of a baby with one of these defects have a 2% to 3% risk of recurrence in a subsequent pregnancy. Ninety percent to 95% of NTD occur in families without such positive histories.

The primary diagnostic test in pregnancies at known increased risk for NTDs is analysis of amniotic fluid α-fetoprotein (AFP), the major fetal serum protein. It is normally present in amniotic fluid, excreted by the fetal kidneys.[91] A ratio between fetal serum AFP and amniotic fluid AFP between 14 and 22 weeks of gestation is maintained at approximately 100 to 1. However, AFP may also cross into the amniotic fluid from exposed membrane surfaces on the fetus, as in anencephaly or open spina bifida. Hence, elevated levels of amniotic fluid AFP can serve as a prenatal diagnostic test for NTDs.*

An association between elevated levels of maternal serum α-fetoprotein and open neural tube defects was first reported in 1973.[92] Only 5% to 10%

*See Chapter 5.

of NTDs occur in families with a previously affected offspring; thus, a method to screen pregnant women to identify the other 90% to 95% is desirable. Measuring the second-trimester concentration of maternal serum α-fetoprotein (MSAFP) has been shown to be an effective means of identifying pregnant women in the general population who are at increased risk of having a fetus with an NTD. A 19-center collaborative study in Britain demonstrated that by screening an unselected pregnant population between the 16th and 18th week of gestation, the prenatal diagnosis of 88% of cases of anencephaly and 79% of cases of open spina bifida could be made.[93] In Great Britain, where the incidence of NTDs is relatively high (5 to 6 per 1,000 births), this approach had been judged practical and cost effective. A number of centers in the United States have now had considerable experience in MSAFP screening,[94-96] and in 1983 the Food and Drug Administration approved wider use of commercial kits for the radioimmunoassay of AFP.[97] However, notwithstanding the routine application of this assay in many centers, some confounding problems exist, and considerable care is required in its use.

As a screening test, MSAFP evaluation does not reveal every fetus with an NTD. Although a variety of programmatic designs have been used to successfully implement MSAFP programs, all share in common multistage testing procedures to optimize sensitivity and specificity. Sufficient data are now available in the United States to describe the results of a uniform MSAFP program applied to the general population of pregnant women.[98, 99]

First Screen.—The initial step is to counsel the couple regarding the voluntary nature, limitations, and implications of the screening process, as well as the possibility that further testing may be necessary. Based upon this information the patient should make her own decision of whether or not to participate in the screening program, and informed consent should be obtained before the first blood sample is drawn.

Experience has shown the optimal time for the first screening is between the 16th and 18th week of gestation as calculated from the first day of the last menses. For each given week of gestation, wide variability exists in normal MSAFP levels. Currently, either the establishment of specific percentiles or median and multiple median levels at each week of gestation has been used in an effort to define suitable cutoff levels. Programs using the 95th to 98th percentile or 2 to 2.5 multiples of the median (MoM) concentration of the MSAFP distribution from unaffected pregnancies can be expected to find approximately 5% to 7% of the screened population demonstrating initially elevated MSAFP.[99] The lower the cutoff level, the greater the sensitivity, but at the cost and risk of reduced specificity, resulting in an increased number of amniocenteses. For example, lowering the cutoff point from 2 times the median (approximately the 96th percentile) to the 92nd percentile would double the number of patients considered at risk for NTDs (from 4% to 8%) and would subsequently double the need for amniocentesis.[99]

Second Screen.—Some programs recommend that patients having an initial elevated MSAFP level be retested. By evaluating a second serum sample, approximately 4% of the screened population will have serially elevated MSAFP levels and require further evaluation. The trend, however, is to proceed directly to further evaluation after a single elevated MSAFP determination.

Evaluation of Serially Elevated MSAFP levels.—If the second MSAFP value is again elevated, the patient is moved into a high-risk category and must receive specific counseling as to possible risks and need for further evaluation. The MSAFP values can be elevated for reasons other than a fetus with an NTD, including: (1) underestimation of gestational age* as values increase as gestation progresses; (2) multiple gestation, with 60% of twins and almost all triplets showing elevations; (3) threatened abortion, presumably due to leakage of fetal blood into the maternal circulation; (4) Rh disease, and (5) other rare but important congenital abnormalities (e.g., congenital nephrosis, omphalocele, upper gastrointestinal atresias, cystic hygromas).[93]

The first step in evaluation of this approximately 4% subgroup of the initial population is a conventional ultrasonographic evaluation. This will show that approximately (1) 20% to 30% will have underestimated gestational age; (2) 5% to 15% will be multiple gestations; (3) 10% will have fetal demise or impending abortion; and (4) a few will have anencephaly or other identifiable major malformations.[100] In approximately 2% of the originally screened population, no explanation is found for the elevated MSAFP, and amniocentesis for amniotic fluid AFP and acetylcholinesterase is necessary.† Approximately 5% to 10% of women who undergo amniocentesis show an elevated amniotic fluid AFP and a positive acetylcholinesterase assay, indicating a fetus with a serious abnormality, most of which will be NTDs. Thus, the overall incidence of NTDs in screened US populations is in the range of 1.1 to 1.5 per 1,000. Depending on the cutoff

---

*The maternal serum concentration of AFP normally rises rapidly between the 10th and 32nd week of pregnancy. Thus, in underestimated gestations the AFP level will appear to be too high; in overestimated gestations, it will appear low.

†See Chapter 5.

chosen, approximately 80% to 90% of the cases of anencephaly and 63% to 90% of the cases of open spina bifida will be detected.[93, 96, 99–101]

Women with one, or certainly those with more than one, MSAFP elevation who have no NTD are still at increased risk for other obstetric complications: low birth weight, preterm delivery, intrauterine growth retardation, fetal demise, bleeding, and possibly placental abruption.[102] These patients therefore warrant more intensive prenatal and intrapartum care, with appropriate biophysical and biochemical monitoring, including repeated ultrasound measurements, to observe fetal growth.[98, 102]

Low Maternal Serum α-Fetoprotein.—Over the last several years, it has become increasingly apparent that *low* maternal serum α-fetoprotein values may be of clinical importance. Specifically, it was determined by some investigators that low MSAFP (≤ 0.25 MoM) may be associated with a dramatic increase in second-trimester fetal wastage, in the range of a 1 in 4 risk.[103] In 1983, data first indicated that pregnancies with fetal chromosome abnormalities, particularly Down syndrome, tended to have lower MSAFP levels than unaffected pregnancies.[104] Other investigators have subsequently made similar observations.‡[105–109]

Cost-Benefit Analysis.—It is the consensus that the actual cost per case detected using MSAFP screening is considerably lower than the cost of medical care of a survivor during the average life span, even if one considers only detected cases of open spina bifida.[110–113] The balance of costs and possible savings depends not only on the sensitivity of the test but also on the prevalence of open spina bifida in the screened population. The favorable benefit-to-cost ratio is notable for countries with a high prevalence of NTDs, but the balance remains positive even for a population with a birth prevalence as low as 1/1,000.

Standard of Care.—Prior to the approval of α-fetoprotein test kits by the Food and Drug Administration (FDA), there was considerable concern about the wisdom of widespread routine MSAFP screening. The major issues that were believed to preclude the recommendation for initiating such programs included (1) problems related to the assay and its interpretation;

---

‡What constitutes a "low" MSAFP has not yet been fully defined, but values lower than 0.4 multiples of the median (MoM) appear to significantly increase the risk of having a fetus that is chromosomally abnormal. The magnitude of increased risk is still uncertain, but a 3-fold to 7-fold increased risk of trisomy 21 over that expected on the basis of age alone seems to exist.[106] For example, a low (≤ 0.4 MoM) value in a 29-year-old woman increases her risk for having a child with Down syndrome from 1/1000 to *at least* 1/133, approximately that of a 35-year-old with normal MSAFP. Such information can be used for counseling couples in considering genetic amniocentesis. See Chapter 5.

(2) the large numbers of false-positive elevations of MSAFP compared with the number ultimately associated with NTD; (3) the insufficiency of patient and physician education; (4) the inadequacy of existing personnel and facilities for the required sophisticated follow-up of positive results; and (5) the substantial unnecessary parental anxiety that such screening programs would engender.[114] Indeed, the American College of Obstetricians and Gynecologists (ACOG) has taken the following position, which we believe is the responsible one: "Maternal serum AFP screening should be implemented only when it can be performed within a coordinated system of care that contains all the requisite resources and facilities to provide safeguards essential for ensuring prompt, accurate diagnosis and appropriate follow-through services. When such coordination and services is not possible, the risks and costs appear to outweigh the advantages and the program should not be implemented."[98]

Nonetheless, with no stated justification other than the 1983 FDA approval of commercial kits for the radioimmunoassay of AFP,[97] ACOG members received a May 1985 "Alert" from the College's Department of Professional Liability entitled "Professional Liability Implications of AFP Tests." The relevant part of the Alert, which is reproduced in its entirety as Figure 3–1, is stated in the second paragraph.

The rationale for this advice was not medical, but legal: to give the physician "the best possible defense" in a medical malpractice suit premised on the birth of a baby with a neural tube defect. While in the long run, this alert may help encourage physicians to provide accurate information about MSAFP testing to their patients, it simply creates confusion in the short run. For example, in September 1985, two physicians wrote incorrectly in the letters section of the *New England Journal of Medicine* that the Alert meant that ACOG had recognized "the value of maternal α-fetoprotein screening."[115] The Alert has also been used by at least one testing kit manufacturer to help justify its product.[116] Such confusion and usage is understandable. It is unprecedented and counterproductive for a professional medical association, dedicated to articulating and promoting sound medical practice, to permit its *legal* department to promulgate *medical* standards. Certainly MSAFP screening should be offered to pregnant women when appropriate counseling and follow-up care are available. But as ACOG has correctly noted in the past, when such care and counseling are not available, "the risks and costs appear to outweigh the advantages."[98]

Setting Standards of Practice

ACOG's Department of Professional Liability has been very agitated about what it sees as a crisis of medical malpractice insurance unavailability

---

Professional Liability Implications of AFP Tests

Now that alpha-fetoprotein (AFP) test kits have been approved by the Food and Drug Administration (FDA) and are becoming more widely available, some professional liability implications should be kept in mind.

It is now imperative that you investigate the availability of these tests in your area and familiarize yourself with the procedure, location and mechanism of the follow-up tests to screen for neural tube defects. It is equally imperative that every prenatal patient be advised of the availability of this test and that your discussion about the test and the patient's decision with respect to the test be documented in the patient's chart. This discussion should include the information you have discovered about the availability, location and mechanism of follow-up tests to screen for neural tube defects in the event of positive AFP test results.

The following ACOG publications should prove to be helpful in fully informing your patients about this test; ACOG Technical Bulletin, No. 67, October, 1982, "Prenatal Detection of Neural Tube Defects;" Patient Education Pamphlets P-010, "Neural Tube Defects," P-019, "Amniocentesis for Prenatal Diagnosis of Genetic Disorders," and P-023, "Genetic Disorders." As with all printed materials, it is important to make sure that the content described therein is commensurate with your mode of practice.

With the availability of prenatal testing for the rare but tragic circumstance of the birth of a child with a neural tube defect, it is important that patients be appropriately counseled. The physician who has fully discussed AFP tests and follow-up testing with his or her patients, who has let the patient make the decision, and who has documented it in the chart should be in the best possible defense position.

May 1985

FIG 3–1.
Department of Professional Liability "Alert" issued by the American College of Obstetricians and Gynecologists.

and unaffordability, a crisis that has reportedly led to about 10% of ACOG's fellows giving up obstetrics altogether and almost 20% dropping high-risk obstetrics. But if malpractice litigation is a problem, letting lawyers set medical standards of care is hardly the solution. Indeed, the general rule has always been that "good medicine is good law." Physicians who follow "good and accepted medical standards" in their practice will be found in compliance with the general standard of "reasonable prudence" for physicians, and thus cannot be found negligent in a malpractice suit. It may also be said of the ACOG Alert that "bad law is bad medicine." If routine MSAFP screening has come of age in the United States, ACOG's scientific committees, not its legal liability department, should so advise its members.[117]

Perhaps ACOG's lawyers were thinking about the famous case of *Helling v. Carey*[118] in which two ophthalmologists were found negligent for not having routinely performed a glaucoma test on a young woman whose glaucoma, when it was finally discovered, had progressed to a point where she had lost her peripheral vision and had her central vision severely reduced. In their defense the physicians argued that it was the standard of care in the ophthalmology community *not* to routinely screen patients for glaucoma under the age of 40 because the incidence of the disease in this population (about 1:25,000) was so small. On appeal from a verdict for the physicians, the Supreme Court of Washington noted that the standard of care is judged on the basis of "reasonable prudence." Even though ophthal- mologists did not routinely offer this test to patients under 40 years of age, the court decided that not to so offer it was a failure of reasonable prudence. The glaucoma screening test, it found, was simple, inexpensive, safe, accurate, and could detect an arrestable and "grave and devastating" disease. The court quoted with approval the past statements of Justices Oliver Wendell Holmes and Learned Hand, both to the effect that while reasonable prudence is usually measured by custom or what is in fact done, custom can never be its sole measure. As Justice Hand put it in the cogent *T.J. Hooper* case:

> [A] whole calling may have unduly lagged in the adoption of new and available devices. It never may set its own tests, however persuasive be its usages. *Courts must in the end say what is required; there are precautions so imperative that even their universal disregard will not excuse their omission* [emphasis added by the Washington court].[119]

But what would this same court have said about MSAFP testing? The initial screening test is relatively inexpensive and safe, but it requires highly trained professionals to do a complex series of follow-up tests, including ultrasound and amniocentesis, to make it accurate. And even with this, there will be false-negatives. Nor can this series of tests be fairly termed "simple." It does detect a serious condition, that can even be described as "grave and devastating," but it is not one that can be "arrested" or "treated" except by aborting the affected fetus. Whether the *Helling* court (or any other court) would require a physician to inform his pregnant patient about the existence of AFP testing would probably hinge on the existence of those factors ACOG identified in its 1982 Technical Bulletin: "a coordinated system of care that contains all the requisite resources and facilities to provide safeguards essential for ensuring prompt, accurate diagnoses and appropriate follow-through services."[98]

In ACOG's September 1985 *Newletter,* its Director of Fellowship Activities, Keith C. White, tried to retreat from the Alert without actually retracting it. The attempt was important, since the Alert itself could be introduced in court as evidence of a standard of care adopted by ACOG. Dr. White stated flatly that "The College has not, and does not recommend routine screening of maternal serum for AFP . . ." He nonetheless concluded with a strangely equivocal statement: "The Department of Professional Liability *does not* set standards; we are trying to 'tell it like it is.' "[120] The problem, of course, is that this does not help either the physician or the patient. Surely no one can take seriously the argument that it is a good defense in a malpractice suit to have documented in the patient's chart that she was advised of the "availability" of MSAFP testing and the patient's "decision" about it, even though ACOG does *not* recommend the test for routine screening, and no facilities for testing and follow-up were reasonably available in the neighboring geographic area. The best defense remains to act in the best interest of the patient, following reasonable medical standards, with the patient's consent. ACOG's lawyers overreacted, and we hope that ACOG will never permit another such "Liability Alert" to be released by their lawyers unless and until its contents are approved by the appropriate scientific committee. Energy should be directed toward setting up an MSAFP screening system that *is* available to all patients regardless of economic status or source of payment, and is based on high professional standards of testing, with solid and helpful counseling at each step along the way.

LEGAL ASPECTS OF GENETIC SCREENING

State Statutes

As noted at the beginning of this chapter, currently 48 states (all except Nevada and North Carolina) and the District of Columbia have statutes pertaining to newborn screening. Only three of these states clearly indicate that their screening program is voluntary, although the majority of states permit refusal on religious grounds.[2] On most other major issues there is far less uniformity. For example, the laws vary considerably on the issue of who is responsible for obtaining the blood sample. Twenty-two states make this the responsibility of the health care institution, although this responsibility is often shared (in 32 states the physician or other birth attendant has the responsibility).[2] Thirty-one states—by statute, regulation, or guidelines—specify the type of laboratory that must do the testing;[2] but only a handful of states require mandatory rescreening to verify test results. The statutes require that the test results be reported to one or more of the following: physician (25 states), the hospital (11 states), the family (12 states), the department of public health (26 states).[2] Only in about half a dozen states are physicians required to notify affected individuals. Although some states do, most state statutes make no provision for recordkeeping, confidentiality, monitoring, counseling, education, or research.[2]

Historical Perspective

Two particular types of genetic screening laws dominated the first dozen years, from 1963 to 1975: PKU and sickle cell. Experience with these two laws, one on newborn screening, the other on potential carriers, continues to play the major role in determining current legal approaches to genetic screening.

In the initial enthusiasm that was created when a screening test for PKU was developed, 41 states passed laws from 1963 to 1967 regarding such testing, and most of these laws made it mandatory for all newborns.[1] Because of some early problems with the test, and side effects caused by treating infants improperly diagnosed as having the disorder (false-positives), this rush legislation has been characterized as "premature biomedical legislation."[121] By the mid-1970s, however, as procedures were regularized and quality control measures introduced, the weight of evidence was clearly on the side of those supporting the test.[122] Physicians were also found negligent in the courts for failure to diagnose PKU in a timely fashion.[123] Nevertheless, we should not forget the important lesson that this initial over-enthusiasm taught us: voluntary programs should be used as long as feasible to gain sufficient information about the efficacy of both the screening test and the planned intervention; mandatory statutes should be enacted, if at all, only if there is a reasonable medical certainty that the measures they prescribe are both necessary for the public health and capable of achieving their legislative purpose. Knee-jerk reaction to implementing screening programs in the laudable hope of preventing some forms of mental retardation may create more problems than it solves by raising unreasonable expectations on the part of the public, and by subjecting certain categories of individuals to testing and treatment with unproved results.[123]

The problem of "premature legislation" with regard to carrier screening is equally well illustrated by our experience with sickle cell screening. In 1970, a simple, inexpensive, and relatively reliable test was made available. By the end of 1972, influenced by the strong lobbying of the Cynthia Foundations, 12 states had passed sickle cell screening laws. What followed was a reaction by the black community on two fronts: the first, pushing for more medical research into the problem; the second, calling for screening on a purely voluntary basis.[123] In partial response, the National Sickle Cell Anemia Control Act of 1972 authorized funds to go only to states with voluntary screening programs. Although no funds were actually appropriated under this act, it did have the effect of more than half the states with mandatory laws replacing them with voluntary ones, and the addition of confidentiality safeguards to such legislation.[124] Mandatory screening of blacks had racist and stigmatizing potential, especially when screening was for a trait for which there was no treatment and the only reasonable advice the clinician could give was either not to have children (if married to a spouse who was also a carrier) or to marry a noncarrier black or a non-black spouse.

One condition that fortunately did not get statutorily mandated screening was 47,XYY, and it, perhaps even better than sickle cell trait, illustrates the potential problems of stigmatization. In the early 1960s it was suggested that this sex chromosome abnormality was associated with a predisposition to antisocial or criminal behavior. Since then, this theory has been widely debated and generally discredited, although no prospective study of the problem has yet been made.[125] In an attempt to do such a study, all newborn males born from 1968 to 1975 at the Boston Hospital for Women were screened for XYY. The plan was to follow up those with this chromosome abnormality, matching them with another male child with a normal XY complement.[123] Putting aside the controversy that later arose over the type of informed consent necessary from the mother to study the infant, both for the initial screening and the follow-up studies, a serious question of stigmatization can be raised.

With most of the scientific community believing that individuals with XYY are no more disposed to violence or antisocial behavior than "normal" XY counterparts, why should parents have it suggested to them that their child is "abnormal" in this regard? Furthermore, what protections must be taken to ensure that this information is not transmitted to the police or school authorities, who may pay more attention to this individual because of his chromosomal makeup? Because of society's profound interest in and fascination with genetics and eliminating "defectives" or deviants, one must be extremely careful in classifying a certain genetic trait as potentially harmful to society, because the pressures to eliminate it (or its carriers) will be intense, whether the thesis is correct or not. No matter what the literature, for example, XYY may be considered a "serious" enough "abnormality" to lead most couples who have undergone amniocentesis for another reason to choose an abortion for this reason alone, even if the child would probably otherwise be normal.*

---

*The XYY karyotype has been raised in a number of criminal trials around the world as a defense. In general, its use has been infrequent and unsuccessful. It was first raised on April 1, 1968, in France in a murder trial. Defendant Daniel Hugon was accused of murdering a 65-year-old prostitute in a Paris hotel. Hugon had an XYY chromosomal complement. He was, nonetheless, found legally sane, convicted of murder, and received a seven-year sentence. In the same year, 21-year-old Lawrence Hannel came to trial charged with the stabbing death of his 77-year-old landlady in Australia. He urged the court to accept an insanity defense based upon the allegation that his behavior was adversely affected by his XYY genotype. After only 11 minutes of deliberation, the jury delivered a "not guilty by reason of insanity" verdict and Hannel was committed to a maximum security hospital until cured. In another

These examples help illustrate the importance of solid scientific evidence and delivery organization prior to launching a mass screening program, as well as the relevance of voluntariness (informed consent) and confidentiality.

Voluntary or Mandatory?

Although almost all state statutes regarding newborn genetic screening are mandatory, this seems to be the result of a historical accident, and not of any reasoned policy decision. Even though it already had a voluntary mass screening program, Massachusetts passed the first mandatory PKU statute in 1963 under the influence of Dr. Robert MacCready of the Massachusetts Department of Public Health. With the aid of the lobbying of the state chapters of the Association for Retarded Children (which in October 1964 voted to advocate "mandatory legislation for the screening of PKU") and Robert Guthrie, the test's inventor, the majority of states adopted statutes that followed the Massachusetts model.[1] At least 23 of them also contained language, like that found in the Massachusetts legislation, that could be construed to authorize a battery of genetic screening tests.[1, 2] It is doubtful that mandatory laws were necessary to ensure

---

case, Ernest D. Beck, a 20-year-old farm worker, was tried in Bielefeld, West Germany, in November 1986 and sentenced to life imprisonment for the murder of three women.

In the United States, XYY's effect in criminal proceedings has been even more limited. In April 1969, Sean Farley of New York, a 6 ft 8 in, 26-year-old man pleaded not guilty by reason of insanity to the alleged brutal murder and rape of a 40-year-old woman in an alley near her home *(People v. Farley,* No. 1827 [Sup. Ct., Queens County, April 30, 1969]). The jury found him guilty of murder in the first degree. Likewise, in *People v. Tanner,* 13, Cal. App. 3d 596, 91 Cal. Rpt. 656 (1970), the XYY defense was held to be insufficient to prove legal insanity under the California version of the M'Naghten Rule. The defendant, Raymond Tanner, had originally pleaded guilty to a charge of assault with intent to commit murder, stemming from a brutal rape. While confined at Atascadero State Hospital for study, he was discovered to possess the XYY chromosomal complement. Thereafter he attempted to change his guilty plea to not guilty by reason of insanity. At a hearing held on this motion, the defense introduced expert testimony and studies attempting to prove to the court that XYY individuals are likely to exhibit certain aggressive behavioral traits. Despite the presentation of considerable expert testimony, supporting evidence, and recent work done at the Atascadero State Hospital in California, the court denied the motion, concluding that there is not sufficient information or knowledge of any relationship between behavior and the XYY karyotype. In 1970, in the Maryland case of *Millard v. State,* 8 Md. App. 419, 262 A. 2d 227 (1970), the XYY defense was again adjudged insufficient to bring the question of insanity before a jury. In that case, the defendant was charged with robbery with a deadly weapon. Using the testimony of a geneticist and the introduction of 40 XYY research papers, an attempt was made to have him declared not guilty by reason of insanity in accordance with Maryland's version of the M'Naghten Rule. The judge ruled as a matter of law that the XYY anomaly as a "mental defect" was not of itself sufficient to show that the defendant lacked substantial capacity to appreciate the criminality of his conduct. The jury found the defendant guilty as charged.

compliance in the first place,[1] and it is time that we reevaluated this issue. The state of Maryland has what has been called by many the best genetic screening law in the country.[1] One thing that makes it a model is the seriousness with which it takes screening and public participation and education. Unlike almost every other law in the country, it is *voluntary*. In a study of the effectiveness of this law, Maryland investigators demonstrated that requiring informed consent for PKU screening was well accepted by the public, improved public knowledge about PKU screening, and did not make the program any less cost-effective.[126] They nonetheless came to the startling conclusion that because 27 parents refused PKU testing since the start of the program, the law should be made mandatory.[127] Just the opposite conclusion is reasonable, and the study should provide the impetus to state legislatures to amend their genetic screening statutes to make them voluntary.

The dilemma for those who want to reduce genetic disease has traditionally been seen as one of governmental effectiveness versus individual freedom. The notion has been that to be effective, individual liberty must be sacrificed. As Daniel Callahan noted more than a decade ago, the real challenge is to find a "way of combining both logics." This will be difficult, he opined, "if only because most people find it easier to cope with one idea than two at the same time." He described what is involved:

> It will mean taking the idea of free choice seriously, allowing parents to make their own choice without penalizing them socially for the choices they make . . . Part of the very meaning of human community, I would contend, entails a willingness of society to bear the social costs of individual freedom.[128]

The most remarkable thing about the Maryland study is that it now seems we can simultaneously protect the values of both beneficence and autonomy. We *can* permit PKU screening programs to be voluntary without running any substantial risk of missing an affected infant. As the authors of the survey note, "the chance of missing a PKU infant at the observed rate of parental refusal (0.05%) is 100 times less than the chance of missing a PKU infant because of a false-negative result."[126] In fact, at the observed rate of refusal, it would take 500 years before one PKU case was missed because of parental refusal of the screening test.[129] Efforts aimed at decreasing the number of false-negatives rather than decreasing the small number of parental refusals would seem more reasonable.

Law can effectively promote the public's health. But in the United States, law also promotes individual liberty. Liberty should be sacrificed only when clearly necessary for the public good. The Maryland study makes clear that PKU testing (and inferentially, all newborn screening) may not necessitate such a sacrifice. Thus, the 1975 recommendations of the National Academy of Sciences regarding genetic screening seem even more relevant today:

> *Genetic screening is appropriate when:* (1) *There is evidence of substantial public benefit and acceptance,* and acceptance by medical practitioners. (2) Its feasibility has been investigated and it has been found that benefits outweigh costs; appropriate education can be carried out; test methods are satisfactory; laboratory facilities are available; and resources exist to deal with *counseling,* follow-up, and other consequences of testing. (3) An investigative pretest of the program has shown that costs are acceptable; *education is effective; informed consent is feasible;* aims have . . . been defined . . . [and] qualified and *effective counselors are available* in sufficient numbers . . . (4) The means are available to evaluate the effectiveness and success of each step in the process [emphasis added].[3]

In regard to mandatory statutes, the Academy's Committee specifically recommended that "participation in a genetic screening program should not be mandatory by law, but should be left to the discretion of the person tested or, if a minor, of the parents or legal guardian."[3]

Similarly, the President's Bioethics Commission, in their 1984 Report, strongly endorsed voluntary screening programs, but noted that mandatory programs "requiring the performance of low-risk, minimally intrusive procedures may be justified if voluntary testing would fail to prevent an avoidable, serious injury to people—such as children—who are unable to protect themselves."[130]

Confidentiality and Other Issues

Because of the ever increasing number of potential screening tests, it seems like a reasonable time for states to "clean up" their genetic screening acts by concentrating on some of their major shortcomings. Ten years ago, Philip Reilly suggested four features that all state PKU statutes should incorporate: (1) public and professional education programs; (2) provision of genetic counseling services; (3) recordkeeping sufficient to track and inform all female PKU-affected infants of their childbearing risks; and (4) quality control in both initial and follow-up testing.[1] All of these suggestions are reasonable. More recently, in 1983, the President's Bioethics Commission underlined the importance of confidentiality by issuing, among other things, the following recommendations:

1. Genetic information should not be given to unrelated third parties, such as insurers or employers, without the explicit and informed consent of the person screened or a surrogate for that person.

2. Private and governmental agencies that use data banks for genetic-related information should require that stored information be coded whenever that is compatible with the purpose of the data bank.[130]

In view of the history of genetic screening and the possible stigmatization that can result from even being identified as a carrier of a recessive gene, these recommendations seem minimal and should be followed. In addition, the Commission recommended that screening programs should not be undertaken at all unless the results that are produced could be routinely relied upon; and a full range of prescreening and follow-up services for the population to be screened should be available before a screening program is introduced. As discussed previously in this chapter, we think these recommendations are reasonable and should be followed as well. It should be noted, however, that primary and follow-up care would be available under any reasonable form of universal health care entitlement, whose existence would not only obviate the need for mandatory genetic screening laws but also provide essential services for all affected infants.

Chapter 4 _____

Prenatal Diagnosis: Indications

Prenatal diagnosis is one of the most dramatic and powerful developments in medical practice. Advancing capabilities in intrauterine detection of genetic abnormalities and monitoring of fetal growth and development have added an entirely new dimension to genetic counseling. Instead of counseling in terms of probabilities, the physician can, in many circumstances, actually determine whether or not a specific fetus is affected for a rapidly growing number of conditions.

In the next three chapters we discuss the indications for prenatal diagnosis, the major techniques available, and the legal and social policy issues in reproductive liberty that permit women and their physicians to consider abortion as an option to carrying an affected fetus to term. Many couples also use prenatal diagnosis for reassurance that their fetus is not affected with a particular disorder; without the availability of this reassurance, a significant number of couples would decide against pregnancy, and many women would choose abortion upon becoming pregnant. In fact, since more than 95% of all prenatal diagnostic tests are negative, the overwhelming majority of such testing helps lead to the birth of children that might not otherwise have been born.

For other couples, the prenatal diagnosis of an abnormality provides them with the opportunity to prepare themselves and their families for the birth of their child. Such advance knowledge may also alter obstetric management and allow time to plan for the care of the abnormal infant. The controversy surrounding prenatal diagnosis centers primarily on a belief by some that routine abortion of abnormal fetuses will lead society to neglect and discriminate against the handicapped even more than it does now.* This is, unfortunately, a real possibility. We believe, however, that prenatal diagnosis should be viewed as the first step in the treatment and prevention of birth defects. This potential for intervention leads ultimately not to discrimination against affected fetuses, but to consideration of the fetus as a patient.†

The division between this chapter on indications for prenatal diagnosis, and the following chapter on techniques, is somewhat artificial, and the discussion in each is necessarily overlapping. This is because new techniques, like DNA sequence analysis, discussed in this chapter, will give rise to new indications for suggesting prenatal diagnosis by their very existence. Nonetheless, because there is so much material to cover concerning prenatal diagnosis, we have found it useful to divide the discussion of this topic into two chapters. This one will discuss indications for attempting prenatal diagnosis in the cases of chromosomal abnormalities, Mendelian abnormalities, DNA sequence variations, and polygenic/multifactorial abnormalities. It will conclude with a discussion of the major legal issues raised by failure to advise parents of the availability of these tests, and negligence in the performance of these tests by physicians and testing laboratories.

CHROMOSOMAL ABNORMALITIES

It is technically possible to determine the chromosomal complement of every fetus. For some couples, however, the risks of amniocentesis or chorionic villus sampling outweigh the potential benefits. Accordingly, it is important to delineate accepted indications for prenatal diagnosis.

Advanced Maternal Age

The increased relative risk of producing children with chromosomal abnormalities, most specifically trisomies, in women age 35 or older is the most common indication for prenatal diagnosis, generally accounting for about 85% of the women tested. The overall incidence of trisomy 21 is approximately 1 in 800 live births. By contrast, a woman 35 years old at the birth of her child has a 1 in 385 risk; at age 45 the risk is 1 in 106 (Table 4–1).[2, 3] Above the age of 30, the rate increases exponentially. Trisomy 21 is not the only chromosomal abnormality that increases with maternal age. Autosomal trisomies (e.g., trisomy 13, trisomy 18) and X chromo-

*See discussion in Chapter 7.
†See discussion in Chapter 10.

TABLE 4–1.

Risk of Having a Live-Born Child With Down Syndrome or
Chromosomal Abnormality by One-Year Maternal Age
Intervals*

MATERNAL AGE	RISK OF DOWN SYNDROME	TOTAL RISK FOR CHROMOSOME ABNORMALITIES†
20	1/1,667	1/526†
21	1/1,667	1/526†
22	1/1,429	1/500†
23	1/1,429	1/500†
24	1/1,250	1/476†
25	1/1,250	1/476†
26	1/1,176	1/476†
27	1/1,111	1/455†
28	1/1,053	1/435†
29	1/1,000	1/417†
30	1/952	1/384†
31	1/909	1/384†
32	1/769	1/323†
33	1/625	1/286
34	1/500	1/238
35	1/385	1/192
36	1/294	1/156
37	1/227	1/127
38	1/175	1/102
39	1/137	1/83
40	1/106	1/66
41	1/82	1/53
42	1/64	1/42
43	1/50	1/33
44	1/38	1/26
45	1/30	1/21
46	1/23	1/16
47	1/18	1/13
48	1/14	1/10
49	1/11	1/8

*Data modified from Hook EB: *Obstet Gynecol* 1981; 58:282, and Hook
EB, Cross PK, Schreinemachers DM: *JAMA* 1983; 249:2034.
†47,XXX excluded for ages 20–32 (data not available).

somal polysomies also show an increased maternal age effect (Table 4–1).
Thus, at age 35 the likelihood that a chromosomal abnormality of any kind
will occur is about 1 in 192; at age 40, the risk is 1 in 66; at age 45, 1 in
21. Some of the latter risk, however, is for sex chromosome polysomies
(e.g., 47,XXX and 47,XYY), which may or may not be associated with significant phenotypic abnormalities.

The frequency of chromosomal abnormalities detected by prenatal amniocentesis is higher than the frequency of such abnormalities among live-born infants. In fact, the prevalence of abnormalities in antenatal studies at 16 to 18 weeks' gestation is about 50% higher than that in live-born infants.[3, 4] The discrepancy between frequencies in live-born infants and in second trimester fetuses is likely accounted for by the disproportionate number of chromosomally abnormal fetuses that abort spontaneously between 16 weeks and term. The excess rate of fetal death (after adjustment for spontaneous loss after amniocentesis) between the time of amniocentesis and live birth is 38% for fetuses with trisomy 21; 67% for trisomy 18; 41% for trisomy 13; 1% for 47,XXX; 1% for 47,XXY; and approximately 30% for other clinically significant chromosomal abnormalities (i.e., 45,X, 47,XYY, unbalanced structural abnormalities).[3]

Therefore, a strict definition of "advanced maternal age" is not appropriate. It is commonly accepted practice in the United States, nonetheless, to counsel all women who will be age 35 or older at the expected date of delivery concerning their risk of producing a child with a chromosomal abnormality and the availability of amniocentesis. However, flexibility is desirable when confronted with inquiries from women less than 35 years of age.*

Prior Child With a Chromosomal Abnormality

Genetic amniocentesis is frequently recommended to couples who have had a prior child with a chromosomal disorder, stillborn, or aborted fetus with either autosomal trisomy or sex chromosomal trisomy, even if parental chromosomal complements are normal. The increased risk in such couples has been attributed to: (1) parental mosaicism; (2) a structural chromosome rearrangement; (3) a Mendelian gene producing a higher risk of nondisjunction; or (4) exogenous factors.[5] However, the risk for a second offspring with Down syndrome or another chromosome abnormality now appears to be increased *only* for mothers aged 29 or less at the time of the birth of a child with a noninherited chromosome abnormality. Data from a collaborative study based on 2,890 cases of prenatal diagnosis from 12 European countries showed that the risk for a chromosomally abnormal fetus at amniocentesis after the birth of a child with abnormality was 1.3% when the mother's age was 34 or less at amniocentesis and 1.8% if the mother was older.[5] The difference between these was not statistically significant.

---

*The issue of whether or not there is an effect of *paternal* age with Down syndrome is controversial. See Chapter 1.

However, for mothers less than 30, the risk for a chromosomally abnormal fetus after a child with noninherited chromosome abnormality was between 10 and 20 times the population risk for Down syndrome for mothers of the same age. The risk was most significant for mothers less than 25 years of age. Nonetheless, because of understandable parental anxieties, prenatal studies should be offered to the parents of such offspring.[6]

Parent With a Translocation or Other Chromosomal Abnormality

Phenotypically normal individuals may unknowingly be balanced carriers (heterozygotes) for a translocation. As briefly introduced in Chapter 1, the clinical significance of translocations can be illustrated by recalling Robertsonian translocations, those involving centromeric fusion of the acrocentric chromosomes 13, 14, 15, 21, or 22. For example, about 3% of individuals with Down syndrome have a translocation, usually between chromosomes 14 and 21. Translocations also occur between 13 and 21, 15 and 21, 21 and 22, 21 and 21, and occasionally between 21 and a nonacrocentric chromosome. Although about 75% of these translocations arise *de novo* in the affected child, in the remainder one parent is found to carry the translocation in a balanced state.[7] In most families this situation is ascertained after the birth of an abnormal child. The likelihood of Down syndrome recurring in parents who have had a child with a *de novo* translocation is probably no greater than that for the general population. On the other hand, in about 25% of individuals who have Down syndrome as a result of a translocation, one parent is found to carry the translocation in the balanced state. If so, the empirical recurrence risk depends on the type of translocation and on the sex of the parent carrying it. If the mother carries a D/G translocation* (usually 14/21), the risk is about 10%.[7] When the father carries the translocation, the risk is less (1% to 2%), presumably because of selection against abnormal sperm. Although lower than theoretically expected, these risks are sufficiently high to justify amniocentesis. A different situation exists if a parent has a 21/21 translocation. Pregnancies lead either to nonviable monosomic zygotes or 21/21 translocation Down syndrome; thus all offspring of a parent with a balanced 21/21 will be abnormal.

Reciprocal translocations are individually rare. They do not involve centromeric fusion and, hence, usually do not involve acrocentric chromosomes. Empirical data for specific translocations are rarely available. Gener-

---

*Prior to the development of banding techniques, chromosomes were categorized into seven groups lettered A through G, based on size and centromere position. D group chromosomes are numbers 13, 14, and 15, and G group chromosomes are numbers 21 and 22.

alizations must usually be made on the basis of pooled data derived from many different translocations. Again, theoretical risks for abnormal (unbalanced) offspring are greater than empirical risks, which are approximately 11%, irrespective of whether the father or mother carries the translocation.[8]†

Fragile X Syndrome

The fragile X syndrome has received an increasing amount of attention since 1969.[9] This X-linked disorder has an estimated overall prevalence of 1:1,000 and accounts for between 6% and 10% of retarded males.[10, 11] These males are usually mentally retarded, have macro-orchidism (enlarged testes), and, less frequently, prognathism (forward-projecting jaw), prominent supraorbital ridges, and large ears. The gene responsible for the condition is linked to a "fragile" site (a secondary constriction) on the distal long arm of the X chromosome.‡ Detection of carrier females may be difficult, for not infrequently they exhibit the fragile site in only a very small fraction of their lymphocytes. Under appropriate laboratory conditions, this marker can be detected in cultured amniotic fluid cells, making prenatal diagnosis feasible.[12, 13]

Parent With a Numerical Chromosomal Abnormality

If a parent has a numerical chromosomal abnormality (aneuploidy), the risk to offspring is increased. For example, approximately 30% (rather than the expected 50%) of offspring of females with trisomy 21 (Down syndrome) also show trisomy 21.[14] Therefore, prenatal diagnosis should be considered in a pregnant female with Down syndrome. Males with Down syndrome are sterile. Approximately 20% of offspring of fertile 45,X, 45,X/46,XX and 45,X/46,XX/45,XXX subjects are said to be abnormal; however, these risks may be biased by the method of ascertainment.[14] Although males with 47,XYY are theoretically also at increased risk for chromosomally abnormal offspring, these men are often sterile. Men with 47,XXY (Klinefelter syndrome) are sterile, but those with mosaicism (e.g., 46,XY/47,XXY) may be fertile. Accordingly, all individuals with a numerical chromosomal abnormality, including mosaics, should be offered prenatal diagnosis.

---

†Prenatal diagnosis should also be considered when other parental chromosomal abnormalities are found. For example, individuals with a chromosomal inversion (a chromosome aberration in which a segment of a chromosome is reversed end-to-end without loss of chromosomal material). Counseling in such situations is usually complex and would best be offered by experienced geneticists.

‡This fragile site has been localized to the interphase between bands Xq27 and q28.

Other Indications

Although less well established as indications for offering prenatal diagnosis, other situations or conditions that have been suggested include the following: (1) previous stillborn or spontaneous abortuses; (2) exposure to irradiation or chemotherapeutic agents; (3) parental metabolic derangements (e.g., maternal antithyroid antibodies or hyperthyroidism); (4) delayed fertilization (i.e., late in the menstrual cycle); (5) pregnancies resulting from ovulation induction; and (6) fetuses manifesting intrauterine growth retardation or decreased activity.[15]

MENDELIAN DISORDERS

Diseases produced by single mutant genes, whether transmitted in dominant or recessive fashion, on an autosome or an X chromosome, are uncommon disorders. Many Mendelian disorders occur only once in 10,000 to 50,000 births. However, although individually rare, mutant genes in aggregate cause abnormalities in approximately 1% of live-born infants, and the risk in certain families for an affected offspring is 25% or 50%, depending on the particular mode of inheritance. Unfortunately, among the more than 3,000 Mendelian disorders, there are relatively few that have an available method for prenatal diagnosis.

Inborn Errors of Metabolism

Most inborn errors of metabolism are transmitted in an autosomal recessive fashion, but a few enzyme abnormalities are inherited in an X-linked recessive, or autosomal dominant pattern. About 0.8% of newborn infants have an inherited disorder of metabolism, one third of which are serious.[12]

The inborn errors of metabolism may generally be subdivided into several categories: (1) mucopolysaccharidoses; (2) mucolipidoses and other disorders of carbohydrate metabolism; (3) lipidoses; (4) amino acid disorders; and (5) miscellaneous biochemical disorders. Physicians who are not geneticists cannot be expected to be informed on all aspects of prenatal diagnosis of these disorders. It is incumbent upon the primary physician to obtain appropriate consultation when a question arises concerning an inborn error of metabolism or to facilitate referral to an experienced geneticist. However, a few generalizations are appropriate. First, couples potentially benefitting from prenatal diagnosis will usually be identified as at risk because they have had an affected child. Occasionally, screening programs identify two heterozygotes at risk for a child with an autosomal recessive disorder (e.g., Tay-Sachs disease). Second, diagnosis of a previously affected offspring must always be verified so that appropriate antenatal tests may be offered. Confirmation is not always easy. If the affected child is no longer alive, confirmation may prove impossible. Third, detection of metabolic errors requires that the enzyme be expressed in amniotic fluid cells or chorionic villus cells. This requirement is not fulfilled by all metabolic disorders—a prominent example is phenylketonuria (PKU). Fortunately, PKU now appears diagnosable by molecular techniques, described later in this chapter. In general, enzymes present in amniotic fluid cells are also expressed in chorionic villi. However, this area is still undergoing investigation. Fourth, metabolic analyses may require more amniotic fluid cells than required for cytogenetic studies. Delays may also occur if the fluid or cultured cells must be transported to a referral laboratory.

Table 4–2 presents a survey of inborn errors that are prenatally diagnosable. This list is under continuous revision; thus, absence of a disorder does not necessarily imply that the inborn error is not diagnosable.

DNA SEQUENCE VARIATIONS*

The number of single gene disorders potentially amenable to prenatal diagnosis has increased dramatically in recent years as a result of advances in recombinant DNA technology. Prior to the development of these techniques, prenatal diagnosis of such disorders was limited to those for which the biochemical or structural defects were known and expressed by cells. Through the use of recombinant DNA technology, all Mendelian disorders are, at least in theory, amenable to prenatal diagnosis.

Virtually every cell in the body contains a complete chromosomal complement. Therefore, each cell contains the full complement of DNA. Even if a gene is not expressed by a particular cell, the DNA coding for that gene product is present. For example, although hemoglobin is expressed only by reticulocytes, the DNA coding for hemoglobin is present in all cells, including amniotic fluid cells and chorionic villi. Furthermore, even if the biochemical or molecular defect is unknown, such as in cystic fibrosis, the DNA coding for the mutant gene is present in each cell.†

*This section is contributed by Carole Ober, Ph.D., Section of Human Genetics, Department of Obstetrics and Gynecology, Northwestern University Medical School, Chicago.

†Another advantage of DNA analysis is that there are virtually unlimited numbers of nucleotide substitutions that result in restriction fragment length polymorphisms (RFLPs). These RFLPs serve as markers for mutant genes that cause disease and allow diagnosis of affected individuals in families, even if the exact genetic defect (i.e., mutation) is unknown. This approach has recently been applied to the prenatal diagnosis of cystic fibrosis and muscular dystrophy. Thus, recombinant DNA technology provides a potentially powerful tool for the diagnosis of genetic disorders.

TABLE 4–2.
Inherited Disorders Diagnosed or Potentially Diagnosable Prenatally*

DISORDER	METHOD OF DIAGNOSIS	MODE OF INHERITANCE†	PRENATAL DIAGNOSIS‡
Conditions with known biochemical defects			
Disorders of amino acid metabolism			
Arginosuccinic aciduria	Deficient arginosuccinase	AR	Yes
Carbamylphosphate synthetase deficiency	Deficient carbamylphosphate synthetase	AR	Probable
Citrullinemia	Deficient arginosuccinic acid synthetase	AR	Yes
Cystathioninuria	Deficient cystathionase	AR	Probable
Cystinosis	Cystine accumulation in amniotic fluid	AR	Yes
Dihydropteridine reductase deficiency	Deficiency of dihydropteridine reductase	AR	Possible
Glutaric aciduria	Deficient glutaryl-CoA carboxylase	AR	Yes
Histidinemia	Deficient histidase	AR	Probable
Homocystinuria	Deficient cystathionine synthetase	AR	Probable
3-Hydroxy-3-methylglutaryl coenzyme A lyase deficiency	Elevated 3-hydroxy-3-methylglutaric acid in maternal urine	AR	Yes
Hyperammonemia	Deficient ornithine transcarbamylase in liver	X	Yes
Hyperargininemia	Deficient arginase	AR	Probable
Hyperlysinemia	Deficient lysine-ketoglutarate reductase	AR	Possible
Hypervalinemia	Deficient valine transaminase	AR	Possible
Isovaleric acidemia	Deficient isovaleryl-CoA carboxylase	AR	Yes
Maple syrup urine disease	Deficient branched-chain ketoacid decarboxylase	AR	Yes
Methylmalonic aciduria	Deficient methylmalonic CoA mutase	AR	Yes
Methyltetrahydrofolate methyltransferase deficiency	Deficient methyltetrahydrofolate methyltransferase	AR	Possible
Methyltetrahydrofolate reductase deficiency	Deficient methyltetrahydrofolate reductase	AR	Possible
Multiple carboxylase deficiency (neonatal)	Deficient carboxylases (biotin responsive)	AR	Yes
Ornithine α-ketoacid transaminase deficiency	Deficient ornithine α-ketoacid transaminase	AR	Probable
Ornithinemia (gyrate atrophy of retina)	Deficient ornithine aminotransferase	AR	Probable

TABLE 4-2. *continued*

DISORDER	METHOD OF DIAGNOSIS	MODE OF INHERITANCE†	PRENATAL DIAGNOSIS‡
Orotic aciduria	Deficient orotidylic pyrophosphorylase and decarboxylase	AR	Possible
Propionic acidemia (ketotic hyperglycinemia)	Deficient propionyl CoA carboxylase	AR	Yes
Tyrosinemia, Type I (tyrosinosis)	Elevated succinyl acetone in amniotic fluid	AR	Yes
Vitamin B₁₂ metabolic defect	Deficient vitamin B₁₂ coenzyme	AR	Possible
Disorders of carbohydrate metabolism			
Aspartylglucosaminuria	Deficient β-aspartylglucosaminidase	AR	Yes
Fucosidosis	Deficient α-fucosidase	AR	Yes
Galactokinase deficiency	Deficient galactokinase	AR	Yes
Galactosemia	Deficient galactose-1-P uridyl transferase	AR	Yes
Glucose-6-phosphate dehydrogenase deficiency	Deficient glucose-6-phosphate dehydrogenase	X	Possible
Glycogen storage, Type I (von Gierke disease)	Deficient glucose-6-phosphatase	AR	Yes
Glycogen storage, Type II (Pompe)	Deficient α1, 4 glucosidase	AR	Yes
Glycogen storage, Type III	Deficient amylo-1, 6 glucosidase	AR	Probable
Glycogen storage, Type IV	Deficient branching enzyme	AR	Yes
Glycogen storage, Type VIII	Deficient phosphorylase kinase	X	Possible
Mannosidosis	Deficient α-mannosidase	AR	Probable
Pyruvate carboxylase deficiency	Deficient pyruvate carboxylase	AR	Probable
Pyruvate dehydrogenase deficiency	Deficient pyruvate dehydrogenase	AR	Yes
Disorders of lipid metabolism			
Abetalipoproteinemia	Deficient apo-β-lipoprotein	AR	Probable
Adrenoleukodystrophy	Accumulation of C26 fatty acids	X	Yes
Cerebellar ataxia (juvenile)	Deficient hexosaminidase A and B	AR	Possible (in some cases)
Cholesterol ester storage disease	Deficient acid lipase	AR	Possible
Fabry disease	Deficient ceramidetrihexoside galactosidase	X	Yes

Disorder	Enzyme/defect	Inheritance	Prenatal diagnosis
Familial hypercholesterolemia	Deficient LDL cholesterol receptors	AR/AD	Yes
Fabry disease	Deficient ceramidase	AR	Yes
Generalized gangliosidosis, GM1 gangliosidosis, Type I	Deficient β-galactosidase	AR	Yes
Gangliosidosis, G$_{M1}$, Type II (juvenile)	Deficient β-galactosidase	AR	Yes
Gangliosidosis, G$_{M2}$ (juvenile)	Partial deficiency in hexosaminidase A	AR	Possible
Gaucher disease	Deficient glucocerebrosidase	AR	Yes
Hypercholesterolemia	Deficient HMG CoA reductase	AD	Yes
Krabbe disease	Deficient galactocerebroside β-galactosidase	AR	Yes
Lactosyl ceramidosis	Deficient lactosyl ceramidase	AR	Possible
Metachromatic leukodystrophy	Deficient arylsulfatase A	AR	Yes
Mucolipidosis, Type I	Deficient α-neuraminidase	AR	Yes
Mucolipidosis, Type II (I-cell disease)	Deficiency of multiple lysosomal enzymes	AR	Yes
Mucolipidosis, Type III	Deficiency of multiple lysosomal enzymes	AR	Possible
Mucolipidosis Type IV (Bermann disease)	Electron microscopy	AR	Yes
Nieman-Pick disease A	Deficient sphingomyelinase	AR	Yes
Nieman-Pick disease B	Deficient sphingomyelinase	AR	Yes
Refsum disease	Deficient phytanic acid α-hydroxylase	AR	Probable
Sandhoff disease	Deficient hexosaminidase A and B	AR	Yes
Tangier disease	Deficient apo-A-l-lipoprotein	AR	Probable
Tay-Sachs disease	Deficient hexosaminidase A	AR	Yes
Wolman disease	Deficient acid lipase	AR	Yes

Disorders of mucopolysaccharide metabolism

Disorder	Enzyme/defect	Inheritance	Prenatal diagnosis
Hunter syndrome (MPS II)	Deficient α-L-iduronic acid-2-sulfatase	X	Yes
Hurler syndrome (MPS I H)	Deficient α-L-iduronidase	AR	Yes
Maroteaux-Lamy syndrome (MPS IV)	Deficient arylsulfatase B	AR	Yes
Morquio syndrome	Deficient N-acetylgalactosamine 6-sulfate sulfatase	AR	Yes
Mucopolysaccharidosis VII	Deficient β-glucuronidase	AR	Probable
Sanfilippo syndrome A (MPS III A)	Deficient heparin sulfatase	AR	Yes
Sanfilippo syndrome B (MPS III B)	Deficient N-acetyl-α-D-glucosaminidase	AR	Yes
Sanfilippo syndrome C (MPS III C)	Deficient acetyl CoA: α-glucosaminide-N-acetyltransferase	AR	Possible

TABLE 4-2. *continued*

DISORDER	METHOD OF DIAGNOSIS	MODE OF INHERITANCE†	PRENATAL DIAGNOSIS‡
Sanfilippo syndrome D (MPS III D)	Deficient N-acetyl-α-D-glucosaminide sulfatase	AR	Possible
Scheie syndrome (MPS I S)	Deficient α-L-iduronidase	AR	Possible
Other metabolic disorders			
Acatalasia	Deficient catalase	AR	Possible
Adenosine deaminase deficiency	Deficient adenosine deaminase	AR	Yes
Adrenogenital syndrome (21-hydroxylase deficiency)	Elevation of amniotic fluid steroids	AR	Yes
α1-antitrypsin deficiency	Deficient α-1-antitrypsin, or restriction endonuclease DNA analysis	AR	Yes
Hyperoxaluria	Increased amniotic fluid oxalate	AR	Yes
Hypophosphatasia	Deficient alkaline phosphatase; ultrasound	AR	Yes (in some types)
Lesch-Nyhan syndrome	Deficient hypoxanthine guanine phosphoribosyltransferase	AR	Yes
Lysosomal acid phosphatase	Deficient lysosomal acid phosphatase	AR	Yes
Menkes disease	Copper incorporation increased	AR	Yes
Nucleoside phosphorylase deficiency	Deficient nucleoside phosphorylase	AR	Probable
Osteopetrosis with renal tubular acidosis	Deficient carbonic anhydrase II	AR	Possible
Placental (steroid) sulfatase deficiency	Deficient placental steroid sulfatase	X	Yes
Porphyria, acute intermittent	Deficient uroporphyrinogen I synthetase	AD	Yes
Porphyria, congenital erythropoietic	Deficient uroporphyrinogen III cosynthetase	AR	Yes
Porphyria, hereditary coproporphyria	Deficient coproporphyrinogen oxidase	AD	Possible
Porphyria, variegate	Deficient protoporphyrinogen oxidase	AD	Probable
Sulfite oxidase deficiency	Deficient sulfite oxidase	AR	Probable
Hematologic and immunodeficiency disorders			
Glucose phosphate isomerase deficiency	Deficient glucose phosphate isomerase	AD	Yes
Hemolytic anemia VII	Deficient triose phosphate isomerase	AR	Probable
Hemophilia A	Deficient factor VIII	X	Yes
Hemophilia B	Deficient factor IX	X	Yes
Sickle cell disease	Restriction endonuclease DNA analysis	AR	Yes

Disorder	Method	Inheritance	Prenatal diagnosis
α Thalassemia	Molecular hybridization DNA analysis	AR	Yes
β Thalassemia	Fetal blood by fetoscopy: decreased synthesis of β-chain	AR	Yes
Von Willebrand disease	Deficient factor VIII	AD	Yes
Connective tissue disorders			
Ehlers-Danlos, Type IV	Deficient type III collagen	AR	Possible
Ehlers-Danlos, Type V	Deficient lysyl oxidase	X	Possible
Conditions with unknown biochemical defects			
Central nervous system disorders			
Cockayne syndrome	Increased sensitivity to UV light	AR	Yes
Dandy-Walker syndrome	Ultrasound	AR	Possible
Fragile X syndrome	X-chromosomal fragility	X	Yes
Meckel-Gruber syndrome	Ultrasound, AFP	AR	Yes
Myotonic dystrophy	Linkage analysis in some families	AD	Yes
Seckel syndrome	Ultrasound	AR	Yes
Aqueductal stenosis	Ultrasound	X/AR	Yes
Hematologic and immunologic disorders			
Bernard-Soulier syndrome	Fetal blood: large platelets	AR	Possible
Chediak-Higashi syndrome	Detection of intracellular inclusion bodies	AR	Probable
Chronic granulomatous disease	Nitroblue tetrazolium slide test; chemiluminescence test	X	Yes
Fanconi anemia	Detection of chromosome breakage	AR	Yes
Severe combined immunodeficiency disease	Fetal Blood: T cell incompetence	X/AR	Yes
Wiskott-Aldrich syndrome	Fetal blood: microthrombocytes	X	Possible
Renal disorders			
Finnish nephrosis	Elevated amniotic fluid AFP	AR	Yes
Polycystic kidneys, adult type	Ultrasound (some)	AD	Yes
Polycystic kidneys, infantile type	Ultrasound	AR	Yes
Skeletal disorders			
Achondrogenesis	Ultrasound, amniography	AR	Yes
Achondroplasia	Ultrasound	AD	Yes
Asphyxiating thoracic dystrophy	Ultrasound	AR	Yes

TABLE 4-2. *continued*

DISORDER	METHOD OF DIAGNOSIS	MODE OF INHERITANCE†	PRENATAL DIAGNOSIS‡
Camptomelic dysplasia	Ultrasound	AR	Yes
Diastrophic dwarfism	Ultrasound	AR	Yes
Ectrodactyly	Ultrasound	AR	Yes
Ellis-van Creveld syndrome	Ultrasound	AR	Yes
Osteogenesis imperfecta congenita (Type II)	Ultrasound: femur growth	AR	Yes
Roberts syndrome	Ultrasound; chromosome analysis	AR	Yes
Thrombocytopenia-absent radii (TAR) syndrome	Ultrasound	AR	Yes
Skin disorders			
Albinism-deafness syndrome	Fetal skin biopsy	X	Possible
Albinism, oculocutaneous (tyrosinase negative)	Fetal skin biopsy	AR	Yes
Ataxia-telangiectasia	Increased spontaneous chromosome breakage	AR	Possible
Bloom syndrome	Increased frequency of sister-chromatid exchange	AR	Possible
Congenital bullous ichthyosiform erythroderma (epidermolytic hyperkeratosis)	Fetal skin biopsy	AD	Yes
Epidermolysis bullosa dystrophica	Fetal skin biopsy	AD	Possible
Epidermolysis bullosa letalis	Fetal skin biopsy	AR	Yes
Epidermolysis bullosa simplex	Fetal skin biopsy	AD	Possible
Hypohidrotic ectodermal dysplasia	Fetal skin biopsy	X/AR	Yes
Ichthyosis, lamellar (harlequin)	Fetal skin biopsy	AR	Yes
Low sulfur hair syndrome	Fetal skin biopsy	AR	Possible
Netherton syndrome	Fetal skin biopsy	AR	Possible
Sjögren-Larsson syndrome	Fetal skin biopsy	AR	Yes
Xeroderma pigmentosum	Defective DNA repair in fibroblasts	AR	Yes

*From Epstein CJ, Cox DR, Schonberg SA, et al: Recent developments in the prenatal diagnosis of genetic diseases and birth defects. *Ann Rev Genet* 1983; 17:49–83. Used by permission.
†AR = autosomal recessive; AD = autosomal dominant; X = X-linked.
‡Yes indicates diagnosis made; probable, gene product present in normal amniocytes; possible, gene product present in fibroblasts.

DNA Analysis

DNA analysis involves three basic technologies: the use of *restriction endonucleases* (restriction enzymes), *Southern blotting,* and *hybridization.* Other techniques, such as DNA sequencing and gene cloning, are not discussed because they are only secondarily relevant to prenatal diagnosis.

Restriction endonucleases are bacterial enzymes that recognize and cut specific nucleotide sequences in double-stranded DNA molecules. These enzymes serve to protect the bacteria against the intrusion of foreign DNA. There are currently more than 200 known restriction enzymes, each of which recognizes and cuts a unique DNA sequence of either 4 or 6 nucleotides. Examples of restriction enzymes are listed in Table 4–3.

The sequences of DNA recognized by specific restriction enzymes are called *restriction sites.* Several different restriction sites may be found within or surrounding any particular gene and are randomly distributed throughout the genome, the full complement of DNA carried by a cell. However, because more than 95% of human DNA does not code for gene products, most restriction sites are, by chance, not within the coded portion of genes. The DNA between two restriction sites is called a *restriction fragment.* The size of a restriction fragment is determined by the distance between two restriction sites and can vary from a few hundred to several thousand base pairs in length. Thus, when DNA is digested with a restriction enzyme, it is cut into many fragments of varying lengths.

One of the remarkable features of the human genome, discovered through DNA analysis, is that nucleotide sequences vary considerably from person to person, particularly within noncoding regions of DNA. In fact, if two chromosomes of any pair are compared, a single base change is found approximately every 100 to 200 base pairs. As a result, individuals will vary with respect to the number of restriction sites that any one particular enzyme will recognize. Because the presence or absence of a restriction site will affect the length of the restriction fragment between two sites, individuals will also vary with respect to restriction fragment lengths. This is illustrated in Figure 4–1. Individuals lacking the second Pvu II restriction site will have one restriction fragment 5,000 base pairs or 5 kilobases (kb) long, whereas individuals with the restriction site will have two fragments, 3 kb and 2 kb long. The variations in fragment lengths among individuals are called *restriction fragment length polymorphisms* (RFLPs). A polymorphism refers to the occurrence in a population of two or more forms of a gene, the least common having a frequency of at least 1%. Classic examples of human genetic polymorphisms are the ABO blood groups, serum transferrin, or the red blood cell enzyme glucose-6-phosphate dehydrogenase (G6PD). However, unlike RFLPs the number of antigen, serum, or red blood cell polymorphisms are limited in the human genome to less than 50

TABLE 4–3.

Examples of Restriction Enzymes
and Nucleotide Recognition Sites

ENZYME	RECOGNITION SEQUENCE*
Pvu II	CAG^CTG
Eco RI	G^AATTC
Mst II	CC^TNAGG
Cvn I	CC^TNAGG
Msp I	C^CGG
Taq I	T^CGA

*^ = cutting site; N = any nucleotide.

loci. On the other hand, RFLPs provide geneticists with a virtually unlimited source of genetic markers through which diseases can be traced in families.

When genomic DNA is digested with a particular restriction enzyme, fragments of many sizes result. The various size fragments can be separated on the basis of size by agarose gel electrophoresis. During electrophoresis larger restriction fragments migrate through the gel more slowly than smaller restriction fragments. After electrophoresis digested DNA appears under ultraviolet light as a smear. To localize a gene of interest within the many different fragments on a gel, the fragments are transferred to a membrane (such as nitrocellulose or nylon) by a method called *Southern blotting.*[17] Prior to the transfer, the DNA is denatured so that it is single stranded. During the transfer, the spatial orientation of the fragments are maintained so that the band patterns on the membrane are identical to

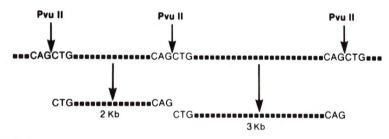

FIG 4–1.
Simplified scheme of the way in which restriction endonucleases cut specific DNA sequences to generate RFLPs. DNA nucleotide sequence is shown as single stranded. Pvu II recognizes the sequence CAGCTG and cuts between the G-C. The length of the restriction fragments generated by Pvu II is determined by the distance between the two sites. In this case, 2 kb and 3 kb fragments are generated. In individuals lacking the middle Pvu II site, a 5 kb fragment only would result from digestion with this enzyme.

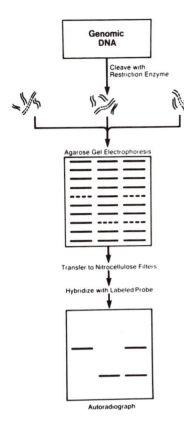

FIG 4–2.
Visualizing RFLPs. DNA is cleaved with restriction enzyme, and the digested DNA is separated by size by using agarose gel electrophoresis. The DNA is then transferred to a membrane, such as nitrocellulose, by a technique called Southern blotting. The orientation of the bands on the membrane is identical to the orientation of the bands in the gel. The membrane is hybridized to a radioactively labeled probe. The DNA fragments that hybridize to the probe are visualized after autoradiography.

those in the gel. The DNA is then hybridized to a specific radioactively labelled probe. The probe contains DNA either from the gene of interest or from DNA very close to (i.e., linked to) the gene of interest. Methods for cloning DNA and making probes are discussed elsewhere.[18, 19]

The probe will hybridize (i.e., pair) to DNA that is complementary to the probe's DNA, because both are single stranded. After the probe hybridizes, the blot is baked dry. Restriction fragments containing the DNA that hybridized to the probe are visualized as dark bands after autoradiography, a method of detecting radioactively labelled molecules on X-ray film. These steps are illustrated in Figure 4–2.

Applications to Prenatal Diagnosis

There are two general approaches to prenatal diagnosis through DNA analysis. The first, the so-called direct method, is the preferred method for prenatal diagnosis. With this approach, DNA from the at-risk fetus is directly tested for the presence or absence of the abnormal gene. There are few potential sources of error with this method, provided the diagnosis is correct. That is, if two different genetic defects result in a similar clinical phenotype, a direct test would not be appropriate for all families with the same phenotype. This potential genetic heterogeneity must always be excluded before direct DNA analysis can be considered. Therefore, the applicability of the direct method is limited to genetic diseases in which the precise molecular defect is known. Although this is considered the ultimate goal for diagnosis of genetic disorders, at this time few genetic diseases can be diagnosed using the direct method of DNA analysis.

The so-called indirect method, based on linkage analysis, is generally applicable to all disorders due to single gene mutations. This approach requires identifying RFLPs that are linked (lie within approximately 1,000,000 base pairs, or 1,000 kb) to the genes that produce disease. The RFLPs are randomly distributed throughout the genome. Thus, it should be possible to identify RFLPs that show linkage to a disease in family studies, even if the abnormal gene itself has not been characterized. The RFLP then can be used to trace the abnormal gene in families. This approach has already been successfully used to prenatally diagnose Duchenne muscular dystrophy, hemophilia A, and cystic fibrosis.

However, because the indirect method does not directly diagnose the defective gene, there are several limitations and sources of error. One limitation is that it requires studying family members, including, in most cases, at least one living relative affected with the disease. A second limitation of the indirect method is that it may not be diagnostic in all at-risk fetuses. Whether or not linkage studies are feasible in any one particular case requires studying the linkage relationship between the RFLP and the disease in each family requesting prenatal diagnosis, a costly and time-consuming process. A third limitation of this approach is the possibility of genetic recombination between the genes that produce disease and the linked marker in one of the parents' gametes. Because this possibility always introduces a potential source of error in the diagnosis, the accuracy of the test is *always* less than 100%.*

The last potential source of error is false paternity. Obviously, if the biologic father is not included in the family studies, erroneous diagnoses may result.

---

*For example, if the recombination rate between an RFLP and the abnormal (mutant) gene is 1%, the accuracy of the test will be 99% (i.e., 1% probability of recombination). In such cases the probability of a false diagnosis is 1%. Because the probability of recombination is proportional to the chromosomal distance between the mutant gene and the RFLP, restriction sites that lie within the gene are the most accurate for diagnosis, and the greater the distance between the site and genes that produce disease, the less accurate the test.

Prenatal Diagnosis Using the Direct Method

The first genetic disorder to be diagnosed prenatally using direct DNA techniques was α-thalassemia,[20] a fairly common disease among Asian and African populations. This disorder, which causes anemia of varying severity, results from a deletion of chromosomal material that includes the α-globin genes. Because normal individuals each have four α-globin genes (two on each chromosome), a spectrum of clinical symptoms results from the deletion of 1, 2, 3, or 4 α-globin genes. The clinical pictures associated with each of these defects are called α-thalassemia-2, heterozygous α-thalassemia-1, hemoglobin H disease, and homozygous α-thalassemia-1, respectively. The clinical spectrum ranges from no symptoms (α-thalassemia-2) to anemia of lethal severity (homozygous α-thalassemia-1).

When genomic DNA is digested with restriction enzyme Eco RI, the α-globin gene is contained within a 13.7-kb fragment of DNA that can be separated and identified using electrophoresis, Southern blotting, and hybridization to an α-globin gene probe. DNA from normal fetuses will reveal one dark band (13.7 kb) after autoradiography. However, DNA from fetuses with homozygous α-thalassemia-1 will not hybridize with the α-globin probe and no bands will appear after autoradiography. Fetuses with only 1 or 2 α-globin genes will show bands of intermediate intensity, which can be quantitated for diagnosis.

This general approach can be applied for diagnosis of any defect due to a gene deletion, provided a probe for the gene is available. A possible error in interpretation of results could arise if the probe is not specific for the precise deletion. Thus, a fetus with a gene deletion may go undetected if the probe hybridizes to DNA around the deleted portion of the chromosome. This may be of particular concern if a defect involves a partial gene deletion. Therefore this approach is applicable only if the probe does *not* hybridize to the gene outside of the deleted area. Furthermore, because diagnosis is based on the absence of a band, an error could result if fetal DNA is accidentally left out of the gel. In this case a normal fetus may be diagnosed as affected. To avoid this potential error, a second probe specific for another gene should always be used to confirm the presence of DNA in the gel.

*Sickle cell anemia** is an autosomal recessive disorder affecting 1 out of 200 black children in the United States. The defect results from a single nucleotide substitution (GAG to GTG) in the sixth codon of the β-globin gene. This *mutation* leads to the transcription of the amino acid valine, in-

*See Chapter 3.

stead of the amino acid glutamic acid. The consequent abnormal β-globin chains cause the red blood cells to assume a characteristic sickle shape.

Two different direct methods of DNA analysis can be used to diagnose this disease. The first utilizes RFLP analysis. Because the mutation causing sickle cell anemia coincidentally resides *within* the recognition sites of restriction enzymes Mst II and Cvn I, an RFLP is created by this mutation. Individuals with the sickle cell mutation lack the restriction site that is present in individuals with normal β-globin genes. The procedure for diagnosing fetuses affected with sickle cell anemia is illustrated in Figure 4–3. The only potential source of error with this procedure is if the disease is caused by a different mutation in a particular family, i.e., genetic heterogeneity. Although the hemoglobinopathies in general are characterized by many mu-

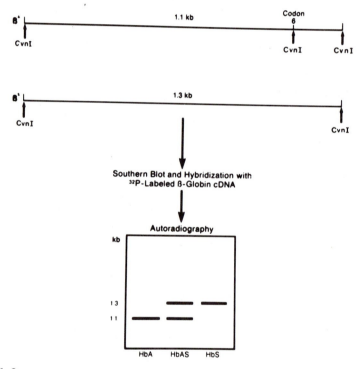

FIG 4–3.
Use of a radioactively labeled β-globin probe to diagnose sickle cell anemia. The mutation causing the disease coincides with a CvnI site. Chromosomes with the sickle mutation lack the site that chromosomes with normal β-globin genes have. After digestion with CvnI and hybridization to a β-globin probe, DNA from individuals with sickle cell anemia yields a 1.3 kb fragment; DNA from individuals with two normal β-globin genes yields a 1.1 kb fragment, and carriers have 1.1 kb and 1.3 kb fragments.

tations causing similar clinical phenotypes, this is less common with sickle cell anemia. However, to avoid this possibility, family studies are usually performed to confirm the presence of the suspect mutation. To date, this simple direct method has only been applied to sickle cell anemia; however, it should be applicable whenever a restriction site coincides with a mutation causing a disease.

A second direct method by which sickle cell anemia can be diagnosed—and one that is more generally applicable to any genetic defect whose molecular basis is known—is through the use of *oligonucleotide probes*. An oligonucleotide probe is a chain of approximately 20 or fewer nucleotides that is synthesized in the laboratory. The usefulness of these short sequences as probes is that unless all nucleotides exactly match the nucleotide sequence in genomic DNA the probe will not hybridize. Therefore, a probe of 18 nucleotides matching the nucleotides in codons 4 through 9 of the β-globin gene will hybridize with DNA from normal fetuses but will not hybridize with the DNA from fetuses with sickle cell anemia. Likewise, a probe made to match the nucleotide sequence in the mutated gene (hemoglobin S) will only hybridize to the abnormal gene and not the normal β-globin gene. Both probes will hybridize to DNA from heterozygous carriers. Thus, this technique is highly accurate because the presence of the normal and abnormal genes can be directly determined. In addition to testing for sickle cell anemia, this approach has also been used to test for α-1-antitrypsin deficiency and certain β-thalassemias in which specific mutations are known.

The only limitation of this approach is that all fetuses tested must have the same molecular defect. If different genetic defects underlie diseases with similar clinical phenotypes (even if the different defects are within the same gene), oligonucleotide probes become less useful. Unfortunately, as our understanding of the molecular bases of genetic disease increases, it is becoming evident that most Mendelian diseases are characterized by extraordinary molecular heterogeneity from family to family. Thus oligonucleotide probes for prenatal diagnosis may not be as valuable a tool for prenatal diagnosis as was once hoped, and linkage-based family studies may be the more appropriate method in most cases.

Prenatal Diagnosis Using the Indirect Method

The indirect method of DNA analysis through linkage-based family studies is, at least in theory, applicable to all genetic disorders. This strategy relies upon finding, through family studies, an RFLP that is linked to the disease of interest. The RFLPs are used as Mendelian codominant markers to follow the inheritance pattern of the disease through families. It has been estimated that if RFLPs are identified on average every 20,000 kb (i.e., 20 million base pairs) throughout the genome, linkage studies will be possible for any genetic trait. Although this concept of a linkage map of the human genome was only first proposed in 1980,[21] the rapid progress in this area has already made prenatal diagnosis of many important genetic diseases possible.

The basic principles and limitations of RFLP linkage analyses are illustrated in *cystic fibrosis* (CF), the most common genetic disorder in the northern European population. Cystic fibrosis is inherited as an autosomal recessive disorder. Approximately 1 in 20 individuals are carriers (i.e., heterozygotes) for the gene, and 1 child in about every 1,500 births is affected with CF. The disease is characterized clinically by chronic obstructive lung disease, pancreatic insufficiency, and elevated sweat electrolytes. Affected individuals rarely live past their 20s and suffer from debilitating illness throughout their lives. Because the biochemical defect causing this disease is unknown, carrier testing and prenatal diagnosis have not been very successful. Despite extensive efforts devoted to identifying the biochemical defect in CF, little progress has been made in this area.

Recently, however, RFLPs have been reported that show close linkage with the CF gene.[22–25] These linked RFLPs can now be used for carrier detection and prenatal diagnosis in most families with an affected child. Because the RFLPs linked to CF are on chromosome 7,[23, 25, 26] it is now known that the CF gene is also on chromosome 7 within approximately 1,000 kb of the RFLPs. These linked sites, however, were found only after extensive testing in many families of linkage between CF and over 100 polymorphic sites located on many different chromosomes. Now that the CF gene has been localized to chromosome 7, it is only a matter of time before the gene itself is located and the molecular defect causing the disease is identified. At that time a direct method of analysis may become available, but until then linkage-based family studies provide many families with reproductive options that were not previously available.

Figure 4–4 illustrates the relationship between the CF gene and a closely linked RFLP in a family with three affected children. The probe used is called Met-H, which is cloned DNA from a gene on chromosome 7. This probe hybridizes to DNA containing two polymorphic restriction sites, one of which results from digestion with restriction enzyme Msp I. The DNA digested with Msp I yields individuals with fragment lengths of 5.5 kb, 2.3 kb, or 1.8 kb, or a combination of any two fragment lengths (recall that each individual has two copies of each gene). The banding patterns are shown in Figure 4–4,A.

Figure 4–4,B shows the pedigree of a family with CF. The parents (I.1 and I.2) are presumed to be heterozygous carriers of the CF gene because they have three affected children. The affected children are assumed to be

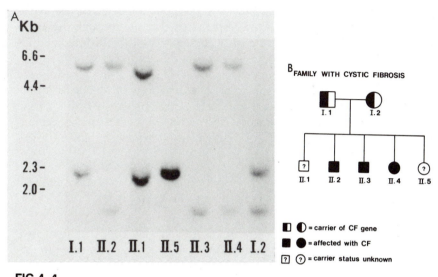

FIG 4–4.
A, DNA studies of family with cystic fibrosis (CF). DNA digested with restriction enzyme MstII and hybridized with probe Met-H. Resulting band sizes are 5.5 kb, 2.3 kb, or 1.8 kb. **B,** family with CF. Children II.2, II.3, and II.4 are affected with CF. Parents are assumed to be carriers of the CF gene because they have affected children. After DNA studies of this family **(A)** it is determined that son II.1 is a carrier of the CF gene and daughter II.5 is homozygous normal.

homozygous for the CF gene. The unaffected children can be either heterozygous carriers of the CF gene or can inherit normal genes from both parents and be homozygous normal. After DNA analysis (Fig 4–4,A), it is determined that the parents are also heterozygous at the Msp I site; the father has 5.5- and 2.3-kb bands and the mother has 2.3- and 1.8-kb bands. The three affected children are also heterozygous (5.5/1.8) at this site. Thus, we can deduce that each affected child inherited the 5.5-kb fragment from their father and the 1.8-kb fragment from their mother and the CF gene must be on these respective parental chromosomes. Both parental chromosomes with the 2.3-kb fragment must carry the normal gene. We can further deduce that the sister with genotype 2.3/2.3 inherited the normal gene from each parent and is not a carrier for CF. The brother with genotype 5.5/2.3, on the other hand, inherited the chromosome with the normal gene from his mother (2.3-kb fragment) and the chromosome with the CF gene from his father (5.5-kb fragment) and is a presumed carrier for CF.

In this family prenatal diagnosis of CF in subsequent pregnancies is possible. Fetal DNA derived from chorionic villi at 9 to 11 weeks' gestation or from amniotic fluid cells at 16 to 18 weeks' gestation could be genotyped for the presence or absence of the Msp I restriction site through the methods described above. The CF status of the fetus could be deduced and reproductive decisions could be made based on this diagnosis.*

Despite its novelty, the indirect method of DNA analysis has already proved to be an invaluable tool for prenatal diagnosis of Mendelian disorders. This general application is currently being applied to many genetic disorders in which the biochemical and molecular defects are as yet unknown, and prenatal diagnosis of any Mendelian disorder should be feasible before long.

POLYGENIC/MULTIFACTORIAL DISORDERS

As discussed in Chapter 1, some disorders result from the cumulative effects of several genes (polygenic) and their interactions with environmental factors (multifactorial). Frequently such disorders involve single organ systems. After the birth of one child with a disorder believed to be inherited in polygenic/multifactorial fashion, the likelihood of recurrence is usually 2% to 5%. Because the recurrence risk is relatively low, most individuals with these disorders have no affected relatives. Examples of defects inherited in polygenic/multifactorial fashion include cleft palate, certain cardiac defects, pyloric stenosis, talipes equinovarus, and neural tube defects (anencephaly and spina bifida).

Neural Tube Defects

Approximately 6,000 infants with neural tube defects† are born each year in the United States. The estimated incidence of NTDs varies from 6 to 8 per 1,000 births in Northern Ireland, Wales, and Scotland to 1.4 to 3.1 per 1,000 births in the United States.[27-31] In the United States, if the

---

*The major potential source of error in linkage studies is the "probability" of recombination between the restriction site and the abnormal gene in the parents' gametes. For example, if there was a meiotic cross-over in one of the father's gametes between the Msp I site and the CF gene, the CF gene would be on the chromosome with the 2.3-kb fragment. If the fetus was determined to have genotype 2.3/1.8, a diagnosis of *carrier* would be made; however, the fetus would be *affected* with CF. Thus results from prenatal testing must always be given as a probability, taking into account the probability of recombination. For example, the recombination frequency between the Msp I site and the CF gene, determined from family studies, is approximately 1%. Thus, if prenatal testing of a subsequent pregnancy in the couple in Figure 4–4 revealed a 2.3/2.3 genotype, they should be counseled that the probability that the fetus does not have CF is 99%. See Chapter 2.

†See also discussion of maternal screening for neural tube defects in Chapter 3.

proband has spina bifida, the likelihood that a first-degree relative (sib, parent, offspring) will have either anencephaly or spina bifida is 1.5% to 2%. If the proband has anencephaly, the total risk to first-degree relatives for either anencephaly or spina bifida is again about 2%.[32, 33] However, there seems to be a relationship between incidence and recurrence risk. For example, in the British Isles couples who have had a child with either anencephaly or spina bifida have a 5% recurrence risk for an NTD occurring in a subsequent offspring. Couples who have had two children with either anencephaly or spina bifida have a 5% (United States) to 10% (British Isles) recurrence risk. If a parent has spina bifida, the likelihood of having a child with NTD is 1.1% (United States) to 5% (British Isles). Even the risk of NTDs in first cousins of affected individuals remains increased over that of the general population. Specifically, the sisters of women with an affected child have a 0.5% to 1% risk for an offspring with NTD.[33, 34] Finally, it is important to attempt to establish a definite diagnosis before offering recurrence risks. Although most NTDs are a consequence of polygenic/multifactorial inheritance, a few may be caused by single mutant genes (e.g., Meckel syndrome, median-cleft face syndrome); chromosomal abnormalities (trisomy 13, trisomy 18, and triploidy); or teratogens (e.g., aminopterin, thalidomide, or valproic acid). In such cases the recurrence risk would be based upon the specific etiologic factor believed responsible for the NTD.

A major advance in prenatal diagnosis was the discovery in 1972 that amniotic fluid α-fetoprotein (AFP) levels were elevated in the presence of fetal NTD.[35] The AFP is the major fetal serum protein during the early weeks of pregnancy, occurring in concentrations as high as 3,000 μg/ml at the 12th week of gestation. Thereafter it falls steadily as albumin levels begin to rise in the fetal serum. It is normally present in amniotic fluid being excreted by the fetal kidneys.[36] Because AFP can also pass by transudation across fetal blood vessels on NTD-exposed membrane surfaces, elevated levels can serve as a basis for prenatal diagnosis. However, it is important to note that 5% to 10% of all NTDs are not open (i.e., the defect is covered with skin) and, hence, would not be detectable using this approach.[33] Also, because the mean AFP concentrations in amniotic fluid normally fall steadily throughout the second trimester, documentation of gestational age is vital before interpreting test results. If the gestational age is incorrectly assigned as being older than the true age, the amniotic fluid AFP may be erroneously considered to be elevated (i.e., false-positive). Conversely, if the age of the fetus is erroneously considered younger than the true age, the amniotic fluid AFP may be interpreted as lower than the true age and an NTD could theoretically be missed (i.e., a false-negative). Gestational age should be determined by three parameters, including: (1) history as determined by the onset of the last menses; (2) physical examination of uterine size; and (3) ultrasonographic measurement of the fetal biparietal diameter. The test is highly sensitive and specific.†

As many as 1% to 2% of all amniotic fluid AFP assays have been reported as false-positives, although most experienced laboratories now report the phenomenon far less frequently (0.1% to 0.2%).[37, 38] Many of these false-positive results can be explained on the basis of admixture of fetal blood with amniotic fluid. Because fetal blood levels of AFP are at least 100 times higher than those normally found in amniotic fluid, even a small amount of contamination may raise amniotic fluid values into the abnormal range. The assay for acetylcholinesterase (AChE) has been demonstrated as being an important complementary test to distinguish between true and false positive results. In a collaborative study in the United Kingdom,[40] AChE measurement by polyacrylamide gel electrophoresis was made on amniotic fluid samples from 1,099 pregnancies with positive AFP results. Of pregnancies with anencephaly, 99.6% (476/478) revealed on AChE band, while of those with open spina bifida, 99.4% (333/335) were likewise positive. Only 6% (8/125) of pregnancies which did not end in miscarriage and in which the fetus did not have a serious malformation showed positive results. In essence this meant that a woman who had an elevated amniotic fluid AFP level and also a positive AChE measurement had a 16 times higher likelihood of having a fetus with a serious malformation than a woman with only an elevated AFP result. Other studies have also demonstrated the value of using AChE as a complementary test to reduce the number of false-positive results from the AFP assay.[41–43] Although the specific AChE band is nearly always present in cases of open NTD and absent in fluids in which fetal blood contamination is the cause of the AFP eleva-

---

†In 1979 the Second Report of the U.K. Collaborative Study was published providing the combined data collected from 19 United Kingdom laboratory centers assessing second-trimester amniotic fluid AFP studies in relation to NTDs.[37] This report included 385 pregnancies in which the outcome was a fetal NTD (222 with anencephaly, 152 with spina bifida, and 11 with encephalocele), and 13,105 in which there was no NTD. Given the different mass unit standards in use at the various laboratories, it became necessary to convert all values into multiples of the median (MoM). Different cut-off levels were selected at various gestational ages: 2.5 times MoM at 13 to 15 weeks, 3.0 times MoM at 16 to 18 weeks, 3.5 MoM at 10 to 21 weeks, and 4.0 times MoM at 22 to 24 weeks. Using these values 98.2% (218/222) of cases of anencephaly and 97.6% (120/123) of cases of open spina bifida gave positive results. Only 0.48% (61/12,804) of the unaffected singleton pregnancies not associated with a spontaneous abortion had elevated values (i.e., a sensitivity of 99.5%). Other large US studies have confirmed the high sensitivity and specificity of this test for the determination of open neural tube defects.[38, 39] Fetal abnormalities other than NTDs have been associated with elevated amniotic fluid AFP, including congenital nephrosis, duodenal atresia, fetal death, gastroschisis, nuchal cysts, omphalocele, severe Rh disease, and teratomas.

tion, the assay is less useful in differentiating between other fetal causes of elevated amniotic fluid AFP (e.g., omphalocele, exstrophy of the bladder, teratomas).[40, 43] Finally, a monoclonal antibody specific for AChE has recently been reported that should greatly simplify the measurement of this enzyme and may allow the test to become more widely available.[44]

LEGAL AND POLICY ISSUES

In recent years there has been a growing expectation on the part of the public that medical science, especially obstetricians and geneticists, can help ensure that only healthy babies are born. As a result of the existence of prenatal testing that can provide relevant information in many cases, the potential types of lawsuits against obstetricians and geneticists have increased to include negligent failure to advise parents of the existence of prenatal diagnostic tests when indicated, and negligence in the performance of these tests. In addition, in some jurisdictions, the child who is born with a handicap that *could* have been detected in utero has been permitted to sue for "wrongful life." The theory is that but for the negligence of the physician or testing laboratory, the child would have been aborted and thus life in a handicapped state would have been prevented. This section outlines some of the major issues involved in "wrongful birth" and "wrongful life" suits.

Wrongful Birth Suits

"Wrongful birth" is a catch-all phrase used to describe, among other actions, those lawsuits brought by parents against physicians, testing laboratories, and others on the basis that their negligence deprived parents of their right to make an informed decision concerning pregnancy or childbirth.[45] Typical kinds of negligence cases include one in which a druggist's negligence in supplying tranquilizers instead of the oral contraceptives called for by the physician's prescription resulted in an unwanted pregnancy,[46] and one in which a negligently performed vasectomy was followed by pregnancy.[47] In both cases, the parents were permitted to recover the costs of raising the unplanned child to the age of majority, with an offset for the benefits the parents derive from raising the child.[48]

In prenatal diagnosis cases in which the physician neglects to inform the parents of the existence of a test applicable to their situation, negligently performs the test, negligently fails to refer to a specialist who could perform the test, or negligently informs the couple about their risks of having an affected child, courts now almost universally permit them to sue their physician for depriving them of their right to make a decision about commencing or continuing a pregnancy.[45, 49] This was not always the case.

In the first case of its kind to reach a state supreme court, the New Jersey Supreme Court in 1967 denied both the parents and their child the right to sue, after the child was born deaf and blind as a result of rubella his mother suffered during the pregnancy.[50] The court reached this conclusion even though the woman's physician knew of the possibility of injury (estimated at 25%), and intentionally withheld this information from the mother. The claim was denied for two reasons: (1) there was no way to measure the child's injury, since the only way to prevent it would have been abortion, and thus the jury would have the impossible task of measuring impaired life versus nonexistence; and (2) in the days prior to *Roe v. Wade*,* the court was able to conclude that abortion would violate society's notion of "the preciousness of human life." The court seemed to conclude that life itself is always, and under all circumstances, a blessing.[51] Twelve years later, in a similar case, the New Jersey court reversed itself as to the parents' claim, concluding that the physician had deprived the parents of the right to make an informed decision concerning continuation of the pregnancy.[52] This conclusion was based almost entirely on the altered public policy regarding abortion.†

The rationale for permitting parents to recover damages in such a case is set forth in typical language by a Texas court:

> It is impossible for us to justify a policy which at once deprives the parents of information by which they could elect to terminate the pregnancy likely to produce a child with a defective body, a policy which in effect requires that the deficient embryo be carried to full gestation until the deficient child is born, and which policy then denies recovery from the tortfeasor of costs of treating and caring for the defects of the child.[53]

We believe this conclusion is correct. Any woman who employs a physician for prenatal care should have the right to have the physician fully inform her of any reason the physician has to believe that her fetus might be handicapped, and to inform her of the existence of diagnostic tests that might identify the precise genetic condition. The physician incurs this duty to disclose because it is this type of information that the pregnant woman seeks prenatal care to discover, i.e., to learn all she can to help her have a healthy child. The physician, of course, does not guarantee a healthy child. But it is entirely reasonable for the pregnant woman to expect her physician

---

*See discussion of *Roe v. Wade* in Chapter 6.

†In 1984, the court reversed itself completely, and permitted children to sue on their own behalf (*Procanik v. Cillo*, 478 A.2d 755 [1984]).

to apprise her of any relevant information regarding her fetus, and options she might have, so that she and the child's father can determine what action to take.[54]

Since we are dealing with handicapped newborns who often require expensive medical care, these cases have the potential for extremely large awards.‡ Even with an impairment as relatively mild as Down syndrome, verdicts can be large. For example, in one case brought on the basis of the birth of a Down syndrome child, the parents were awarded $1,533,000 by a federal trial judge.[55, 56] The case involved a young couple whose son was born with Down syndrome in 1977. The woman, who was 23 years old at the time, had had one previous pregnancy which had resulted in a spontaneous abortion. She also gave a family history that indicated she had a sister who had Down syndrome. Nonetheless, she was neither given counseling nor offered any genetic testing. There was uncontradicted testimony that the child had an IQ of 56 and had a life expectancy of 50 years, during which he would need "twenty-four hour care and supervision." The parents asked that the award be put into trust for the exclusive benefit of their child during his lifetime.

A pair of New York cases serve to complete our discussion of wrongful birth and introduce our discussion of wrongful life. These two cases were consolidated by New York's highest court and decided together.[57] The first case involved Dolores Becker, who in 1974, at the age of 37, became pregnant. She was under the exclusive care of her obstetrician from the tenth week of her pregnancy until the child's birth. The child was born with Down syndrome. Mrs. Becker alleged that she was not advised of the availability of amniocentesis, and that if she had been so advised, she would have aborted the fetus if the test indicated that the child was affected. The plaintiffs in the companion case, Hetty and Steven Park, had had a child in 1969 afflicted with polycystic kidney disease who had died five hours after birth. Following this tragedy, Mrs. Park asked her obstetrician what the chances were of future children being similarly affected. The obstetrician allegedly replied (incorrectly) that the chances were "practically nil." Based on this reassuring information, Mrs. Park again became pregnant and again gave birth to a child with polycystic kidney disease. Unlike her first child, however, this one lived for 2½ years. Neither case had actually been tried before they were heard by the New York Court of Appeals, so the only question before the court was, *assuming everything the plaintiffs alleged was true,* did they have a right to present their case to a jury and possibly recover money damages?

The court upheld the right of both sets of parents to sue. Accepting

‡The medical treatment of handicapped newborns is addressed in Chapter 7.

their version of the facts (which the court had to do), the court found that the parents had stated a proper malpractice claim. Specifically, in order to prevail in a medical malpractice action, the plaintiff must prove four elements: duty, breach of duty, damages, and causation. In this case, the parents would have to prove that the physician owed them a duty to disclose the information (usually proved by medical testimony based on "good and accepted medical practice" but often by exploring the duty to disclose inherent in the fiduciary nature of the doctor-patient relationship). Further they must prove that the physician's failure to provide this information directly caused the plaintiff monetary damages (in this case, the cost of raising a handicapped child that would have been aborted had the parents been given the opportunity). Unlike some other courts, however, the New York court refused to permit recovery for emotional or psychiatric damages suffered by the parents. It thought awarding such damages would "inevitably lead to drawing artificial and arbitrary boundaries" such as balancing the emotional trauma with the parental "love that even an abnormality cannot fully dampen."[57]

The court thus ruled that if the Beckers could prove all of their allegations in a trial, they could recover the sums expended for long-term institutional care of their Down syndrome child. Likewise, if the Parks could prove their case, they could recover the money expended for care and treatment of their child until death. Although these two cases produced almost hysterical commentary in the press, many predicting million dollar verdicts, they are unremarkable cases from a legal perspective,[58] and each ended anticlimactically. The jury apparently did not believe the Parks' story. It returned a verdict in favor of the physician (instead of awarding them the $67,000 both sides agreed was the cost of caring for their child). The Beckers, on the other hand, gave their child up for adoption. Since they then had no financial obligation to the child, their case was eventually settled out of court for the money they had previously spent on foster care, reportedly $2,500.

This settlement raises an extremely important issue: while the New York court required the damages awarded to be measured in terms of the cost of long-term care, the parents were not obligated to spend any of it for the child's actual care. Accordingly, had the Beckers waited until after obtaining a million dollar verdict to put the child up for adoption, the parents could have become rich, while the adopting parents would have no claim to funds awarded on the basis of the child's need for special care. This potential outcome could be eliminated by legislation requiring that the award be placed in a trust fund for the exclusive use of the child, or by permitting the child to bring suit on the child's own behalf.[51] This latter type of lawsuit has been termed one for "wrongful life."

Wrongful Life

The New York Court of Appeals rejected both the Beckers' and Parks' request to permit their handicapped children to sue on their own behalf for "wrongful life." Following closely the logic of the original New Jersey decision on damages,[50] the court ruled that the children had not suffered any "legally cognizable injury." In the court's words:

> Whether it is better never to have been born at all than to have been born with even gross deficiencies is a mystery more properly to be left to the philosophers and the theologians.[57]

The court thought that recognition of an action in "wrongful life" would raise the possibility of a lawsuit every time a child was born less than "perfect." Finally, the court decided it was impossible to place the child in the position he would have been in but for the negligent act, since the child would not have existed at all:

> Simply put, a cause of action brought on behalf of an infant seeking recovery for wrongful life demands a calculation of damages dependent upon a comparison between the Hobson's choice of life in an impaired state and nonexistence. This comparison the law is not equipped to make.[57]

Many courts and commentators have found this logic entirely persuasive. The notion that there can be something like a "wrongful birth" seems to some to suggest that individuals with various genetic handicaps would be seen as second-class citizens, citizens who should not have been born. The danger, it is suggested, is the creation of a living underclass who are shunned or discriminated against by the rest of society. Nietzsche's polemic in *Thus Spoke Zarathustra* seems to these commentators to be coming true:

> Many die too late, and a few die too early. The doctrine still sounds strange: 'Die at the right time!' Die at the right time—thus teaches Zarathustra. Of course, how could those who never live at the right time die at the right time? *Would that they had never been born! Thus I counsel the superfluous* [emphasis added].

Viewing the genetically impaired as "superfluous" or less worthy of life than other citizens is not, of course, a necessary consequence of either prenatal diagnosis or permitting wrongful life lawsuits. Late 20th century United States is neither late 19th century nor World War II Germany. The foundation of our legal system is radically different: in the United States the state exists to enhance the liberty of its citizens, citizens do not exist for the sake of the state. One can actually view wrongful life lawsuits as equalizers of a sort. At least in cases in which the child's parents are unable to sue (e.g., because the statute of limitations has run out, or because they have given their child up for adoption), this type of lawsuit gives the handicapped child a chance to recover money to pay for medical and custodial care, whereas in the absence of such a remedy, the child would have no recourse against anyone.

Just as the tort of wrongful birth went from absolute rejection to virtually universal acceptance in less than 20 years, the tort of "wrongful life" will likely find, if not universal, at least increasing acceptance over the coming years. The reason is that the wrong complained of by the child has been imprecisely stated by most courts, just as the wrong to the parents had been improperly stated in wrongful birth cases. This is because most courts continue to focus on the impossibility of conceptualizing the comparison between nonexistence and impaired existence from the viewpoint of a child that exists. But this is an imprecise conceptualization. As Professor Alexander Capron has quite properly pointed out, there is nothing illogical in the child saying, "I would have preferred not to exist. But since I'm here, I want to be compensated for my handicap." The real harm is the "deprivation of choice" that has been denied to the child, just as it was denied to its parents.[58, 59] This claim may seem strange at first, but it rests on a firm foundation, and only if it is rejected should wrongful life suits be rejected. We permit parents to make decisions for their children, at least as long as they are in the "best interests" of the child. The wrongful life claim is valid for any parent who concludes that it is in their potential child's best interests not to be born. We think many parents will qualify, and that many reluctantly opt for abortion, even though they believe they can handle a handicapped child, because they don't think it would be fair to the child. Such parents choose abortion because they wish to protect their potential child from a life of unbearable burdens.

For example, it seems perfectly possible that the Parks might have decided to abort their second fetus (had they known it had polycystic kidney disease) to spare it a brief life of inevitable and severe pain and suffering, because they believed that this decision would be in the best interests of their potential child. It is, of course, a fiction to pretend a fetus can have thoughts and preferences, but it may be a useful one. Assuming the fetus understood its situation and could communicate to us, and assuming it was afflicted with polycystic kidney disease that doomed it to a brief, horrible life, it would probably decide itself that it was better off not coming into existence than being born to endure that life.

The first crack in the wall of court refusals to hear wrongful life cases occurred in California. As with most landmark cases, the facts were compelling and made it almost impossible for the court to deny the child an opportunity to present her case to a jury.[60]

The plaintiff, Sauna Tamar Curlender, was born with Tay-Sachs disease. Her parents had previously retained the laboratory named as defendant to administer tests to determine whether or not they were carriers for Tay-Sachs disease. The tests were reported to have been negative. The parents relied upon these tests. Because of the alleged negligence in the laboratory's performance, they had a child with Tay-Sachs disease, subject to severe suffering, and a life expectancy of only approximately four years.

The child's lawsuit sought damages for emotional distress and the deprivation of 72.6 years of life. She sought an additional $3 million in punitive damages on the grounds that the defendants knew their testing procedures were likely to produce a substantial number of false-negatives and yet proceeded to use them "in conscious disregard of the health, safety, and well-being of the plaintiff. . ." The court could not determine whether the parents relied upon the test to conceive a child or to forego amniocentesis; nor did the court seem to care.

The court began its inquiry with a worthwhile excursion through the history of so-called "wrongful life" cases. On the basis of this history, and the court's own view of what the law should be, it made a number of important observations concerning the handling of "the 'wrongful life' problem" by previous courts. The court concluded that there is a major difference between a child who is unwanted or illegitimate, but healthy (the type of children involved in the original cases in which the courts first coined the term "wrongful life")* and a child who is born with a severe deformity or disease. Unlike a severe deformity, illegitimacy is simply not an injury.

Second, the court noted a trend in the law to recognize that there should be recovery when an infant is born defective and its "painful existence is a direct and proximate result of negligence by others."

Third, the court observed that children have continued to sue for wrongful life because of the seriousness of the wrong, the increasing understanding of its causes, and "the understanding that the law reflects, perhaps later than sooner, basic changes in the way society views such matters."

Given these observations, the court was determined to recognize the right of the child to sue for the negligent acts of others that led to her birth:

**Zepeda v. Zepeda*, 41 Ill. App. 2d 240, 190 N.E. 2d 849 (1963), *cert. denied*, 379 U.S. 945 (1965) (illegitimate child's action against his father for illegitimacy dismissed because of the court's belief that granting relief would create too sweeping a precedent and therefore the decision was more properly one for the legislature); *Williams v. State*, 18 N.Y. 2d 481, 223 N.E. 2d 343, 276 N.Y.S. 2d 885 (1956) (child born as a result of a sexual assault on a woman confined as a patient in a state mental institution; suit brought against the state dismissed because of difficulty in measuring damages for illegitimacy, and the potential far-reaching effects of granting relief); *Pinkney v. Pinkney*, 198 So. 2d 52 (Fla. Dist. Ct. App. 1967) (an action by a daughter against her father for having caused her birth out of wedlock and for having shot her mother; action dismissed citing *Zepeda* as precedent).

The reality of the "wrongful life" concept is that such a plaintiff both exists and suffers, due to the negligence of others. It is neither necessary nor just to retreat into meditation on the mysteries of life. We need not be concerned with the fact that had defendants not been negligent, the plaintiff might not have come into existence at all. The certainty of genetic impairment is no longer a mystery . . . a reverent appreciation of life compels recognition that the plaintiff . . . has come into existence as a living person with certain rights.

This remarkable statement dealt with the major imponderable in wrongful life cases by dismissing it with the phrase, "We need not be concerned [about it]." All the court's major points are addressed by permitting the parents to recover damages. Certainly they have been injured; expecting a normal child, they must deal with an abnormal one. Expecting full and accurate information during the pregnancy, they have received neither. There are both emotional and monetary costs. But what about the child, Sauna Curlender? She expected nothing, not even birth. She never had the possibility of being born healthy—only the chance of being either aborted or not conceived at all. From one way of looking at it, she could not be damaged by the testing laboratory's negligence, because without the negligence she would not have existed. The argument is not that any life is better than none, no matter what the suffering; but rather that to be damaged one must be worse off after the negligent act complained of than before it. It cannot be said, *in this sense,* that Sauna is worse off existing than not existing if one assumes that nonexistence is a state in which there are no rights and no rightful expectations.

On the other hand, for policy reasons we may want to ignore this troublesome issue and deal with the reality of the existence of a handicapped child who needs care and attention. It is correct to say that the testing laboratory did not cause the child's disease, but it is also correct that the child would not exist, suffering from the disease, if the testing laboratory had not been negligent. Without permitting Sauna to recover damages, there could be a wrong without a remedy. The court's position is no more difficult to sustain than the traditional one.

Concerning damages, the court denied recovery based on a 70-year life expectancy, and instead required that damages be based on Sauna's actual life expectancy of four years. Though one can quarrel a bit with this, it seems a fair compromise. After all, she never had any opportunity for a 70-year life span: it was no life or a four-year life. Under these circumstances, limiting damages for medical expenses and pain and suffering for her actual life span seems reasonable. This may be especially so in light of the court's decision to permit the plaintiffs to proceed with their $3 million claim for punitive damages. The case was reportedly settled for $1.6 million.

Two years later, in 1982, the California Supreme Court became the first state supreme court to recognize the tort of wrongful life and did so based on Professor Capron's view of the injury suffered.[59] The case involved a young couple who consulted an expert in hearing disorders for their daughter.[49] They were incorrectly advised that her hearing was within normal limits, when in fact she was "stone deaf" as a result of a hereditary ailment. Had the diagnosis been properly made, her parents would not have conceived a second child. They did, and the second child, Joy, was also born deaf. Joy's ability to sue on her own behalf was the only issue before the California Supreme Court.

The Court determined that the *Curlender*[60] analysis was faulty because it concentrated on injury at the time of birth and thereafter. The real injury occurs prior to birth or conception, at a time when the parents are prevented from making an informed decision to conceive a child or continue a pregnancy. While this is fundamentally an injury to the parents, it can also be considered a simultaneous injury to the child. In the court's words:

> Although in deciding whether or not to bear such a child parents may properly, and undoubtedly do, take into account their own interests, parents also presumptively consider the interests of their future child. Thus, when a defendant negligently fails to diagnose an hereditary ailment, he harms the potential child as well as the parents by depriving the parents of information which may be necessary to determine whether it is in the child's own interest to be born with defects or not to be born at all.[49]

As previously discussed, this analysis seems correct.* The court also seems correct in concluding that in a case like Joy Turpin's, in which the only affliction is deafness, "it seems quite unlikely that a jury would ever conclude that life with such a condition is worse than not being born at all."

Although much debate continues to swirl around the notion of wrongful life, the California Supreme Court seems to have the proper focus: wrongful life claims should be cognizable only for *serious* impairments, like polycystic kidney disease and Tay-Sachs disease, in which fetuses, if they could speak, would agree with an objective societal consensus that their own best interests would be served if they were aborted. Cases like deafness

---

*Other state supreme courts have joined California in recognizing lawsuits for wrongful life, but have also limited damages to "special" damages. E.g., *Harbeson v. Parke-Davis, Inc.*, 656 P. 2d 483 (Wash. 1983) (involving failure to warn of possibility of fetal hydantoin syndrome resulting from use of Dilantin during pregnancy); and *Procanik v. Cillo*, 478 A. 2d 755 (N.J. 1984) (involving failure to diagnose German measles contracted during the first trimester, and resulting birth of child with multiple impairments). It should be noted, however, that the Washington case is *not* a wrongful life case *per se* since in the absence of negligence, the child would have been born healthy, an option never open to the child in a "real" wrongful life case.

would clearly not qualify. Cases like Down syndrome represent the "hard case," in which the real injury is probably much more to the parents than to the child, since the child would almost always consider a life with Down syndrome better than no life at all.

The second portion of the California opinion is more problematic: limiting damages to medical and caretaking expenses (so-called special damages), but denying damages of "pain and suffering" (general damages). There is, as the dissent properly notes, no conceptual basis for this strange division, and it seems simply an arbitrary compromise that permits the courts to do justice to the injured child (by making sure it has the funds to be cared for during its life), without opening up the possibility of extremely high awards based on emotion rather than any logical attempt to value impaired existence versus nonexistence. It may also recognize the paradox that the more extreme the damage to the child, the stronger the claim for a large monetary award becomes, but the less likely it becomes that the award can actually compensate the infant in any meaningful way for existing. As one commentator has put it, "There is something troubling in awarding huge sums to infants whose lives cannot be improved by any amount of money while denying it to those infants whose lives might benefit."[61] We should note, however, that even if damage assessments are made on admittedly arbitrary grounds, such damages might better serve the ends of justice than no damages at all.[62]

Public Policy Considerations

All this may seem a bit frightening to obstetricians and genetic counselors, but legal developments in wrongful life should be placed in perspective. First, in almost all cases, the parents will be able to recover the amount of money projected for the care of an impaired newborn under traditional tort principles (wrongful birth cases). Thus, since courts have limited direct recovery by the child (wrongful life) to these out-of-pocket expenses, the child's independent right to sue will only be useful to it or its parents when, for some reason, the parents have lost their right to sue. Such reasons would include failure to file a suit under the applicable statute of limitations (assuming the child has a longer period of time to file such a suit), and cases in which the parents have given the child up for adoption or otherwise relinquished their parental rights in the child. Therefore, while wrongful life discussions are inherently interesting, they are rarely relevant.

More importantly, what seems to be going on in the courts' discussion of both wrongful birth and wrongful life suits is essentially a discussion of providing a method of paying for the care of handicapped newborns. The handicapped newborn, of course, did not cause its own condition—nor did the physician. But the physician could have prevented the existence of the handicapped child by giving the parents sufficient information for them to refrain from pregnancy or terminate the pregnancy. The question can thus be restated as an insurance question: between the physician who negligently or willfully withheld relevant information from the parents, and the child, which party should bear the financial burden of medical and caretaking costs required by the handicap? We believe the proper answer is actually neither, and that a just society would provide governmentally-financed payment mechanisms to properly treat and care for *all* handicapped newborns throughout their lives, whether they are the result of wanted or unwanted pregnancies or births, or whether they resulted from accurate genetic counseling or negligent genetic counseling. Until such a social insurance scheme is devised, however, it seems reasonable to hold those who have the legal obligation to provide accurate information to the parents financially responsible for the consequences of their negligent acts.

This analysis leaves out the parents as possible culprits, and we think this is as it should be. The *Curlender*[60] court, on the other hand, suggested that if the physician properly informed the mother of the child's handicapped condition, but she nonetheless decided to continue the pregnancy, then the child should be able to sue its mother for negligence. Remarkably, the *Curlender* court concluded, we find "no sound public policy which should protect those parents from being answerable for the pain, suffering, and misery which they have wrought upon their offspring." Others have made similar suggestions. Geneticist-lawyer Margery Shaw, for example, has suggested that women who "abandon their right to abort" upon being informed that their fetus is affected with a disorder, should incur a "conditional prospective liability" for negligence toward the fetus should it be born alive. She would permit handicapped children to sue their mothers for failure to abort them, and also go further to permit children harmed by fetal alcohol syndrome or drug addiction to sue their mothers on the basis that they have a "right to be born physically and mentally sound."[63]

While this might seem a logical extension of the notion of wrongful life, it is neither a necessary nor desirable one. It converts a woman's *right* to have an abortion into a *duty* to have an abortion in certain circumstances, and thus misses the point of all of those cases and rationales that focus on procreational liberty and informed *choice* as the critical issue. Such a "right" could almost immediately turn into a duty on the part of potential parents and their caretakers to make sure that no defective, different, or "abnormal" children are born. This could lead to drastic deprivations of the liberty of pregnant women, especially after fetal viability.*

---

*See, e.g., the discussion of maternal-fetal conflicts in Chapter 10.

Moreover, there is no such thing as a "right to be born physically and mentally sound" any more than there is a right to be born rich, white, or urban. Nor is there, we believe, any such thing as a "right not be be born." The nature of the right is the right to have one's parents make the decision to have children based on accurate and complete information.† Finally, unless the parents relinquish the child, the financial resources they have will likely be used for the child's benefit in any event, so such a lawsuit is only likely to occur *if* the parents have some form of health insurance that would pay the child's expenses only if the parent negligently injured the child. It was for these, and other reasons, that the California legislature, after the *Curlender* decision,[60] passed a statute that relieves the parents of any liability for deciding to conceive a child or failing to abort a handicapped child.[49]

Parents should be permitted, as they now are, to make good-faith procreative judgments. Some children will suffer, but this seems a less onerous result than the massive curtailment of liberty of adults implicit in the "right to normalcy" notion. Health care providers have the legal obligation to provide parents with accurate information on which to base decisions; they do not have the right to make decisions for them. Only by keeping this distinction firmly in place can we help to assure that increases in genetic knowledge will lead to increases in human liberty, rather than to its destruction.

†A more precise argument is proposed by philosopher Joel Feinberg who, while rejecting the notion of children being "dragged struggling and kicking into their mother's wombs" from "a strange never-never land," nonetheless proposes what he terms a "plausible moral requirement that no child be brought into the world unless certain very minimal conditions of wellbeing are assured."[62] The notion is that this "basic minimum" is the child's birthright, and if it cannot be supplied, the child has been wronged by being born. Feinberg argues that even though the child has not been *harmed* (since the child's initial position was a "harmed" condition, and the physician did not make it worse), the child can nonetheless be *wronged* by being brought into existence under conditions that any rational being would prefer nonexistence to.

Chapter 5 _____

Prenatal Diagnosis: Techniques

Having discussed when it is appropriate to offer prenatal diagnosis,* this chapter concentrates on the actual performance of various prenatal diagnostic techniques and their follow-up. Some of the techniques that will be examined, like chorionic villus sampling, are still experimental. All of the techniques require specific skills, and consistently reliable and safe prenatal diagnosis requires an experienced team to provide the necessary expertise.

Ideally, couples should have the opportunity to discuss their genetic risks and the available diagnostic tests prior to pregnancy.[1, 2] The counselor should elicit an accurate history, confirm the diagnosis of any abnormality in question, be aware of diagnostic capabilities, and be cognizant of psychological defenses (e.g., denial, guilt reactions, and blame) engendered during genetic counseling.† Couples must understand the risks of the diagnostic procedure itself, accuracy and limitations of prenatal diagnosis, time required before results become available, technical problems potentially necessitating additional procedures, and, rarely, the inability to make a diagnosis.[3]

The obstetrician performing the diagnostic procedure must also be prepared to deal with any resultant complications. If an abnormality is detected and the couple elects to terminate the pregnancy, the obstetrician must either perform the abortion or refer the patient to another obstetrician who will. In this chapter we review the prenatal diagnostic techniques of amniocentesis, chorionic villus sampling, fetoscopy, and level II ultrasound.

*See Chapter 4.
†See Chapter 2.

AMNIOCENTESIS

Technical Aspects

Amniocentesis, the aspiration of amniotic fluid, is currently the most commonly utilized technique for prenatal diagnosis. The procedure is best performed around 15 to 16 weeks' gestation (menstrual weeks), at which time the ratio of viable to nonviable cells is the greatest.[4] In addition, the uterus at this time is technically accessible by an abdominal approach and there is a sufficient volume of amniotic fluid (200 to 250 ml) to allow an adequate sample (20 to 30 ml) to be removed safely.[1, 5, 6]

Amniocentesis may be performed in an outpatient facility. In preparation for the procedure, the patient empties her bladder so that inadvertent aspiration of urine does not occur. An ultrasound examination should be performed immediately prior to amniocentesis in order to (1) detect multiple gestation; (2) document fetal viability by visualizing cardiac movements; (3) confirm the gestational age (by measurement of the fetal biparietal diameter or femur length); (4) localize the placenta; (5) determine fetal position; (6) select the optimal pocket of amniotic fluid; (7) detect very obvious fetal malformations, or molar pregnancies; and (8) detect uterine or adnexal abnormalities.[3, 7] The umbilical cord and insertion site should be identified, if possible, and avoided.

The procedure is performed under strict aseptic conditions; the patient's lower abdomen is cleansed with an antiseptic (Betadine) and draped with sterile towels. A local anesthetic (1% lidocaine hydrochloride) is infiltrated into the skin at the preselected needle insertion site.[8] Amniocentesis performed concurrently with ultrasonographic monitoring enables visualization of the needle during the entire procedure. With this approach a sterile ultrasound scanning gel is applied adjacent to the insertion site. An ultrasound transducer is placed inside a sterile bag or glove containing gel, and held in position by an assistant such that the ultrasound beam is directed parallel to the planned needle track (Fig 5–1). A 20- or 22-gauge, 3½-in. spinal needle with stylet is then directed into the amniotic cavity under ultrasound guidance. The tactile perception of the needle passing through the various tissues is also important in confirming proper needle placement. After the stylet is removed, several milliliters of amniotic fluid are aspirated through a syringe. The first few milliliters are theoretically most likely to contain maternal cells (from vessels, the abdominal wall, or the uterine muscle); therefore, this sample is often not analyzed.

Twenty or 30 ml of amniotic fluid are next aspirated into sterile, disposable plastic syringes. If there is any question that urine rather than amniotic fluid has been inadvertently aspirated, the crystalline arborization test, which confirms that amniotic fluid has been withdrawn, should be done.[9]

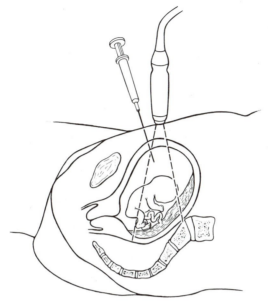

FIG 5–1.
Genetic amniocentesis under continuous ultrasound guidance.

The amniotic fluid specimen must be carefully labeled and transported at ambient temperatures to the laboratory.

Following amniocentesis, the fetal heart motions may be again documented by ultrasonographic visualization. The patient should be observed briefly following the procedure and should be instructed to report any fluid loss per vagina, bleeding per vagina, uterine cramping, or fever. Reasonably normal activities may be resumed following the procedure; however, strenuous exercise (e.g., jogging or aerobic exercises) and coitus should be avoided for a day.*

Multiple Pregnancies

Multiple gestation may be suspected if uterine size is larger than expected by the date of the last menstrual period, but the diagnosis is usually

---

*Rh-immune globulin should be administered to all unsensitized Rh-negative women following amniocentesis unless documentation can be provided that the father is also Rh-negative.[3] This is a prophylactic measure based on the possibility that disruption of the feto-placental circulation might have an immunizing effect.[10] However, the propriety of administering Rh-immune globulin is controversial, and the safety has been questioned by some investigators.[11, 12]

made at the time of ultrasonography. If multiple gestations are detected, the patient may still be offered prenatal diagnosis. However, amniocentesis of each sac is necessary to determine the status of each fetus.

If twins are detected, separate sacs may be distinguished by injecting a dye, such as indigo carmine, after aspiration of the first fluid sample (Fig 5–2). The second amniocentesis is performed in the ultrasonographically determined location of the other fetus. Visualization of the membrane separating the two sacs is generally possible. Aspiration of colorless fluid indicates that the second sac was entered, whereas aspiration of fluid colored with the dye indicates that the first sac was reentered. Triplets (and presumably gestations of greater multiplicity) can be managed by sequentially injecting dye into successive sacs, again following withdrawal of clear amniotic fluid. The number of aspirations of clear amniotic fluid should equal the number of fetuses. Using such a regime or a variation thereof, experienced investigators have successfully performed amniocentesis in more than 90% of twin pregnancies.[3, 13, 14]

Discordance for a fetal abnormality is a real possibility in multiple pregnancy, and should be discussed prior to amniocentesis. In such circumstances, three options exist: (1) continuing the pregnancy; (2) terminating the entire pregnancy; and (3) attempting selective feticide of the abnormal fetus. Selective feticide carries a number of potential risks: spontaneous abortion of the normal twin, premature labor, disseminated intravascular coagulopathy, infection, and psychological problems. Moreover, it may be difficult to select the correct fetus for termination should there be no structural abnormality that can be delineated by ultrasonography or fetoscopy.[15] Conceptually, selective feticide performed either by fetoscopic or ultrasonographic guidance is relatively straightforward. In practice, however, it may be quite difficult to accomplish, particularly if the woman is obese or the abnormal fetus is in an unfavorable position. Nonetheless, successes have been reported.[16–20]

The legal and ethical aspects of selective feticide have never been dealt with entirely satisfactorily. Even though the physician will rarely be confronted with this issue, we pause here to discuss it because it highlights why prenatal diagnosis is controversial and presents the limits of the usefulness of the woman's right to abortion in this case. The "easiest" case will be a prenatal diagnosis of a devastating disease, like Tay-Sachs, prior to fetal viability. Assuming the woman wishes to attempt to abort the fetus with Tay-Sachs and continue the unaffected fetus to term, does she and her physician have the legal right to attempt this procedure? The answer to this question hinges on two others: (1) is the procedure experimental?, and (2) does the mother have the right to consent to the selective abortion?[21]

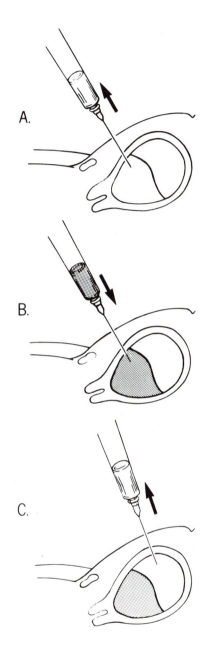

FIG 5–2.
Technique for amniocentesis in twin gestations, procedure performed under continuous ultrasound guidance. **A,** fluid aspirated from the first amniotic sac. **B,** indigo carmine dye injected into the first amniotic sac. **C,** second tap in the ultrasonographically determined location of the second fetus. Clear fluid confirms that the second amniotic sac was successfully aspirated. (From Elias S, Gerbie AB, and Simpson JL, et al: Genetic amniocentesis in twin gestations. *Am J Obstet Gynecol* 1980; 138:169. Used by permission.)

Since there are no accepted protocols for such a procedure, and since very little is known about its risks to the healthy fetus, the procedure is properly classified as experimental to both fetuses.[21, 22] This raises two problems: (1) as with any experimental procedure, it should be reviewed and approved by the hospital's institutional review board (IRB) to ensure that the risks are outweighed by the possible benefits, that proper prior research on the procedure has been done to make it a reasonable one to attempt, and that informed consent can be obtained;[22] and (2) fetal experimentation must be permissible under state law.† Assuming that these two hurdles can be cleared, the next question is the mother's consent. Can the mother agree to put her healthy fetus at risk by permitting the attempted selective destruction of its twin? The initial question is whether the woman would have the right to abort her fetus if it was a singleton. Assuming we are in a stage in the pregnancy prior to viability, the answer to this question is yes.‡ The conclusion that the woman has the right to have one (if a singleton) or both (if twins) fetuses aborted, however, does *not* necessarily mean she can risk the life and health of the one she plans to carry to term by attempting to abort the other. For example, in states like Massachusetts, where fetal experimentation is prohibited, a woman cannot consent to have experimental procedures performed on her fetus, whether or not it is the subject of a planned abortion. Likewise, we may have the legal right to have our pets destroyed humanely, but that does not mean we can be cruel to them or perform painful experiments on them.[23] The point is simply that the right to destroy a creature does not carry with it the right to do anything to it short of destruction.

How then do we decide if the mother can properly consent to attempted feticide that endangers the healthy fetus? If we treated the newborn the same as the fetus, the "easiest" answer from the perspective of the healthy fetus would be to permit both to go to term, and then kill the affected child. Although this "solution" has some ardent supporters, we believe the live-birth boundary is one that should not be tampered with and that handicapped newborns have a right to live that cannot be extinguished solely for the sake of others.*

Another way to approach the question is to suggest a hypothetical conversation between the in utero twins; let's call them Joe and Jane. Jane is the healthy fetus and Joe the one with Tay-Sachs. The conversation might go something like this:

---

†See state law discussion in Chapter 10.
‡See Chapter 6.
*See Chapter 7.

Jane: Mother has decided that she cannot handle having a child with Tay-Sachs, and that is why she sought prenatal diagnosis. She has now discovered that we are twins and has decided to abort both of us unless she is permitted to try to just abort you.

Joe: I don't have much sympathy for that position, unless my life is likely to be so horrible that I am actually better off never having been born.

Jane: I can understand that. But since you do have Tay-Sachs, you probably are better off left unborn. Moreover, since you will not be born in any case, it would be really nice if you agree to be aborted, because it will both save you from a horrible life and permit me the chance to live a healthy one.

Joe: I really don't have any good choices; but at least I'll know that someone with a genetic makeup very close to my own will be living if I agree to this. OK, I'll do it.

This conversation is, of course, entirely hypothetical, and it may even be misleading by imputing to the fetuses knowledge that they could never have. On the other hand, it is useful in viewing the matter from their perspectives. This helps determine what action might be in their respective "best interests." Obviously, the unaffected fetus will always have an interest in being born. The mother's interests in reproductive liberty to make her own decisions will, nonetheless, outweigh this interest *legally* prior to fetal viability. But, since no physician is obligated to perform an abortion, and since in the case of selective feticide the woman *wants* to give birth to the healthy fetus if possible, this situation is much more complex than the situation with a single, affected fetus.

Our hypothetical case actually makes it as easy of resolution as possible by assuming that the affected fetus would actually be "better off not being born" (essentially paralleling our previous discussion of "wrongful life"†), and also giving the affected fetus some "benefit" by having a portion of its genes live on in its twin. This benefit is, of course, one about which the twin will never actually know and could apply similarly to any future pregnancy of its parents. Therefore, we should not take it terribly seriously. Nonetheless, in a situation like this, in which the defect is extremely serious, and in which the mother is firm in her decision to abort both fetuses if she cannot attempt to have the affected fetus alone aborted, we can conclude that selective feticide can be a reasonable option.

It should be noted, however, that the reasonableness of it will vary with the likelihood of success. If there is a high probability that the healthy fetus will be injured, then the procedure is much less reasonable. This is because it could result in the birth of one (or two) severely injured fetus(es), a

†See discussion of wrongful life in Chapter 4.

situation actually worse than simply continuing the pregnancy. Likewise, if the condition that afflicts the affected fetus is relatively minor, like XXX, the justification for attempting selective feticide almost evaporates.

Looked at more abstractly yet, one could view Jane and Joe in conversation *before* prenatal diagnosis was performed, and thus before they knew which, if either, of them was affected with Tay-Sachs disease. In this case, if neither is affected (56% probability), they will both be born, and if both are affected (about 6% probability), they will both be aborted. Assume without selective abortion, if only one is affected, they will also both be aborted (38% probability). Might Jane and Joe agree *in advance*, that if only one of them was affected, the affected twin should be aborted to "save" the other one (assuming, again, that their mother would abort both before having one child affected with Tay-Sachs)? The answer is yes, at least if we assume that selective feticide carries minimal risks to the healthy fetus. The reason is that if Tay-Sachs is considered a life not worth living, then the only interest each fetus has is to maximize its chance to live a normal life. With no selective abortion option, its chances to live a normal life are only 56% (i.e., neither affected), since both fetuses will be aborted if either or both is affected. But with the option of selective abortion, the odds of a normal life for *each* fetus are raised to 75%, the same as they would be for a singleton pregnancy. Thus, *each fetus* maximizes its probability of living a normal life by agreeing in advance to be selectively aborted if it is affected and its twin is not. Again, we conclude that, at least under some circumstances, the availability of selective abortion is in the best interests of fetuses in that it can actually increase the probability of their being born at all.*

We conclude that selective abortion of previable fetuses is legal and ethical, at least in cases in which the procedure is medically reasonable, and the condition afflicting the affected fetus is so devastating as to lead to an objective conclusion that the fetus itself is better off not being born. Attempting selective feticide under other conditions is much more problematic. Although it is currently legal to attempt it prior to viability, *if* the procedure is medically reasonable and has been approved by an institutional

---

*If we did the same analysis after fetal viability, the state could prohibit abortion altogether, and if it did, selective abortion would not be an option. On the other hand, if there were an in utero treatment for the defect, the law would probably permit the woman to consent to the treatment, even if it put the healthy fetus at risk so long as "the potential benefit to the affected fetus outweighed the risk to the healthy one."[21] This is primarily because the law is likely to view this difficult and tragic choice-type decision as a personal, *family* one, and so will permit, in such extreme situations, families to take reasonable risks to save the life or health of other family members, at least so long as inherently unfair criteria are not used by the family to justify favoring the life or health of one child over another.[22] See Chapter 10 for a discussion of fetal experimentation.

review board, the real danger is that the healthy fetus could be severely injured and survive, or that both an injured healthy fetus and the affected fetus could survive.

Accordingly, we believe physicians should not offer the option of selective feticide unless at least two minimum conditions exist: (1) the physician concludes that this is a reasonable medical procedure, is personally comfortable performing it, and is willing to abort both fetuses if the attempt is unsuccessful; and (2) the pregnant woman is fully informed of the risks of the procedure to her healthy fetus and is willing to agree to abort both fetuses if the healthy fetus is injured in the attempt to kill the affected fetus. This scenario requires *both* the physician and the woman to seriously contemplate the real potential for disaster and to decide whether, given the fact that both fetuses may be destroyed (*either* by directly aborting them or by attempting selective feticide), it may not be a reasonable option to continue the pregnancy of both to term. It is suggested that continuing the multiple pregnancy will be preferable unless the fetal handicap is a devastating one, one that might lead a "reasonable fetus" to conclude that it would rather see itself aborted and its twin live, than see both of them aborted, or neither aborted.

Risks of Amniocentesis

The risks of amniocentesis may be divided into those affecting the mother and those affecting the fetus. Maternal risks are quite low. Intra-amniotic infection occurs in approximately 1 per 1,000 cases.[24] This usually leads to fetal loss, and only rarely causes a serious problem for the mother. An international workshop identified only one maternal death due to complications of amniocentesis from over 20,000 procedures.[25] Additional potentially serious complications include hemorrhage, injury to an intra-abdominal viscus, and blood group sensitization. Minor maternal complications (e.g., uterine cramping, transient vaginal spotting, minimal amniotic fluid leakage) occur more often, but still infrequently.[26]

Potential fetal risks include spontaneous abortion, injuries due to needle puncture, placental separation, intra-amniotic infection, premature labor, injury due to withdrawal of amniotic fluid (e.g., joint contractures), or injury due to defects in the amniotic membranes (e.g., amniotic bands). Rare but reported major needle injuries include ileocutaneous fistula, gangrene of an arm, corneal perforation and blindness, ileal atresia, porencephalic cysts, patellar disruption, peripheral nerve injury, and umbilical cord hematoma.[27–32] Some of these problems are more logically attributed to amniocentesis than others. Four major collaborative studies have attempted to assess the risks of amniocentesis.‡ When the study designs are taken into account, differences among these studies are minimized, justifying the following conclusions: (1) the increased risk of fetal loss following amniocentesis is in the range of 0.5%; (2) the maternal risk appears to be minimal; (3) the risk of major fetal injury is minute; and (4) the fetal risk of a small needle mark is low. Finally, these collaborative studies establish amniocentesis as a medical diagnostic procedure, with an overall accuracy rate of 99.5% or greater.

CHORIONIC VILLUS SAMPLING

Amniocentesis cannot be safely performed prior to about 15 weeks' gestation. Thus, fetal diagnosis of chromosomal, biochemical, or DNA abnormalities can rarely be established prior to 18 weeks' gestation. Couples awaiting results frequently undergo considerable psychological stress. More-over, if a genetic disorder is detected and the couple elects to terminate the pregnancy, an abortion must be performed in the late second trimester.

‡The first major prospective study was coordinated by the National Institute of Child Health and Human Development and comprised 1,040 subjects and 992 controls (the NICHHD Amniocentesis Registry).[26] The incidence of immediate complications (e.g., leaking of amniotic fluid, bleeding) was 2.4%; 3.5% of women who underwent amniocentesis experienced fetal loss subsequent to the procedure, whereas an almost identical percentage (3.2%) of pregnant controls experienced fetal loss. A fetal loss during a previous pregnancy did not increase the risk for another fetal loss in the amniocentesis group. Neither the volume of amniotic fluid removed nor the number of amniocentesis procedures performed before obtaining fluid (i.e., on different days) correlated with frequency of fetal loss. Newborn evaluations of case and control infants showed similar mean birth weights, incidence of prematurity, and 5-minute Apgar scores. One newborn in the amniocentesis group had a single mark on the back which could have been caused by the amniocentesis needle. No other injuries were found in the US collaborative study, nor were there differences in the number of physical anomalies in the amniocentesis group as compared with that of the controls. Repeated examinations at 1 year of age showed no difference in infant growth, neurologic findings, or developmental status between the two groups.
A prospective Canadian collaborative study[33] showed a similar frequency of pregnancy loss among women undergoing midtrimester amniocentesis (3.2%); matched controls were not studied. The incidence of immediate amniocentesis complications exclusive of spontaneous abortion (e.g., bleeding, cramps, fluid leakage) was 3.6%. Most of these pregnancies did not terminate in spontaneous abortion. Newborns were not evaluated for injuries caused by the amniocentesis needle.
In contrast to the US and Canadian studies, a British collaborative study[34] showed a significantly higher fetal loss rate among the study group (2.6%) than among controls (1.1%), and an unexplained increase in infants with respiratory distress syndrome. Some control bias may be suspected in this study, because the controls were significantly older and of greater parity than the study subjects.
Most recently, a randomized controlled trial of genetic amniocentesis in 4,606 low-risk women (aged 25–34 years) conducted in Denmark showed a 1.7% spontaneous abortion rate following amniocentesis compared to a 0.7% spontaneous abortion rate in the control group (relative risk 2.3).[35] The amniocenteses were performed under real-time ultrasound.

These circumstances impose greater maternal risk, expense, and psychological stress compared with an outpatient first-trimester abortion. Accordingly, accurate first-trimester diagnosis would be of significant benefit to couples.

Although still an investigative procedure, the new obstetric technique of chorionic villus sampling (CVS) permits the diagnosis of genetic disease in the fetus at 9 to 11 weeks' gestation. Tissue aspirated via a catheter transcervically placed into the developing placenta is suitable for various genetic studies. This is possible because shortly after fertilization, the zygote differentiates first into the blastocyst, which contains an inner cell mass that develops into the fetus, and an outer trophoblast layer, which develops into nonfetal structures such as the amnion, chorion, and placenta. The genetic complement of the trophoblast reflects the inner cell mass (i.e., fetal cells) because they both are derived from the same zygote. It follows, therefore, that chromosomal, DNA, and biochemical analysis on trophoblast cells should yield comparable information to that obtained by amniocentesis. The only major difference is that assays requiring amniotic fluid liquor, namely α-fetoprotein, cannot be performed using CVS. First-trimester sampling of fetal tissues was initially attempted in 1973 in Sweden.*

In 1975, Chinese researchers transcervically aspirated chorionic villi for X-chromatin studies.[37] Even though ultrasound was not employed, only 4 of 100 subjects aborted following the procedure. Thirty patients terminated their pregnancies after the sex became known, but the remaining 66 pregnancies continued uneventfully. Fetal sex was accurately predicted in 94% of these 66 cases. Other first-trimester techniques were subsequently attempted, but CVS became practical only after the advent of improved ultrasonographic techniques.† The first large sample was studied in Milan.[39]

The National Institutes of Health are currently funding seven US centers to investigate the safety and accuracy of CVS: Yale University; Mount Sinai Medical School; Jefferson Medical College; Michael Reese Medical Center; The University of Tennessee, Memphis;‡ Baylor University; and the University of California, San Francisco. Results will be available in several years. Other collaborative studies have been initiated in Canada and Europe.

---

*The study involved 39 Swedish women undergoing pregnancy termination. Subjects between 8 and 20 weeks' gestation underwent transcervical chorionic biopsy utilizing a 5-mm endoscope.[36] Chromosomal studies were completed in 20 cases, all of which were consistent with sex of the abortus. In 19 cases, pregnancy termination was delayed between 7 and 43 days; the only complications observed were two infections. Further attempts were abandoned with the demonstration that amniocentesis was relatively safe and highly reliable.

†In 1982, British researchers described 63 patients in whom chorionic villus sampling was performed by transcervical aspiration ultrasonographically directed.[38]

‡This center was transferred from Northwestern University, Chicago, in July 1986.

The ethical rationale for a randomized clinical trial was developed by the medical ethicist John Fletcher.[40] He noted that the primary objection to the study was one based on the notion that abortion was wrong because (1) it violates the primary purpose of medicine, to save life; and (2) it unfairly and unequally discriminates against certain fetuses. Fletcher concedes that selective abortion violates the equality principle by discriminating against affected fetuses, and thus seems to make our moral judgments inconsistent and to decrease our compassion for handicapped individuals. He nonetheless finds the arguments favoring the study more persuasive. The arguments supporting the CVS studies are that not to do them would increase the suffering of parents and families; allow great harm in the case of some potential children; encourage passivity and resignation toward inherited diseases; and potentially obstruct the development of meaningful fetal therapy. In addition, he argues persuasively that a strict application of the equality principle "unnecessarily restricts the diversity of ethical principles required to resolve many types of moral conflict in abortion cases and research with human fetuses."[40, 41]

Another major objection was that a randomized clinical trial would itself encourage abortions. Fletcher doubted this and noted that in any event no woman would be required to choose abortion as a prerequisite to entering the study. In addition, subjects would be given the clear choice to refuse to enter the study, and yet retain the right to select the prenatal diagnostic method of their choice. Subjects may also withdraw from the study at any time without penalty.

On balance Fletcher concluded (as did the institutional review boards at the seven major US institutions involved in NIH's nonrandomized study) that even though it was nontherapeutic for the fetus, it was justified because of the potential benefits it could bring to other fetuses "in the very near and distant future." This may seem a slender reed on which to brace this study, but we believe, although difficult to articulate, the justification is genuine:

> *The long term consequences of a trial may help to reduce over-reliance on abortion in prenatal diagnosis.* Perhaps fetal therapy will eventually be enhanced by safer, accurate, and earlier fetal diagnosis. Fetal therapy is now impossible for the chromosomal disorders to be found in the most likely trial. However, long range consideration of fetal interests should not dismiss the role of this trial in many steps toward such therapy. Fetal therapy is slowly growing as an integral specialty in medicine. Anyone who wants to reduce the incidence of abortion for genetic disorders in the future would surely favor fetal therapy. But *the risks of learning must precede the benefits of treatment* [emphasis added].[40]

Finally, it was noted that federal regulations limit such fetal research to that involving only "minimal risk," and based on the studies outlined in this chapter, it was concluded that "the most probable risks in a trial will be less than the current risks of amniocentesis, when one considers the background risks of spontaneous abortion in each period of pregnancy."[40]

The optimal time for performing CVS is between 9 and 11 weeks from the onset of the last menses.[42] Gestational age is confirmed by ultrasonographic measurement of crown-rump length. Although CVS has been performed in multiple gestations, some investigators believe restriction to singleton pregnancies is warranted because of the uncertainty of successfully monitoring each fetus. Patients should be excluded if they show signs of threatened abortion (cramping and/or bleeding per vagina); active cervical, vaginal, or vulvar infection; or undiagnosed cervical lesions. Most centers screen for *Neisseria gonorrhoeae* by cervical culture.

The CVS may be temporarily delayed if a uterine contraction is ultrasonographically visualized prior to sampling. Although a contraction may occasionally facilitate the procedure, it more frequently prevents proper catheter placement. A respite of about 30 minutes is usually sufficient to allow the contraction to end.

Chorionic villus sampling can be performed in an ambulatory surgery unit that provides facilities required to handle any immediate obstetric complication that may result and offers a sterile environment to minimize the risk of infection. Initially, a bimanual pelvic examination is performed to ascertain uterine position. After a speculum is inserted, the vagina and cervix are then cleaned with an antiseptic solution and blot-dried with gauze. The anterior lip of the cervix is grasped with a single-toothed tenaculum, and the CVS catheter is transcervically introduced and directed toward the site of the developing placenta under continuous ultrasonographic (sector) guidance. If additional attempts are required to obtain an adequate specimen, a fresh catheter is used each time.

When the catheter tip is appropriately directed to the placental site (Fig 5–3), the stylet is removed and a 30-cc syringe containing culture media is attached to the end of the catheter. Five to 10 cc of intermittent negative pressure is applied as the catheter is slowly withdrawn. The aspirated specimen is transferred to a Petri dish and inspected through a dissecting microscope ($\times 50$). The quantity of tissue is judged adequate if at least 5 mg of villi is obtained. The optimal sample weighs between 20 and 40 mg. The quantity of tissue can be estimated by comparison to reference photographs. The best quality specimens show distinct arborization of villi capillaries and multiple buds. Edematous or degenerating villi are generally unsatisfactory for analysis. The tissue specimen is immediately transported to the laboratory for processing.

Upon completion of CVS, the cervix is observed for bleeding either from the cervical canal or from the site of tenaculum placement—the most common source. Rh-negative unsensitized patients are given 300 μg of Rh

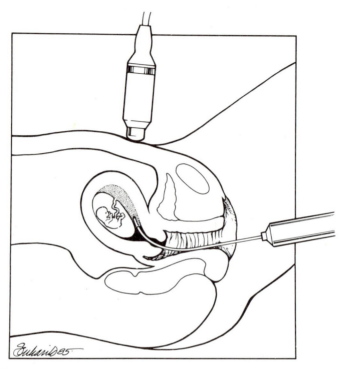

FIG 5–3.
Chorionic villus sampling procedure. (From Elias S, Simpson JL: Chorionic villus sampling, in Sabbagha RE (ed): *Diagnostic Ultrasound Applied to Obstetrics and Gynecology,* ed 2. Philadelphia, JB Lippincott Co, 1986 (in press).

immunoglobulin following the procedure. The patient is observed over 30 to 60 minutes for any untoward effects. At 16 to 18 weeks' gestation, maternal serum α-fetoprotein is determined.

An alternative approach to transcervical CVS that is gaining in popularity, is transabdominal CVS. This procedure involves aspiration of villi through a needle that is ultrasonographically guided into the placenta. The main advantage of transabdominal CVS is that it avoids the potentially infected endocervical canal and should thereby reduce the risks of maternal and fetal complications as compared to the transcervical approach.[43]

For cytogenetic analysis CVS specimens may be processed in one of two ways: (1) the so-called "direct method," whereby chromosome preparations are obtained from spontaneous mitoses freed from the cytotrophoblast, and that permits cytogenetic analysis within 24 hours; or (2) culturing villi, which provides a greater number of metaphases and permits cytogenetic analysis in five to seven days.[44] For biochemical studies and DNA analysis, extracts of chorionic villi may be prepared by the same methods used to prepare fibroblasts or cultured amniotic fluid cells.

The diagnostic accuracy of CVS has not yet been fully established. Aspirated cells could be of maternal origin, clearly an issue if the CVS complement is 46,XX. Furthermore, trophoblastic cells may not necessarily reflect fetal status. Indeed, in vitro aberrations occur in amniotic fluid cells and could even be more frequent using chorionic villus techniques.[44] Substantially more data must become available before assuming that the procedure has the same diagnostic accuracy as amniotic fluid cell culture.

Despite worldwide experience with more than 20,000 procedures, precise data with respect to safety are not yet available.[44, 45] Most large studies cite an *uncorrected* spontaneous abortion rate following CVS in the range of 2.0% to 4.5%.* However, such absolute rates must be corrected for a host of confounding variables: (1) accuracies in the identification and timing of spontaneous fetal loss rates; (2) maternal history of prior induced abortions; (3) parental cytogenetic factors (recurrent aneuploidy, translocations, inversions); (4) maternal age; (5) gravidity; (6) smoking; (7) alcohol consumption; and (8) environmental factors (e.g., exposure to infectious agents, drugs, nutrition, chemical toxins).[46]

Given the unknown complication rates and unknown diagnostic accuracy, a cautious approach is to assume that at the present time chorionic villus biopsy represents an experimental technique. Although many workers are quite enthusiastic about it, CVS does not represent a clear option to amniocentesis, an accepted procedure whose diagnostic accuracy and complication rate have been known for a decade. Chorionic villus sampling should be performed under an experimental protocol, approved and monitored by an institutional review board. This, together with careful attention to informed consent, will protect patient, geneticist, and obstetrician. Patients must understand that neither the complication rate nor diagnostic accuracy is yet known. Because for many patients the procedure is likely to prove an extremely attractive alternative to amniocentesis, added efforts must be used to emphasize both its experimental nature and its possible risks and complications.

---

*In this context the initial experience of SE and colleagues with CVS at Northwestern University was encouraging.[46] Among the first 109 women who underwent CVS, a specimen adequate for analysis was obtained in 94.5%. Only one fetal loss occurred among these cases. An ultrasound scan was normal two weeks after CVS; however, fetal demise became evident three weeks later. In four (3.7%) cases the pregnancies were terminated because of abnormal results, and in one (0.9%) case the pregnancy was electively terminated after normal results. There were two premature deliveries; one of these two infants died shortly after birth following premature rupture of the membranes at 29 weeks' gestation.

FETOSCOPY

The techniques most commonly used to obtain information about fetal status for prenatal diagnosis involve analysis of amniotic fluid (cells or liquor) or chorionic villi. Many genetic disorders, however, are not amenable to diagnosis using these methods. In such cases fetoscopy may prove useful. Fetoscopy is the introduction of an endoscope transabdominally into the amniotic sac, allowing direct visualization of the fetus and sampling of fetal tissues, including blood and skin, for the prenatal diagnosis of certain genetic disorders.[47, 48]

Technique

Fetoscopy is best performed between the 17th and 20th weeks of gestation based on the onset of the last menses. A preliminary ultrasonographic examination is required to (1) confirm fetal viability; (2) diagnose multiple gestation; (3) confirm gestational age by measurement of the fetal head, biparietal diameter, and femur length; (4) localize the placenta, especially the umbilical cord insertion site; and (5) determine the fetal lie. High resolution real-time ultrasonography should be employed concurrently with the procedure. The fetoscope produces a distinctive echo separate from the fetus, umbilical cord, placenta, and uterine wall. This greatly facilitates the procedure, especially tissue sampling.

Fetoscopy must be performed under strict aseptic conditions, preferably in an ambulatory surgical suite with standby anesthesia. After the entry site is selected based upon the ultrasound examination, the abdomen is prepared with a povidone-iodine solution and alcohol, and appropriately draped. The patient may be sedated with 10 mg of intravenous diazepam. This is particularly useful for fetal skin sampling, because diazepam crosses the placenta into the fetal circulation and causes a reduction of fetal activity. The skin is infiltrated with 1% lidocaine hydrochloride for local anesthesia, and a 5-mm stab incision is made with a scalpel blade. The trochar, housed in the cannula, is percutaneously inserted into the amniotic cavity. The trochar is withdrawn, and insertion in the amniotic cavity is verified by the return of amniotic fluid. A syringe may be attached to the cannula to withdraw amniotic fluid for additional studies (e.g., chromosomal analysis, α-fetoprotein analysis). The fetoscope (2 to 4 sq cm) orientation may be difficult, and ultrasound is therefore used to help direct the scope.

For fetal skin sampling, the cannula is placed against a stationary part of the fetus (e.g., thorax, back, buttocks, scalp) which can be preselected to provide optimum information depending on the disorder in question. The fetoscope is removed from the cannula, the biopsy forceps inserted, and a specimen taken. Multiple specimens can be obtained in a very brief period of time, and, if desired, more than one anatomical site can be sampled.

If fetal blood sampling is desired and the placenta is posterior, a blood vessel on the chorionic plate of the placenta can usually be visualized. Recently, fetoscopists have more frequently elected to obtain blood samples directly from the umbilical vein at the insertion of the cord into the placenta. This has resulted in improved success in obtaining pure fetal blood uncontaminated with maternal blood or amniotic fluid. Either a 25- or 27-gauge flexible needle is directed through the trochar channel, which is parallel and contiguous with the fetoscope. Under direct visualization, the aspirating needle is advanced into the chosen vessel and 50 μl to 1 ml of blood is withdrawn into a heparinized syringe containing an anticoagulant.

Fetoscopy has been successfully performed in twin gestations.[20] Depending upon the indication, fetal positions, and placental sites, fetoscopy can be performed using either two uterine insertions or only one uterine insertion, with the second fetus studied by passage of the fetoscope through the septum dividing the sacs.

Indications

The indications for fetoscopy have been limited. Until recently, fetoscopy was most commonly employed for fetal blood sampling for the prenatal diagnosis of hemoglobinopathies, e.g., sickle cell disease, α-thalassemia, and β-thalassemia.* Such diagnosis is feasible because reticulocytes of affected fetuses manifest effects of the mutant genes early in gestation, and heterozygotes can be accurately distinguished from homozygotes. However, recent developments in molecular genetics now permit the diagnosis of sickle cell anemia and many other hemoglobinopathies, using amniotic fluid fibroblasts or chorionic villi rather than fetal blood.[51] These techniques allow diagnosis not on the basis of gene products (for example, hemoglobin), but on the basis of the DNA that codes for the gene in question.† Many other disorders that have depended upon fetal blood sampling for prenatal diagnosis are also now amenable to DNA analysis, at least in some families. Such disorders include hemophilia A (factor VIII deficiency), hemophilia B (factor IX deficiency), and Duchenne muscular dystrophy. Nonetheless,

---

*Recently many centers have abandoned fetoscopy altogether for fetal blood sampling. Fetal blood samples have been obtained from the umbilical vein at the placenta insertion site with use of a fine needle guided by ultrasound. The fetal loss rate using this technique has been in the range of 1%, which is appreciably safer than fetoscopic blood sampling (see above).[49] Similar methods have been applied in intrauterine exchange transfusions for severe erythroblastosis fetalis.[50]

†DNA techniques are discussed in detail in Chapter 4.

there are still conditions in which fetal blood sampling is required for prenatal diagnosis. These include chronic granulomatous disease, hereditary congenital neutropenia, severe combined immunodeficiency disease, and determination of IgM levels in cases of suspected fetal infections (e.g., rubella).

Fetoscopy was originally conceived of as a technique to directly visualize the fetus for the diagnosis of various morphologic abnormalities. However, with improved technology in ultrasonography many such physical defects can be visualized through this noninvasive method. Nonetheless, fetoscopy may be a useful adjunctive procedure when ultrasonographic findings are equivocal. An example of a disorder that would not be detectable by current ultrasound capabilities, yet would be possibly detectable by direct fetal visualization through fetoscopy, is the Smith-Lemli-Opitz syndrome. This autosomal recessive syndrome is characterized by failure to thrive, mental retardation, microcephaly, low-set ears, ptosis, broad nose with upturned nares, micrognathia, high arched palate, broad alveolar ridge, clubbed feet, and cryptorchidism with or without hypospadias. A distinctive marker for this syndrome is syndactyly between the second and third toes, which should be detectable via fetoscopic visualization.

Recently, significant advances have been made in the prenatal diagnosis of hereditary skin disorders (genodermatoses). Fetoscopy and fetal skin sampling have been successfully utilized for the prenatal diagnosis of a number of genodermatoses including harlequin ichthyosis, epidermolysis bullosa letalis, and epidermolytic hyperkeratosis.[52–54] The list of genodermatoses detectable by such methods will undoubtedly increase.

Finally, pure fetal blood samples can be obtained for rapid chromosomal analysis in pregnancies complicated by ultrasonographically demonstrable fetal anomalies. Cytogenetic analysis of fetal lymphocytes can be obtained in two to four days.‡

Although fetoscopy carries a greater risk of fetal mortality than amniocentesis, it has the advantage of providing accurate results rapidly, thereby alleviating parental anxiety associated with a long delay, and allowing the option of pregnancy termination should any major abnormality be found in cases of advanced gestational age, usually greater than 20 weeks. Rapid chromosomal analysis could also be appropriate in the third trimester of pregnancy, because knowledge that the fetus is cytogenetically normal

‡In a 1986 series of 118 pregnancies studied for such indications, Nicolaides and colleagues[55] found chromosomal abnormalities in 12 of 37 fetuses with nonhemolytic hydrops fetalis, 8 of 12 with exomphalos, 1 of 3 with duodenal atresia, 9 of 39 with obstructive uropathy, 1 of 3 with unilateral pleural effusion, 2 of 10 with severe growth retardation and oligohydramnios, 2 of 9 with isolated hydrocephalus, and 3 of 4 with choroid plexus cysts (of the last 4, 1 also had obstructive uropathy and 1 exomphalos). Three fetuses with gastroschisis were cytogenetically normal.

would allow parents and the health care team to discuss alternatives and choose the appropriate time, mode, and place of delivery, and to prepare for optimum postnatal care. Alternatively, if the fetus is chromosomally abnormal, the parents and the health care team may decide that obstetric intervention, such as delivery by cesarean section for fetal distress, should be avoided. Whether amniocentesis or fetoscopy would be the preferred diagnostic test in late pregnancy would depend upon the gestational age and a careful weighing of the risks and benefits of each procedure.

Safety

Application of fetoscopy requires a balance between potential diagnostic benefits and potential fetal and maternal risks. Risks of fetoscopy include (1) spontaneous abortion; (2) leakage of amniotic fluid per vagina; (3) infection; (4) prematurity; (5) hemorrhage from injury to a blood vessel either in the anterior abdominal wall or the uterus; (6) maternal bowel or bladder injury; (7) fetal injuries; and (8) placental injuries.

Data from the 1982 International Fetoscopy Group, which tabulated the experiences of 24 fetoscopy programs, allow some evaluation of the safety of the procedure.[56] The spontaneous abortion rate was calculated as the total number of fetal losses (intrauterine demises and abortions) before 28 weeks' gestation divided by the number of completed pregnancies, and was 6.8% (128/1,875) for fetoscopy for fetal blood sampling, 7.9% (16/203) for visualization, and 16% (4/25) for fetal skin sampling.*

*The relatively high spontaneous abortion rate in the skin sampling group was probably reflective of the small sample size. The risk of the fetoscopy procedure per se is best assessed by looking at the total experience. It should be pointed out that baseline spontaneous abortion rate from 13 to 28 weeks' gestation for women not undergoing any prenatal diagnosis has been estimated at 1.1% to 2.3%.[57] The perinatal loss rate was calculated as the number of perinatal losses divided by the number of completed pregnancies continuing past 28 weeks' gestation and was 1.4% (24/1,747) for fetoscopy for fetal blood sampling; 11.2% (21/187) for visualization; and 4.8% (1/21) for fetal skin sampling. Although the findings have not been tabulated and controlled, there is a question of an increase in preterm delivery associated with fetoscopy in the range of 10%.[58]

At the Seventh International Meeting, "Prenatal Diagnosis and Fetal Treatment," held in Giessen, Germany (Sept 11–12, 1985), the experience with fetal skin sampling in a total of 132 patients ascertained from 13 fetoscopy programs was tabulated: 25 therapeutic abortions (i.e., abnormal results); 3 fetal losses within 20 days of the procedure; 1 loss between day 21 and the 28th week of gestation; 2 losses after 28 weeks' gestation; and 60 infants had been delivered and survived at least 7 days. Because of the relatively small number of patients who have undergone fetal skin sampling, additional data will have to be collected before any definitive statements can be made regarding the frequency of procedure-related fetal losses and neonatal mortality.

With respect to fetal skin sampling, there is also the concern that cosmetically or functionally significant injuries could occur. Because the experience with biopsy examination of fetuses that have been allowed to go to term is limited, the magnitude of such risks is unknown. What experience there is would suggest that such injuries will probably be uncommon.[59, 60]

As with most specialized procedures, all investigators have reported a decrease in the complication rate and an increase in the success rate with experience. However, it is unlikely that the procedure-related abortion rate will ever be substantially lower than 3% to 5%. In order to minimize the complication rate, it has been recommended that individuals desiring to attain proficiency in fetoscopy perform the procedure in volunteers undergoing elective midtrimester abortions, although this is illegal in states like Massachusetts, which prohibits experimentation on fetuses that are the subject of a planned abortion.[22, 61] The exact number of such cases that would be necessary before performing fetoscopy in continuing pregnancies will vary with the general experience the investigator has performing in utero procedures.

ULTRASONOGRAPHY

Over the past decade advances in ultrasonic instrumentation, particularly the advent of high-resolution real-time scanners, have made possible a high degree of diagnostic accuracy in the evaluation of both normal and pathologic fetal anatomy.[62] Ultrasound is not, however, used in all pregnant women as a screening tool for the detection of birth defects.† Detailed ultrasonic targeted imaging for fetal anomalies, or level II ultrasound, is primarily intended for pregnant women at high risk for birth defects, because of the following reasons: (1) the cost-benefit ratio of routine use is not established; (2) prolonged exposure to ultrasound required for targeted imaging examinations is deemed unnecessary in the face of a low yield of anomalies in normal pregnancy; and (3) the accuracy of targeted ultrasonic imaging is not fully established.[63]

Because of the rapid development of new biomedical technologies, clinical decisions are sometimes based on data derived from a new modality prior to full appreciation of its limitations. Such is the case with ultrasonography. Numerous reports have appeared in the medical literature describing the prenatal diagnosis of various structural malformations, and the list will undoubtedly continue to grow (Table 5–1). An example of a condition in which ultrasound is commonly used for prenatal diagnosis is open spina bifida (Fig 5–4). However, the predictive value, sensitivity, and specificity of ultrasonography for the prenatal diagnosis of structural abnormalities have only recently begun to be evaluated in a meaningful scientific fashion.[63, 64] In the best of tertiary centers, predictive values of abnormal and normal ultrasound targeted imaging examinations have been in the range of

†See discussion in Chapter 3.

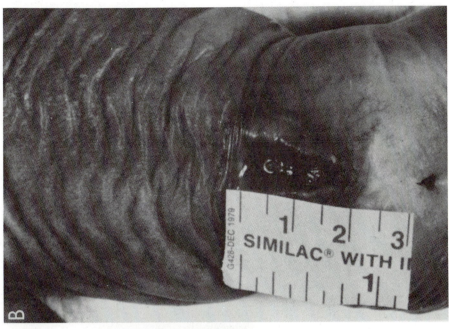

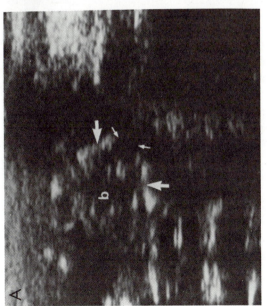

FIG 5-4.

A, scan showing cross section of fetal trunk in sacral area. The iliac wings are shown *(large arrows)* and the open spina bifida *(small arrows)*. Neural tissue *(two white echoes)* is seen in the center of the defect. The bladder *(b)* is anterior. B, spina bifida lesions in aborted fetus. (From Sabbagha RE, Sheikh Z, Dalcampo S, et al: Predictive value, sensitivity, and specificity of ultrasound targeted imaging for fetal anomalies in gravid women at high risk for birth defects. *Am J Obstet Gynecol* 1985; 152:822–827. Used by permission.)

TABLE 5–1.
Selected Fetal Malformations Potentially
Prenatally Detectable by Ultrasonography*

Central nervous system
  Anencephaly
  Hydrocephalus
  Microcephaly
Genitourinary system
  Polycystic kidney
  Multicystic kidney
  Renal agenesis
  Ureteropelvic junction obstruction
  Ureterovesical obstruction
  Urethral obstruction
Gastrointestinal system
  Duodenal atresia
  Gastrointestinal obstruction below duodenum
  Omphalocele
  Gastroschisis
  Diaphragmatic hernia
  Hirschsprung disease
Skeletal system
  Limb reduction defect
  Split hand syndrome
  Arthrogryposis
Cardiac system
  Ventricular septal defect
  Hypoplastic left ventricle
  Tetralogy of Fallot
  Transposition of great vessels
  Arrhythmias
Other
  Cystic hygroma
  Conjoined twins
  Hydrops fetalis
  Asphyxiating thoracic dystrophy

---

*Modified from Sabbagha RE, Shiekh Z, Tamura RK, et al: Predictive value, sensitivity, and specificity of ultrasonic targeted imaging for fetal anomalies in gravid women at high risk for birth defects. *Am J Obstet Gynecol* 1985; 152:822.

95% and 99%, respectively. In general the accuracy will depend upon: (1) expertise of the examiner; (2) prevalence of the anomaly in specific geographic locations; (3) whether the population undergoing examination was screened by history, biochemical tests, basic ultrasound scans, or for other pregnancy complications; and (4) period of follow-up, since subtle, nonlethal anomalies may be undetected at birth.[63]

Chapter 6 _____

Reproductive Liberty

The most significant recent development in constitutional law has been explicating the individual's right to decide whether or not to bear or beget a child.[1] Over the past two decades, the US Supreme Court has enunciated this right as part of a citizen's "right to privacy," and defined it to include not only decisions about contraception, but also decisions regarding termination of a pregnancy and involuntary sterilization. This same privacy right to make important personal decisions free from governmental interference (sometimes called "the right to be left alone"), has been used by many courts in other areas of medical care, such as the right to refuse treatment. In this chapter we review the major legal milestones in defining the individual's right to reproductive liberty, a right that permits individuals and their physicians to make use of the medical procedures discussed in this book.

CONTRACEPTION

An individual's right to use contraceptive drugs and devices is protected by the US Constitution. Two major cases enunciated this right. The first, and most important, *Griswold v. Connecticut*,[2] involved a challenge to the Connecticut law against contraception by the Planned Parenthood League of Connecticut. The Connecticut law provided that:

> Any person who uses any drug, medicinal article or instrument for the purpose of preventing conception shall be fined not less than fifty dollars or im-

prisoned not less than sixty days nor more than one year or be both fined and imprisoned.[2]

We might smile at this quaint law from 1879, but it was still in effect in 1961 when members of Planned Parenthood were arrested, tried, and convicted of aiding and abetting this crime.* They were fined $100 each, and appealed. The Supreme Court reversed the criminal convictions and found the statute itself unconstitutional. In so doing, the Court enunciated a constitutional right to privacy, suggested by "penumbras" that emanate from the specific guarantees in the Bill of Rights. Defining a particular "zone of privacy," the Court focused on sexual relations in marriage:

> We deal with a right of privacy older than the Bill of Rights—older than our political parties, older than our school system. Marriage is the coming together for better or for worse, hopefully enduring, and intimate to the degree of being sacred. It is an association that promotes a way of life, not causes; a harmony in living, not political faiths; a bilateral loyalty, not commercial or social projects. Yet it is an association for as noble a purpose as any involved in prior decisions.[2]

And to nail down the argument, Justice William Douglas, who wrote the opinion of the divided Court, made it clear that the statute could not be enforced without massive and unthinkable governmental intrusion into people's lives and homes: "Would we allow the police to search the sacred precincts of marital bedrooms for tell-tale signs of the use of contraceptives? The very idea is repulsive to the notions of privacy surrounding the marriage relationship."[2] No governmental interest was suggested or found that could permit such an intrusion.

Strictly speaking, this case applied only to married couples. Might unmarried individuals be protected as well? This question was presented to the Court in 1972 in the case of *Eisenstadt v. Baird*.[1] It resulted from a speech that William Baird gave at Boston University in 1967, during which he exhibited and distributed various contraceptive devices to his college audience. He was arrested and jailed under a Massachusetts statute that made it a felony to sell, lend, give away, or exhibit "any drug, medicine, instrument, or article whatever for the prevention of conception . . ." After the *Griswold* decision, the statute had been amended to provide an exception for

---

*Twenty-six states passed laws relating to birth control after a federal law that prohibited the mailing, importation, or furnishing of contraceptives was enacted in 1873. Eight states, including Connecticut and Massachusetts, attempted complete suppression. In the 1930s, the Connecticut legislature refused to amend the statute to exempt prescriptions by physicians to married women whose health would be endangered, and the Connecticut Supreme Court upheld its constitutionality in 1940, on the grounds that the state's police power "may be exerted to preserve and protect the public morals." (*State v. Nelson*, 126 Conn. 412, 425 [1940]).

contraceptives provided to married couples by prescription. When the statute came before the Supreme Court in 1972, Justice William Brennan, writing for the Court, struck it down under the equal protection clause of the Constitution.

The question, as the Court defined it, was whether the state had a reasonable basis for treating unmarried citizens differently than married ones in the area of contraception. The Court reviewed all of the reasons for unequal treatment set forth by the Commonwealth of Massachusetts and found them woefully inadequate. For example, the Commonwealth had argued that it had the right to discourage premarital sex and fornication. But, the Court noted, fornication was a Massachusetts crime punishable by only a $30 fine or 90 days in jail, while the anticontraceptive statute was a felony punishable by up to 2½ years in prison. Its real purpose, the court found, was to prohibit contraception itself, and to punish premarital sex by pregnancy. The Court concluded that individual sexual relationships, not marital relationships, were the critical issue in deciding about the right to privacy in human reproduction:

> If under *Griswold* the distribution of contraceptives to married persons cannot be prohibited, a ban on distribution to unmarried persons would be equally impermissible. It is true that in *Griswold* the right of privacy in question inhered in the marital relationship. Yet the marital couple is not an independent entity with a mind and heart of its own, but an association of two individuals each with a separate intellectual and emotional makeup. If the right to privacy means anything, it is the right of the *individual,* married or single, to be free from unwarranted governmental intrusion into matters so fundamentally affecting a person as the decision whether to bear or beget a child.[1]

This was an extremely important decision. Obviously, the Court's restatement of the right to privacy as broad enough to encompass the individual's decision whether "to bear or beget a child" went much further than the Court had to go to decide a case that dealt only with "begetting" a child. This can be explained by the fact that at the same time the Court was deciding this case, the Justices were attempting to fashion an opinion in the most significant reproductive rights case in history: *Roe v. Wade.*[3, 4]

ABORTION

There is no more contentious issue in medical ethics, politics, or health law than abortion.[5] Prenatal genetic screening and counseling today presuppose and depend upon the existence of high-quality, safe, legal abortions, including late second trimester abortions. Without this availability and legality, most prenatal screening would be irrelevant since there are no known cures or treatments for the vast majority of conditions that can be diagnosed in utero. The coming of age of fetal surgery and other interventions will hopefully change this in the future,* and ultimately we must continue to work for the day when the conditions discovered by diagnostic methods can be treated in ways other than by destroying the affected fetus.

As controversial as elective abortion is, the use of abortion when a woman is carrying a fetus with a severe genetic defect is very well accepted by a vast majority of both the public and physicians. For example, in a 1981 public opinion poll, 87% approved abortion for this indication (compared with 88% approval for pregnancies resulting from rape, and 86% for pregnancies resulting from incest).[6] Similarly, a 1985 survey of 1,300 members of the American College of Obstetricians and Gynecologists found that more than 90% believed fetal abnormalities a legitimate reason for a first trimester abortion. Beyond the first trimester, 84% found fetal abnormalities an acceptable reason, and this was *followed* by the woman's physical health (75%), rape or incest (68%), the woman's mental health (56%), economic difficulties (36%), and personal choice (36%). Although these surveys show exceptionally strong support for a woman's choice for abortion of genetically abnormal fetuses, there is much less support for purely "elective" abortions for any reason the pregnant woman might have. Only about 25% of the public and about 35% of obstetricians/gynecologists seem to support this position. A much higher percentage of both the public and physicians appear to believe that abortion is morally wrong, even though they do not believe that it should be forbidden by law.[6] This view seems to be based on a tacit acceptance of the United States as a free society of pluralistic values and on a notion that our society should tolerate diversity even in areas where a majority of the population believes that a certain practice is morally wrong. The most fundamental notions in our legal system are individual liberty and the injunction that the government not interfere with one's fundamental constitutional rights unless it can demonstrate a compelling state interest. It was because the Supreme Court concluded that the decision to continue or interrupt a pregnancy was part of a woman's fundamental "right to privacy" that the current law on abortion came to have its current shape and limitations.

Roe v. Wade

The US Supreme Court's 1973 decision in *Roe v. Wade*[4] is the most important, most controversial, and most well-known US Supreme Court

---

*See Chapter 10.

decision in recent history. In the 13 years following this decision, the Court has decided more than a dozen major abortion cases, all aimed at delineating the precise contours of *Roe v. Wade.* The decision remains under constant attack from organized "right to life" groups and from President Ronald Reagan, who describes abortion as "murder" and has adopted as a litmus test for new judges their abortion position. Nevertheless, *Roe* has consistently been reaffirmed by a majority of the Court. With the possibility of a significant shift in Court personnel, however, parts of the decision could be reversed, and the criminalization of abortion could reappear in some states. No matter what the future holds, however, it is critical for the welfare of patients and the effectiveness of physicians that the current state of the law on abortion in the United States be understood and appreciated.

In *Roe v. Wade,* and in all of the abortion cases that followed it (other than the funding cases), the Court has been faced with a *criminal* statute. In *Roe,* the Texas statute it was reviewing made it a crime to "procure an abortion" or to attempt one, except to save the life of the mother. Justice Harry Blackmun, formerly legal counsel to the Mayo Clinic, wrote the opinion of the Court. One of his major goals was to prevent the government from interfering with the practice of medicine and in the doctor-patient relationship.[3]

Building on a series of cases that described a "right to personal privacy, or a guarantee of certain areas or zones of privacy," the Court determined that a "right to privacy" existed "in the Fourteenth Amendment's concept of personal liberty and restrictions upon state action . . ." The Court went on to hold that this right "is broad enough to encompass a woman's decision whether or not to terminate her pregnancy":

> The detriment that the State would impose upon the pregnant woman by denying this choice altogether is apparent. Specific and direct harm medically diagnosable even in early pregnancy may be involved. Maternity, or additional offspring, may force upon the woman a distressful life and future . . .

The Court, however, stopped short of declaring that a woman's right to an abortion was always absolute. Instead, the Court recognized that the state may have some interests that may at times be "compelling" enough to limit abortion. The Court identified two such interests: the protection of maternal health, and the protection of viable fetuses. The protection of maternal health has always been a legitimate state interest. In the case of abortion, however, the Court ruled that this interest could never be so "compelling" as to prohibit abortion prior to the stage in pregnancy when it is less dangerous for the woman to carry the fetus to term than to have an abortion (about the end of the first trimester). The Court decided that during the first trimester the state could only regulate abortions to protect the woman's health by requiring that they be performed by a physician. Thereafter it could only regulate on this basis in ways reasonably calculated to enhance the woman's personal health (rather than to protect the fetus or to discourage abortions).

The second state interest remains the most divisive: the interest in "protecting the potentiality of human life." The Supreme Court did not decide that the fetus is not human, but only that a fetus is not a "person" as that term is used in the Fourteenth Amendment. The Court also properly noted that "the pregnant woman cannot be isolated in her privacy"; but rather, her interests in privacy must be weighed against the state's interest in the life of the fetus. The question is: When does this interest become so "compelling" that the state can justifiably interfere with the woman's constitutional right to have an abortion? No satisfactory answer to this question can be garnered from science, and any line of demarcation is inherently arbitrary. The Court decided to choose viability, the interim point between conception and birth, at which the fetus "is potentially able to live outside the mother's womb, albeit with artificial aid."[4] The choice of viability as the constitutionally significant line has been the subject of much debate and criticism.* Constitutional scholar John Hart Ely for example, thought the Court should have chosen the more traditional "quickening" line, the point at which the fetus begins to make movements independent of the mother, and which usually occurs closer to the beginning than the end of the second trimester.[8] He also thought that the Court tried to explain its choice of viability simply by defining it, rather than by presenting a logical argument for the choice. In his oft-quoted but imprecise criticism, "The Court's defense [of viability as its choice] seems to mistake a definition for a syllogism."[8]

After viability, which occurs near the end of the second trimester, but whose actual determination is a function of medical technology and skill,

---

*There are two primary avenues of attack on *Roe v. Wade.* The first is that the "right to privacy" that is broad enough to encompass abortion appears nowhere in the Constitution, and is thus "legislatively created" by the Court. The second is that the "viability" line is arbitrary and undefinable. The undefinable quality of the term "viability" does seem inherent in it, and the term appears to have been chosen to enhance the discretion of physicians to act in what they see as the best interest of their patients without state interference. This is because estimates of gestational age are basically professional guesses, based on the woman's last menstrual period, clinical examination of uterine size, and perhaps ultrasound. Moreover, physicians' own opinions about what constitutes the threshold of viability range from a 5% chance of survival upwards. *Colautti v. Franklin,* 439 U.S. 379 (1979). Since there is no professional consensus on this issue, the functional definition of viability itself remains unsettled. It should be noted, however, that other possible lines, such as completion of the neural connections in the fetal brain, and sleep and wake brain activity, occur near "viability" at 28- to 32-weeks' gestation.[7] Similar line-drawing problems abound in deciding when to permit research on human embryos. See Chapter 10.

the state "may, if it chooses, regulate, and even proscribe, abortion except where it is necessary, in appropriate medical judgment, for the preservation of the life or health of the mother." Although states can regulate abortions after viability (or, more accurately, restrict birth inductions), only about half the states have enacted laws that attempt to restrict abortions since *Roe*.

Roe v. Wade was a 7–2 decision, with Justices Byron White and William Rehnquist dissenting. They have continued to consistently dissent to post-*Roe* decisions, and have been recently joined by Justice Sandra O'Connor, and even former Chief Justice Burger on one occasion. Most of the reaction to *Roe* in the political and legal arena has concentrated on two areas: (1) eliminating public funding for abortions for poor women; and (2) restricting availability of legal abortions by statute as much as possible.

Funding for Abortion

The initial set of decisions involving abortion funding were rendered in 1977. In the first case, the Court upheld a state Medicaid regulation that refused to pay for "unnecessary" or "nontherapeutic" abortions, while at the same time funding childbirth for indigent women, as consistent with the federal Medicaid Statute (Title XIX of the Social Security Act).[9] In the second, the Court held that the Constitution did not require a state participating in the Medicaid program to fund nontherapeutic abortions if it paid for childbirth.[10] And in the third opinion, the Court concluded that the Constitution did not require public hospitals to perform elective abortions, even though these hospitals provided care for childbirth.[11]

The most important of this trilogy was the second, *Maher v. Roe*.[10] Writing for the majority, Justice Lewis Powell concluded that funding for childbirth but not abortion was not a denial of equal protection because (1) poverty is not a "suspect class" (like race or religion), and (2) failure to fund abortions does not "impinge upon" the woman's fundamental right to have an abortion. The reason for the latter conclusion is that by failing to fund abortions for poor women, the state "places no obstacles in the pregnant woman's path to an abortion," i.e., the state did not create the woman's poverty that prevents her from obtaining an abortion. This makes the regulation constitutional as long as it rationally furthers a legitimate state purpose. The Court concluded that the regulation accomplishes this by furthering the state's "strong interest in protecting the potential life of the fetus," and its "strong and legitimate interest in encouraging normal childbirth." Justice Blackmun, in dissent, argued that the Court's disregard for poor women was "disingenuous and alarming, almost reminiscent of 'let them eat cake.'" There does seem to be an inherent inconsistency in permitting the government to interfere with a woman's choice by selective funding (i.e., of childbirth), but not by penalties.[12] Although one can conclude that as long as the woman is not actually *forced* by government policy to have a child, her *choice* is still at least theoretically "protected."

The latest Supreme Court opinion on funding was a 5–4 decision in the 1980 case of *Harris v. McRae*.[13] This case involved the constitutionality of the "Hyde Amendment," named after its Congressional sponsor, and used in various versions to restrict federal funding of some therapeutic abortions. The version of the amendment under consideration by the Court forbade the use of federal funds for abortion except where

> the life of the mother would be endangered if the fetus were carried to term; or except for such medical procedures necessary for the victims of rape or incest when such a rape or incest has been reported promptly to a law enforcement agency or public health service.[13]

Justice Potter Stewart, writing for the majority, viewed the case as a simple extension of *Maher,* ruling that the amendment was constitutional for the same reasons the Medicaid regulation in *Maher* was constitutional. The difference between medically necessary and elective abortions was seen as constitutionally irrelevant; the government need fund neither. This opinion seems to conclude that the federal government could deny funding for abortions even for women who would suffer severe and long-lasting physical harm, and even death, if it was not performed. Effective choice is available only to those with the money to pay for abortions.[14]

This put an end to the funding argument. The government is not required by the Constitution to fund *any* medical care for poor people, no matter how vital it is to their health or welfare, as long as this refusal is "rationally related to a legitimate government interest." Funding is a matter for the Congress and the legislatures of the individual states to determine. We believe this is an extreme position and are in agreement with the four-judge minority. Justice John Paul Stevens, who switched from the majority in *Maher* to the minority in *Harris,* is, we believe, correct in arguing that once the government decides to alleviate some of the hardships of poverty by providing "necessary medical care," the government should be required to use neutral criteria in distributing benefits, not criteria that penalize those indigents in need of an abortion. Justice Thurgood Marshall also seems to be correct in arguing that the Hyde Amendment actually serves *no* legitimate governmental interest. He notes that the amendment refuses funding even where normal childbirth will *not* result, e.g., where the child will die shortly after birth. Since this is the result, he argues that the only rational basis of the amendment is that it was "designed to deprive poor and minority women of the constitutional right to choose abortion, and this, of course, is not a constitutionally permissible purpose for legislation."[10]

Writing Restrictive Laws

The second line of cases involves attempts to limit the availability of legal abortions by state legislatures. The first such statute to reach the Supreme Court was from Missouri and was reviewed in the 1976 decision of *Danforth v. Planned Parenthood of Missouri*[15] written by Justice Harry Blackmun. *Roe v. Wade* defined the woman's right to an abortion broadly, but left many specific issues unresolved. In *Danforth,* the Court decided many of them, holding inter alia that:

• The application of the definition of fetal viability must be left to the "judgment of the responsible attending physician;"

• A state *may* constitutionally require a woman to give her informed, voluntary, and written consent to abortion;

• A state *may not* outlaw a method of abortion that is safer than carrying a child to term;

• A state *may* require certain records to be kept "for the advancement of medical knowledge" so long as they are kept "confidential;"

• A state *may not* require the consent of a spouse to a first trimester abortion; and

• A state *may not* require the consent of a minor's parent or parents to a first trimester abortion.[15, 16]

The primary rationale for striking down both the spousal and parental consent requirements was that if the state cannot directly forbid abortion, it should not be permitted to delegate "veto power" to someone else. Justice White, joined by two others, would have upheld spousal consent on the grounds that the father has an extremely strong interest in the potential child:

> A father's interest in having a child—perhaps his only child—may be unmatched by any other interest in his life. It is truly surprising that the majority finds in the United States Constitution, as it must in order to justify the result it reaches, a rule that the State must assign a greater value to a mother's decision to cut off a potential life by abortion than a father's decision to let it mature into a live child.[15]

But the issue of parental consent divided the Court much more deeply. The state, under the *parens patriae* doctrine, has a duty to protect the welfare of minors. There was evidence before the Court that girls as young as 10 and 11 years old had sought abortions. Moreover, the counseling at one abortion clinic was done in groups of both minors and adults who were strangers to one another, not done by a physician, and concerned mainly abortion procedures, complications, and birth control methods. The lower court had found a compelling state interest sufficient to justify parental consent to safeguard "the authority of the family relationship." The majority of the Court disagreed, noting that "Constitutional rights do not mature and come into being magically only when one attains the state-defined age of majority. Minors, as well as adults, are protected by the Constitution and possess constitutional rights." Regarding the state's interest in the family, Justice Blackmun wrote:

> It is difficult to conclude that providing a parent with absolute power to overrule a determination made by the physician and his minor patient will serve to strengthen the family unit. Neither is it likely that such veto power will enhance parental control where the minor and the nonconsenting parent are so fundamentally in conflict and the very existence of the pregnancy already has fractured the family structure.[15]

Somewhat hedging this statement, Justice Blackmun noted that the Court was *not* holding that "every minor, regardless of age or maturity may give effective consent to an abortion." In fact, the holding was that such consent was valid only if the minor was capable of giving an informed consent to the procedure, i.e., capable of understanding the abortion, its options, and the risks and benefits of each.*

There have been two other major decisions that outline the limits of tolerance of the majority of the Court toward state "tinkering" with abortion laws to reduce the number of abortions performed within the state: *Akron v. Center for Reproductive Health*[20] in 1983 and *Thornburgh v. ACOG*[21] in 1986.

Akron was a 6–3 decision written by Justice Lewis Powell. It is an extremely strongly worded opinion in which the Court goes out of its way to reaffirm *Roe v. Wade* and to note that *Harris* did not signal any retreat from *Roe:*

> Arguments continue to be made . . . that we erred in interpreting the Con-

---

*In another case, the Court examined a Massachusetts statute and decided to return it to the Massachusetts Supreme Judicial Court for interpretation.[17] When it later came back to the Court, eight justices agreed that it was unconstitutional.[18] Four of them, however, indicated that a hypothetical statute that gave a minor an option of seeking court approval *or* parental approval would be constitutional, so long as the only role of the court would be to determine if the minor was mature enough to give her informed consent. If the minor was not mature, then, and only then, could the judge decide what course would be in the minor's best interests. Three other cases involving parental consent have reached the Court to date, but as a result of split voting and conflicting rationales, "the constitutional dimensions of the right of a minor to obtain an abortion have still not been conclusively dealt with by the Court."[19]

stitution [in *Roe v. Wade*]. Nonetheless, the doctrine of *stare decisis*, while perhaps never entirely persuasive on a constitutional question, is a doctrine that demands respect in a society governed by the rule of law. We respect it today, and reaffirm *Roe v. Wade.*

At issue in *Akron*, and a companion case, *Planned Parenthood v. Ashcroft*,[22] were the constitutionality of the following provisions of the Akron City Ordinance (1–5) and the Missouri abortion statute (6–8):

1. A requirement that all abortions after the first trimester be performed in a hospital accredited by the Joint Commission on the Accreditation of Hospitals;

2. A requirement that a physician inform a woman of the status of her pregnancy, the development of the fetus, the date of possible viability, and the physical and emotional complications that might result from an abortion; the physician was also required to state that "the unborn child is a human life from the moment of conception," and describe the anatomical and physiological characteristics of the fetus in detail;

3. A requirement that the physician inform the woman of "the particular risks associated with her own pregnancy and the abortion technique to be employed . . .;"

4. A requirement of at least a 24-hour waiting period between the time the woman signed the consent form and the performance of the abortion;

5. A requirement that physicians performing abortions were required to dispose of fetal remains in a "humane and sanitary manner;"

6. (Similar to 1) A requirement that abortions after 12 weeks must be performed in a hospital;

7. A requirement that a pathology report be done for each abortion;

8. A requirement that a second physician be present during abortions performed after viability.

The Court struck down all of the provisions of the Akron ordinance, and the similar hospital provision of the Missouri statute. It did, however, uphold provisions 7 and 8, which were part of the Missouri statute.

The Court went to some length to explain its reasoning in each case. The provisions requiring that all abortions after the first trimester be performed in hospitals, for example, were struck down as out of touch with current medical practice and knowledge. Noting that the medical evidence in 1983 indicated that dilation and evacuation abortions were safer than childbirth up to a gestational age of 16 weeks, the Court nonetheless continued to draw the line for the state's interest in maternal health at about "the end of the first trimester." But this no longer justifies a blanket hospital rule because: (1) the safety of second trimester abortions has "increased dramatically" since *Roe;* (2) the American Public Health Association and the American College of Obstetricians and Gynecologists both agree that second-trimester abortions using dilation and evacuation can be safely performed in nonhospital facilities; and (3) the additional cost of an in-hospital abortion, $850 to $900, versus $350 to $400 for a clinic abortion, "places a significant obstacle in the path of women seeking abortion."

A number of points merit discussion. First, cost is a major issue with the Court, and regulations that significantly increase the cost of abortion without significantly increasing its safety will be struck down. In this regard we can compare requirements 1 and 6 with requirement 7, the pathology report requirement. The pathology requirement was upheld because it related directly to the woman's health, and added only a "comparatively small cost" (estimated at $19.40). Similarly, the 24-hour waiting requirement (requirement 4) was struck down because of the added cost burden it put on the woman in terms of requiring a return trip, and also its interference with medical judgment.† Apparently small costs with health rationales are permissible; burdensome and unnecessary added costs are not. It is also important to underline that the Court placed great weight on "accepted medical practice" and deferred to it in determining what types of second trimester abortions could be safely performed outside of hospitals. Thus, as medical practice changes, the contours of permissible restrictive state legislation may also change.

The detailed consent requirements were struck down as well, even though the Court had previously approved general informed consent rules in *Danforth.*[15] The ordinance required the physician to personally inform the pregnant woman of a number of specific items, including the statement that "the unborn child is a human life from the moment of conception;" a description of the "anatomical and physiological characteristics of the particular unborn child . . . including appearance, mobility, tactile sensitivity, including pain, perception, or response . . .;" the warning that "abortion is a major surgical procedure, which can result in serious complications . . . and can result in severe emotional problems;" and the suggestion that "numerous public and private agencies are available to assist her during pregnancy and after the birth of her child if she chooses not to have an abortion. . ."[20]

---

†It would probably have been preferable to strike it down on the grounds that such a waiting period is not required for any other medical procedure.

The Court reasonably concluded that these requirements were not intended to inform the woman at all, "but rather to persuade her to withhold consent altogether." In short, the provision was not designed to protect the woman's health or enhance her decision-making ability. Instead, it intrudes "upon the discretion of the pregnant woman's physician . . . [when it insists] upon the recitation of a lengthy and inflexible list of information."

The Court likewise rejected the requirement that the physician personally obtain informed consent because it did not believe this rule was reasonably designed to further the state's interest in maternal health. The "humane and sanitary" disposal of fetuses requirement was struck down because it was vague, a fatal flaw in a criminal statute. Finally, the second physician rule was upheld because the state has a compelling interest in the life of the fetus after viability, and could even prohibit most abortions altogether during this period.

Justice O'Connor issued a strong dissent, in which she was joined by the two dissenters in the original *Roe v. Wade* opinion, Justices White and Rehnquist. Not surprisingly, perhaps, her dissent was really addressed to *Roe v. Wade* rather than *Akron*. She argued that the trimester system is "completely unworkable" because it requires the courts and legislatures "to continuously and conscientiously study contemporary medical and scientific literature; to determine the acceptability of current practice, the safety of abortion at a given period in pregnancy, and the point of viability. This, she argued, turns the Court into a "science review board" and violates a primary principle of judicial decision-making: the application of neutral principles "sufficiently absolute to give them roots throughout the community and continuity over significant periods of time. . ." Her central argument was that *Roe's* trimester scheme "is clearly on a collision course with itself" and therefore should be abandoned.[23]

The most recent Supreme Court opinion on abortion was decided in mid-1986, *Thornburgh v. American College of Obstetricians and Gynecologists*.[21] This opinion sent tremors of fear through the pro-choice community because it was a 5–4 decision, with Justice Burger joining the three dissenters in *Akron*. For the first time since 1976, Justice Blackmun again delivered the opinion of the Court on a major abortion decision. At issue in the case were six specific provisions of the Pennsylvania Abortion Control Act: (1) informed consent; (2) printed information; (3) reporting requirements; (4) determination of viability; (5) degree of care required in postviability abortions; and (6) second opinion requirement. Relying heavily on *Akron*[20] and *Ashcroft*,[22] the Court invalidated all six of these provisions.

The "informed consent" and "printed information" provisions required that certain information be given to the woman by the referring physician or the physician who would perform the abortion at least 24 hours prior to the abortion, and certain other information be provided by the physician or his agent at least 24 hours prior to the abortion. *The physician information* included the name of the physician who would perform the abortion; the fact that there "may be detrimental physical and psychological effects which are not accurately forseeable;" the medical risks associated with the particular method to be used; the probable gestational age of the "unborn child"; and the medical risks associated with carrying a fetus to term. The required information (that could be conveyed by the physician's agent) included: that medical assistance benefits may be available for prenatal care, childbirth, and neonatal care; that the father is liable to assist in the support of the child; and that the pregnant woman has a right to review printed materials (which she shall be orally informed "describe the unborn child and list agencies which offer alternatives to abortion"). Prior to the abortion, the woman must certify in writing that all of this information was provided to her.

While not exactly the "parade of horribles" struck down in *Akron*,[20] the majority struck down these requirements using the *Akron* rationale that the information is designed not to obtain the woman's informed consent, "but rather to persuade her to withhold it altogether." In addition, the Court objected to the "rigidity" of the requirement that imposed an "undesired and uncomfortable straitjacket" on the physician. In an overstatement, the Court concluded, "All this is, or comes close to being, state medicine imposed upon the woman, not the professional medical guidance she seeks, and it officially structures—as it was obviously intended to do—the dialogue between the woman and her physician." Giving some examples, the Court described as "cruel" requiring this information in a case of a "life-threatening pregnancy," and "gratuitous" in the case of a rape victim having to be told about the theoretical financial responsibility of the rapist.

The "reporting" and "determination of viability" provisions required the physician to determine whether or not the fetus was viable. If viable, the physician was required to report the basis for the determination that the abortion was necessary to preserve maternal life or health. If not viable, the physician had also to report the basis for this determination. In addition, the physician was required to report to the state department of health the following information: the identification of the physician and facility involved in the abortion and the referring physician; the political subdivision and state in which the woman resided; the woman's age, race, and marital status; the number of prior pregnancies; the date of last menstrual period; the type of procedure used; complications; the length and width of "aborted unborn child"; the basis for medical emergency; the date of consultation examination; and whether the abortion was paid for by the patient, medical assistance, or medical insurance. These reports were required to "be made available for public inspection and copying within 15 days of receipt in a form that will not lead to the disclosure of the identity of any person filing a report."

As previously noted, in *Danforth*[15] the Court had approved recordkeeping requirements designed to "preserve maternal health" so long as patient confidentiality was maintained. The court found these rules, however, to go "well beyond" maternal health care interests, especially information related to payment period, personal history, and basis for medical judgment. The court found that maintenance of privacy seemed problematic, and the possibility of a breach would "necessarily" make a woman and her physician "more reluctant to choose an abortion," and thus potentially "chill the exercise" of her constitutional right:

> Pennsylvania's reporting requirements raise the spectre of public exposure and harassment of women who choose to exercise their personal, and intensely private, right, with their physician, to end a pregnancy. Thus, they pose an unacceptable danger of deterring the exercise of that right, and must be invalidated.[21]

The "degree of postviability care" and "second physician" provisions were considered separately. The first required that the physician exercise the same care delivering a viable fetus that he would in delivering "an unborn child intended to be born and not aborted;" and that "the abortion technique employed shall be that which would provide the best opportunity for the unborn child to be aborted alive unless . . . this would present a significantly greater medical risk to the life or health of the pregnant woman." Violation of this standard was a felony, punishable by up to seven years in jail. The Court found the provisions "facially invalid" because the phrase "significantly greater medical risk" required the physician to "trade-off" the woman's health and fetal survival without providing that maternal health was to be the physician's "paramount consideration."

The second physician provision required that another physician be present at the abortion to "take control of the child . . . and provide immediate medical care for the child . . ." when viability is possible. Violation of this provision was also a felony. Again, although in *Danforth* the Court had upheld a general second physician requirement, the *Thornburgh* Court struck this one down. The reason was that unlike the more general Missouri statute, which could be read to contain an emergency exception, the Pennsylvania statute could not be read to make an exception for a medical emergency in which the health of the mother might be endangered as a result of the delay in the arrival of the second physician.

The Court might have gone either way on some of these provisions (informed consent, and the second physician rule), but chose to strike them all down by reading *Akron*[20] and *Danforth*[15] strictly. The Court apparently took this route because the majority was frustrated at having to continually review very restrictive state abortion statutes, and because it believed that the *criminal* nature of these statutes required that they be very precisely drawn in order not to frighten physicians from performing abortions altogether. Accordingly, Justice Blackmun's majority opinion made it clear that neither he nor the majority of the Court has backed down one inch from *Roe v. Wade,* and that the states should recognize it as the law of the land and respect it:

> Again today, we affirm the general principles laid down in *Roe* and in *Akron.* In the years since this Court's decision in *Roe,* states and municipalities have adopted a number of measures seemingly designed to prevent a woman, with the advice of her physician, from exercising her freedom of choice. *Akron* is but one example. But the constitutional principles that led this Court to its decisions in 1973 still provide the compelling reason for recognizing the constitutional dimensions of a woman's right to decide whether to end her pregnancy. 'It should go without saying that the vitality of these constitutional principles cannot be allowed to yield simply because of disagreement with them.' . . . *The States are not free, under the guise of protecting maternal health or fetal life, to intimidate women into continuing pregnancies* [emphasis added].[21]

Concluding the opinion, Justice Blackmun argued that the promise "that a certain sphere of individual liberty will be kept largely beyond the *reach of government*" is one that "*extends to women, as well as to men.*" Regarding the abortion decision, he wrote, "few decisions are more personal and intimate, more properly private, or more basic to individual dignity and autonomy than a woman's decision—with the guidance of her physician and within the limits specified in *Roe*—whether to end her pregnancy.

This 5–4 decision brought three written dissents. Justice O'Connor mainly restated her *Akron* dissent. Now retired Chief Justice Burger based his dissent (a new position for the Chief Justice) on his own apparent misreading of *Roe v. Wade.* Justice White wrote a detailed dissent, which he seemed to be using as a warm-up exercise to write what he hopes someday will be a majority opinion overruling *Roe v. Wade.* Justice White dissented in all but the funding cases involving abortions and is not prepared to change his mind, even after 13 years of unbroken majority opinions upholding *Roe.* He explained that following precedents, the doctrine of *stare decisis* is a critical "principle of law" that prevents the exercise of "judicial will" from becoming "arbitrary and unpredictable." Nonetheless, he asserted that cases that determine statutes unconstitutional "call other considerations into play." Specifically, he objected to "decisions that find in the Constitution principles or values that cannot fairly be read into the document" because these decisions "usurp the people's authority, for such decisions represent choices that the people have never made and that they cannot disavow through corrective legislation." Accordingly, he argued, the Court should correct constitutional decisions that "on reconsideration are found to be mistaken."

Justice White then presented his arguments for overruling *Roe v. Wade.* He first restated his argument that a woman's right to an abortion is not a "fundamental" constitutional right, and therefore the state need show only a "rational basis" for legislation in restricting its exercise, rather than a "compelling state interest." Justice White accordingly accused the majority of "engaging not in constitutional interpretation, but in the unrestrained imposition of its own, extraconstitutional value preferences."

Justice White then argued that the "viability" rule is "entirely arbitrary." In his view, the governmental interest at stake is "in protecting those who will be citizens if their lives are not ended in the womb." This interest, he argued, is not contingent upon medical science or other factors, but "is in the fetus as an entity in itself, and the character of this entity does not change at the point of viability under conventional medical wisdom." Justice White correctly noted that if these views are accepted, states may adopt "a broad range of limitations on abortion (including outright prohibition) that are now unavailable."*

Justice Stevens limited his concurring opinion to addressing Justice White's dissent, and reviewing Justice White's previous pronouncements in related cases. His commentary is devastating to White's argument. On the issue of the fetus having the same interest throughout pregnancy, for example, Justice Stevens noted:

> I should think it obvious that the state's interest in the protection of an

*Two weeks after deciding *Thornburgh,* the Court, again split 5–4, refused to expand the Constitutional protection of the "right to privacy" beyond "family, marriage, or procreation," to protect any intimate sexual relationship, including sodomy, even when performed in the privacy of a bedroom. *Bowers v. Hardwick,* 92 L. Ed. 2d 140 (1986). Justice White, this time writing for the majority, stated simply and simplistically that there is "no fundamental right to engage in homosexual sodomy"; and that the morality of the majority of a state's legislature is sufficient governmental rationale to criminalize sodomy. Justice Blackmun, writing for the four dissenters, said that he believed the privacy line of cases stands for the proposition that all individuals have a fundamental interest "in controlling the nature of their intimate associations with others . . . Indeed, the right of an individual to conduct intimate relationships in the intimacy of his or her own home seems to me to be the heart of the Constitution's protection of privacy." As to legislative majority morality being sufficient legal justification for an anti-sodomy statute, Blackmun correctly notes that "the legitimacy of secular legislation depends on whether the State can advance some justification for its law beyond its conformity to religious doctrine." The case is disturbing not only because it is so clearly anti-gay (Justice Burger wrote, for example, "To hold that the act of homosexual sodomy is somehow protected as a fundamental right would be to cast aside millennia of moral teaching"), but also because its simplistic structure could be directly applied to limit *Roe v. Wade.*

embryo . . . increases progressively and dramatically as the organism's capacity to feel pain, to experience pleasure, to survive, and to react to its surroundings increases day by day. The development of a fetus—and pregnancy itself—are not static conditions, and the assertion that the government's interest is static ignores this reality . . . there is a fundamental and well-recognized difference between a fetus and a human being; indeed, if there is not such a difference, the permissibility of terminating the life of a fetus could scarcely be left to the will of the state legislatures.[21]

Combining the cases of *Danforth,*[15] *Akron*[20] and *Thornburgh,*[21] we can construct a list of state regulations concerning abortion that have been upheld and contrast it with a similar list of regulations that have been struck down (Table 6–1). On the basis of a similar table that he constructed before *Thornburgh,* Boston University Health Law Professor Leonard Glantz

TABLE 6–1.
State Abortion Regulations Struck Down and Upheld by the US Supreme Court Since *Roe v. Wade*

REGULATIONS STRUCK DOWN	REGULATIONS UPHELD
Requiring detailed "informed consent" provisions designed to discourage consent	Requiring pathologic examination of fetal tissue
Requiring use of detailed material on fetal development and child placement services	Mandatory record-keeping and reporting, related to maternal health and kept confidential
Mandatory hospitalization in the second trimester	General informed consent requirements
Mandatory 24-hour waiting period	Mandatory presence of a second physician at postviability abortions if there is an exception for emergencies
Legislative determination of fetal viability	
Mandatory spousal consent	
Ban on saline abortions	
Requiring the physician to personally obtain informed consent	
Requiring record-keeping and reporting not directly related to maternal health	
Mandatory reporting basis for determination that the fetus is not viable	
Requiring physician to trade off maternal health for fetal life in postviable abortion	
Requiring presence of second physician at postviability abortion without express or implied exception for emergencies	

derived a series of five "not necessarily independent tests" that the Court has used in various combinations to invalidate or uphold regulations on abortions:

1. Has the state placed an obstacle in front of the woman or otherwise significantly burdened the pregnant woman's ability to choose or obtain an abortion?
2. Is abortion treated differently than other similar medical or surgical procedures?
3. Does the regulation interfere with the exercise of professional judgment by the attending physician?
4. Does the regulation conflict with, or is it stricter than, accepted medical and scientific standards?
5. Is the regulation reasonably designed to protect maternal health in an area where no less restrictive or less expensive regulation will do?

To this list can be added a sixth,

6. Does the regulation protect the fetus without putting the mother in jeopardy (if it is a postviability requirement)?

Using this scheme, we can see that the four approved regulations all produce a positive answer to one of the last two questions and negative answers to all of the first four questions. A similar, converse, observation can be made of the 12 items that have been struck down; all produce a negative answer to both of the last two questions, and a positive answer to at least one of the first four questions. It can also be argued that the more "yes" answers to the first four questions (even if one of the last two is answered "yes"), the more likely the regulation will be struck down. What can be concluded from this list is that, "Over the past decade it is quite remarkable how consistent the Court has been in protecting a woman's right to obtain an abortion and a physician's right to perform one."[19]

All this consistency could, of course, be thrown into disarray if there are additional personnel changes in the Court that result in a reversal or modification of *Roe v. Wade*. In this regard, Justice Stevens' remarks in response to Justice White on *stare decisis* are useful to remember:

> [T]he fact that the doctrine of *stare decisis* is not an absolute bar to the reexamination of past interpretations of the Constitution [does not] mean that the values underlying that doctrine may summarily be put to one side. There is a strong public interest in stability, and in the orderly conduct of our affairs, that is served by a consistent course of constitutional adjudication. Acceptance of the fundamental premises that underlie the decision in *Roe v. Wade*, as well as the application of those premises in that case, places the primary responsibil-

ity for decision in matters of childbearing squarely in the private sector of our society. The majority remains free to preach to evils of birth control and abortion and to persuade others to make correct decisions while the individual faced with the reality of a difficult choice having serious and personal consequences of major importance to her own future—perhaps to the salvation of her own immortal soul—remains free to seek and obtain sympathetic guidance from those who share her own value preferences.[21]

Justice Stevens concluded that, "In the final analysis, the holding of *Roe v. Wade* presumes that it is far better to permit some individuals to make incorrect decisions than to deny all individuals the right to make decisions that have a profound effect upon their destiny."

Perhaps any concentration on the possibility of reversing or revising *Roe v. Wade* is overalarmist. As Harvard Law Professor Lawrence Tribe has noted, *Roe v. Wade* is only "part of a series of decisions allocating to the woman the essentially unfettered choice of whether to bear a child." As part of this series it "represents less a decision in favor of abortion than a decision in favor of leaving the matter, however it might come out in particular cases, to women rather than to legislative majorities . . ."[12]*

We now turn to the first case in the "series" to which Professor Tribe refers, the sterilization case of *Skinner v. Oklahoma*.[24]

STERILIZATION

In the most notorious case involving involuntary sterilization, the Supreme Court upheld a Virginia statute that was used as the basis for sterilizing Carrie Buck, whom the Court described as a "feeble-minded eighteen-year-old" who was "the daughter of a feeble-minded mother and the mother of an illegitimate feeble-minded child."[25] Oliver Wendell Holmes, speaking for the Court, argued:

> It is better for all the world, if instead of waiting to execute degenerate offspring for crime, or let them starve for their imbecility, society can prevent those who are manifestly unfit from continuing their kind . . . Three generations of imbeciles are enough.

This case, decided in 1927, was the capstone of almost three decades of the eugenics movement in the United States. Even though it continues

---

*Tribe also notes, "Whatever might be said of a consistent commitment to helpless unborn life, the argument for preferring majority rule over the woman's choice in matters of reproduction seems thin to the vanishing point. Among other things, the argument at least suggests, though it does not logically compel, the conclusion that majority rule should prevail over the woman's choice even when her preference is for life and the majority's is for death."[12]

to be cited by the Court without comment, *Buck v. Bell*[25] is not good law today, and was decided on incorrectly stated facts, even in 1927.* Most importantly, it was decided without any discussion of Ms. Buck's rights. It is tragic that the case was so poorly presented and brutishly decided, because it resulted not only in the sterilization of Carrie Buck, but also of more than 8,300 inmates of the Virginia state mental institutions from 1927 to 1972, and helped set the stage for the involuntary sterilization of more than 60,000 US citizens.[26–29]

It was not until 1942, in the case of *Skinner v. Oklahoma*,[24] that the Supreme Court examined the issue of sterilization again. The case dealt with the constitutionality of an Oklahoma statute that provided for the sterilization of "habitual criminals." It applied to larceny, but specifically exempted persons convicted of embezzlement, even though these crimes are of the same nature. Justice William Douglas, writing for the Court, ruled that the statute violated the equal protection clause of the Fourteenth Amendment, and along the way affirmed the fundamental "value of reproductive autonomy over a majoritarian decision in favor of sterilization."[12] In the Court's words:

> We are dealing here with legislation which involves one of the basic civil rights of man. Marriage and procreation are fundamental to the very existence and survival of the race. The power to sterilize, if exercised, may have subtle, far-reaching and devastating effects. In evil or reckless hands it can cause races or types which are inimical to the dominant group to wither and disappear.[24]

Nonetheless, the Court did not explicitly overrule *Buck v. Bell*. Indeed in a concurring opinion, Justice Stone suggested that, "Undoubtedly, a state may, after appropriate inquiry, constitutionally interfere with the personal liberty of the individual to prevent the transmission by inheritance of his socially inferior tendencies."

---

*Neither Carrie, nor her mother Emma, for example, were ever described as "imbeciles" at the trial. They were each alleged to have a mental age of 8 or 9 years, which placed them in the category of low to middle-grade morons, Carrie's classification. More to the point, although little is known about Emma Buck, whose misfortunes seem to have stemmed as much from poverty as lack of intelligence, enough is known about Carrie and her daughter Vivian to refute Justice Holmes's conclusion. Carrie, who had progressed to the sixth grade after five years in grade school, left the mental institution immediately after she was sterilized. She married and lived with her husband for 24 years, until he died. She later met and married again. In 1970, suffering from ill health, she and her husband returned to Carrie's hometown, where they lived in poverty until 1980, when she was hospitalized. She died in a nursing home at the age of 76 in 1983. It is reported that "through her adult life she regularly displayed intelligence and kindness . . . she was an avid reader, and even in her last weeks was able to converse lucidly, recalling events from her childhood." Her daughter, Vivian, who was used to "prove" that her mother's "defects" were "hereditary," lived barely eight years; and in her two years in school, she "performed quite well, at one point earning a spot on the school's 'Honor Roll.' "[26]

No other sterilization case has come before the Court since World War II, but numerous states have considered the question of both voluntary and involuntary sterilization of the mentally incompetent person in the 1970s and 1980s. Some states have specific statutory provisions; in others only the court can permit sterilization; and in still others, there is no clear law on the subject.[30-33] Probably the leading state decision on the subject, and the one that serves well to summarize the major issues involved, is the decision of the New Jersey Supreme Court in the case of Lee Ann Grady.[34, 35]

The Case of Lee Ann Grady

At the time that her case came before the New Jersey Supreme Court, Lee Ann Grady was a 19-year-old who had Down syndrome.[35] She was the oldest of three children, lived at home with them and her parents, and had never been institutionalized. Her IQ was in the "upper 20s to upper 30s range." She could converse, count to some extent, and recognize letters of the alphabet. She could dress and bathe herself. Her life expectancy and physical maturation were normal; however, her mental deficiency prevented the normal emotional and social development of sexuality. If she became pregnant, she would not understand her condition, and she would not be capable of caring for a baby alone.

Because of her sexual development, her parents had provided her with birth control pills for four years, although there was no evidence that she had ever engaged in sexual activity or had any interest in it. At the age of 20, she would leave her special class in the public school system. Her parents wanted to have her placed in a sheltered work group, and eventually in a group home for retarded adults so that she could begin more independent life and have a place to live after they died. They believed that dependable and continuous contraception was a prerequisite to this change, and they and their physician sought to have her sterilized, using a tubal ligation, at the Morristown Memorial Hospital. The hospital refused to perform the surgery without court approval, and a lawsuit followed.

The lower court granted the parents' application, and the public advocate and attorney general appealed. The New Jersey Supreme Court began its analysis by recognizing that "sterilization [destroys] an important part of a person's social and biological identity" and rejected any notion that might assign fewer rights to the mentally retarded than to other citizens. The court declined to classify the proposed sterilization as either voluntary (since she could not understand the problem or the proposed solution) or compulsory (since no one was actually objecting to the procedure on her behalf). Instead it defined a new category: a procedure "lacking personal consent because of a legal disability."

The court concluded that the right to prevent conception through sterilization is one of the privacy rights protected by the US Constitution and declined to discard it for the mentally retarded "solely on the basis that [their] condition prevents conscious exercise of the choice." The court also refused to permit the person's parents and a court-appointed guardian to make the decision. Instead it insisted that only the court can make this decision for an incompetent person. The court noted that similar decisions in adoption and child custody cases are routinely made by courts, and held that, under its inherent *parens patriae* power, the courts have the authority to protect incompetents who cannot protect themselves because of an innate legal disability.†

The court understood that its decision was *not* Ms. Grady's but

> . . . is a genuine choice . . . designed to further the same interests she might pursue had she the ability to decide herself. We believe that having the choice made in her behalf produces a more just and compassionate result than leaving Lee Ann with no way of exercising a constitutional right. *Our Court should accept the responsibility of providing her with a choice* to compensate for inability to exercise personally an important constitutional right [emphasis added].[35]

Having decided that a court is the proper decision maker, the court considered the standards and procedures to be employed. The court stopped short of requiring a showing of "strict necessity," but enunciated very strict criteria that must be met before sterilization can be authorized. The court must appoint a guardian *ad litem* to represent the interests of the ward, and "should receive" independent medical and psychological evaluations by qualified professionals. The trial judge must personally meet with the individual before making a decision that the person lacks the capacity to make a decision about sterilization and that the incapacity is unlikely to change. This incapacity must be proved by clear and convincing evidence. Finally, the court must be persuaded, also by clear and convincing evidence, that the sterilization is in the person's *best interests*. In making this determination, the court must consider the following:

- Possibility of pregnancy;
- Possibility of physical and mental harm from pregnancy and from sterilization;
- Likelihood of sexual activity;

---

†This power has been applied in medical cases, including authorizations to treat children over parental objection, and in kidney and bone marrow transplant cases involving minor donors.[36]

- Inability of the person to understand contraception;

- Feasibility of a less drastic means of sterilization (e.g., tubal ligation versus hysterectomy);

- Possibility of postponing sterilization;

- Ability of the person to care for a child, or the possibility of marriage at a future date with ability of the couple to care for the child;

- Evidence of relevant medical advances;

- Demonstration that the proponents of sterilization are seeking it in good faith for the primary concern of the person and not their own or the public convenience.

This list is not meant to be inclusive, and "the ultimate criterion is the best interest of the incompetent person." Because the trial court did not apply the stringent "clear and convincing" standard of proof (it used the more traditional "preponderance of the evidence" standard) to the best interests conclusion, the case was remanded for further proceedings.

The court thus found that incompetent persons had a substantive right to sterilization and sought to protect incompetent persons from its arbitrary use by demanding strict due process protections. This is far superior to a blanket prohibition against sterilization, and much more protective of individual rights than permitting families to make this decision on their own.

If a structural problem exists with the decision, it is in the role of the guardian *ad litem*. The court defined the guardian's role as "representing the interests of his ward." This seems inappropriate for a proceeding in which the judge, not the guardian, will make the judgment as to whether the sterilization is in the person's best interests. Since the petitioners will always be arguing in favor of the sterilization, it would make more sense if the guardian *ad litem* were required to present all of the arguments against sterilization to the best of his ability, so that both sides of the issue are considered. As Boston College Law Professor Charles Baron has argued, "Without advocates on both sides of the issue to develop the record, the court is too likely to face mental set and path-of-least-resistance pitfalls . . . [A] general pattern will seem to emerge from the evidence; an accustomed label is waiting for the case, and without awaiting further proofs, this label is promptly assigned to it."[28]

The New Jersey model is as good as anything that exists, but it stands almost alone in the country. Since most courts will not act without explicit statutory authority, statutes should be enacted in each state. They should prohibit sterilization of the mentally retarded and other incompetent individuals except when a court finds, after an adversary hearing, that the sterilization is in the best interests of the individual. Such a procedure permits sterilization in cases in which a compelling case can be made, and protects potential victims from abusive sterilization performed for the benefit of others.

Chapter 7 _____

Treatment of Handicapped Newborns

In his Pulitzer prize winning play, *Buried Child*, Sam Shepard depicts the moral disintegration of an American family following the intentional drowning of an unwanted child. The mother's husband, who was not the father of the child, states simply, "I killed it. I drowned it. Just like the runt of a litter." The image of a defective newborn as an animal is not unique to art. Philosopher Peter Singer suggested in a *Pediatrics* commentary that, "Only the fact that the defective infant is a member of the species *Homo sapiens* leads it to be treated differently from a dog or a pig. Species membership alone, however, is not morally relevant."[1] This drew 50 negative letters, and only 1 that supported the editor's decision to publish the commentary.

It is facile to contend that we should treat all infants equally simply because they are alive. Traditionally dealt with privately, the questions of how we view handicapped infants and what rights we afford them have been at the center of a political debate in the United States since the beginning of the Reagan presidency.[2] The answers, of course, are related to the abortion debate, and "right to life" groups have been the prime movers in encouraging governmental intervention. Questions concerning who should make what decisions, and on what basis, remain unresolved. The outer limits of parental authority regarding treatment decisions for their handicapped infants are vague, and the role of physicians is disputed. We may be tempted to throw up our hands like the drunken minister in *Buried Child* and try to escape the situation by saying, as he did, "I don't know what to do. I don't know what my role is." We may not know our "role," or what the government's role should be, but a decision not to decide is a decision for the status quo. This chapter reviews the policy debate on treatment of severely handicapped children and concludes that after all the lawsuits, regulations, and statutes that have been passed, we have legally returned to the place where we began our journey. Nonetheless, the experiences of the past five years ensure that decision making involving handicapped newborns will never be the same, and that parents and physicians will properly be required to consider more factors than many had in the past before deciding not to treat.

THE "BABY DOE" DEBATE

In general, parents have a legal obligation to provide their children with "necessary medical care." When alternative modes of treatment are available, and each is consistent with generally accepted medical practice, parents may choose among them. However, when the only alternative is nontreatment, parents may lawfully choose this option only if it is consistent with the "best interests" of the child. To deny the child beneficial treatment can be child neglect, and the state has an obligation to exercise its *parens patriae* power to protect children from such neglect.[3]

So important is society's view of the sanctity of human life that when a duty to treat exists, and treatment is withheld, both parents and the physician could be charged with homicide.[3] Only one such case has ever been brought in the United States, however. That case involved a charge of attempted homicide for the initial failure to treat Siamese twins born in Danville, Illinois, but it was dropped for lack of evidence.[4] The children were eventually successfully separated, and at last report they were "faring moderately well."[5] The "best-interests" standard has a long legal pedigree, but it is often extremely difficult to apply in the neonatal intensive care unit. Sometimes decisions are made that are not in the best interests of the child, but rather in the interests of the parents. Sometimes decisions are made against treatment because insufficient or biased information is presented to the parents. Examples of both types of decisions are described in the famous 1973 Duff and Campbell article, in which treatment was withheld from 43 infants with the concurrence of their parents.[6] In a more recent University of Oklahoma myelomeningocele classification study, all 24 infants relegated to a "supportive care only" category died within 189 days.[7] Quality of life was used as a major criterion in classification.

The most notorious nontreatment cases have involved the withholding of life-saving corrective surgery from Down syndrome children. The story of an unnamed baby who was born at Johns Hopkins in the early 1970s with duodenal atresia and not treated is the subject of the film, "Who Shall Survive?" Based on a composite of six similar actual cases, the film has been widely used in schools and hospitals for the past decade. The child starved to death. Another famous Down syndrome baby, known only as Baby Doe, died in Bloomington, Indiana, on April 15, 1982, at the age of six days, following a court-approved decision that routine life-saving surgery be withheld. The infant had a tracheoesophageal fistula that was not repaired; instead the child was medicated with phenobarbital and morphine and allowed to starve to death. The court believed that if there was a dispute among physicians regarding treatment, the parents should be able to withhold treatment.* Given existing legal principles, however, that require treatment if it is in the child's best interests, it seems that legally and ethically, Baby Doe should have been treated. The public, accordingly, was properly outraged that he was not.[8]

On the strength of the Baby Doe case, the Department of Health and Human Services (HHS) wrote a letter to approximately 7,000 hospitals, on May 18, 1982, putting them on notice that it was

> unlawful [under sec. 504 of the Rehabilitation Act of 1973] for a recipient of Federal financial assistance to withhold from a handicapped infant nutritional sustenance or medical or surgical treatment required to correct a life-threatening condition if: (1) the withholding is based on the fact that the infant is handicapped; and (2) the handicap does not render treatment or nutritional sustenance contraindicated.

The penalty for noncompliance was the possible loss of federal funds. In announcing the policy, then Secretary Richard Schweiker said: "The President has instructed me to make absolutely clear to health care providers in this nation that federal law does not allow medical discrimination against handicapped infants."[9]

The Original "Baby Doe" Regulations

This policy statement set off a continuing nationwide political, legal, medical, and ethical debate over the proper role of government regarding

---

*In an interview after the fact, Judge John Baker of the Monroe County Court said, "I knew what I was going to decide while it was still being argued. The problem was I just didn't know how to say it." What he reportedly decided was that if there were two divergent medical opinions, i.e., if one physician recommended treatment, and another recommended against it, then the parents had the right to choose either course. The judge believed this was true, apparently, even if the physician who recommended against treatment did so solely on the basis of his personal assessment of the child's potential quality of life.[5]

medical treatment of handicapped infants. About ten months after the letter was sent, and shortly after the tenth anniversary of the US Supreme Court's abortion decision, the White House instructed HHS to issue more detailed follow-up regulations. In emergency regulations published in March 1983, HHS required the conspicuous display of the substance of the May 1982 letter in each delivery ward, maternity ward, pediatric ward, nursery, and intensive care nursery (Fig 7–1). Included in the notice was a toll-free, 24-hour "hotline" number that individuals with knowledge of any handicapped infant being discriminatorily denied food or customary medical care were encouraged to call. The HHS officials were given authority to take "immediate remedial action" to protect the infant, and hospitals were required to provide access to their premises and medical records to agency investigators.[10]

The American Academy of Pediatrics and others brought suit against HHS and its new Secretary, Margaret Heckler, to enjoin the "interim final rule" on March 18, four days before it was to become effective. In early April 1983, US District Court Judge Gerhard Gesell ruled the regulation invalid because HHS had failed to follow the Administrative Procedures Act in promulgating it.[11] Judge Gesell also added some personal comments on the regulation, noting that he saw its primary purpose as requiring "physicians treating newborns to take into account wholly medical risk-benefit

NOTICE

DEPARTMENT OF HEALTH AND HUMAN SERVICES
Office for Civil Rights

DISCRIMINATORY FAILURE TO FEED AND CARE FOR HANDICAPPED INFANTS IN THIS FACILITY IS PROHIBITED BY FEDERAL LAW. SECTION 504 OF THE REHABILITATION ACT OF 1973 STATES THAT

"NO OTHERWISE QUALIFIED HANDICAPPED INDIVIDUAL SHALL, SOLELY BY REASON OF HANDICAP, BE EXCLUDED FROM PARTICIPATION IN, BE DENIED THE BENEFITS OF, OR BE SUBJECTED TO DISCRIMINATION UNDER ANY PROGRAM OR ACTIVITY RECEIVING FEDERAL FINANCIAL ASSISTANCE."

Any person having knowledge that a handicapped infant is being discriminatorily denied food or customary medical care should immediately contact:

Handicapped Infant Hotline
U.S. Department of Health and Human Services
Washington, D.C. 20201
Phone 800-368-1019 (Available 24 hours a day) - TTY Capability

In Washington, D.C. call 863-0100

OR

Your State Child Protective Agency

Federal Law prohibits retaliation or intimidation against any person who provides information about possible violations of the Rehabilitation Act of 1973.

Identity of callers will be held confidential.

Failure to feed and care for infants may also violate the criminal and civil laws of your state.

FIG 7–1.
HHS's March 1983 Notice for display in each hospital delivery ward, maternity ward, pediatric ward, nursery, and intensive care nursery.

considerations" and to prevent parents from having an influence upon decisions as to whether further medical treatment is desirable. Without a definition of the required "customary medical care," the judge noted that the regulation is "virtually without meaning beyond its intrinsic *in terrorem* effect."[11, 12]

First Revised "Baby Doe" Regulations

Instead of pressing an appeal of Judge Gesell's ruling, HHS reissued the regulations in early July 1983, as proposed rules, following proper procedure and giving interested parties 60 days to comment on them. The revised proposal was identical with the original with four exceptions: (1) The hotline notice need only be posted at "each nurse's station"; (2) the minimum size requirement for the notice was reduced to 8.5 × 11 in.; (3) the state child protective agency's telephone number had to be added to the poster; and, most significantly, (4) an entirely new section mandated that each state's child protective services agency establish procedures designed "to prevent medical neglect of handicapped infants."[13, 14]

The Department of Health and Human Services received 16,739 comments (many based on letter-writing campaigns) on its July proposal, of which it categorized 97.5% as supportive. This aggregate precisely reflected the breakdown of the 322 nurses who responded, but 72% of 141 pediatricians opposed the regulations, as did 77% of hospital officials and health-related organizations. The Department took at least some of these comments into account in issuing its final regulations in January 1984.[15]

Final "Baby Doe" Regulations

Only two substantive changes were adopted: (1) The notice was changed to require that "nourishment and medically beneficial treatment (as determined with respect for reasonable medical judgments) should not be withheld from handicapped infants solely on the basis of their present or anticipated mental or physical impairments"; and (2) the size ("no smaller than 5 by 7 inches") and the location ("where nurses. . .will see it") of the notice was changed, and an alternative notice of compliance adopted.[15]

The first change inadequately addressed the most conspicuous deficiency of the original regulation: it provided no guidance at all to physicians as to their legal obligations, but simply mandated that they follow "custom." But this remains the central regulatory problem in the neonatal setting. Because the alternative treatments for extreme prematurity and other now treatable conditions are relatively new, no "medical custom" or standard of care has developed or been defined. That is why the original regulations offered no useful guidance to physicians. As Judge Gessel argued, they had the effect of frightening physicians into always treating everything, thereby often resulting in "overtreating" at the expense of increased suffering on the part of incurable and dying infants.[11] Surgeon General C. Everett Koop had earlier argued that it was not the Administration's intention to prolong the dying process, and the "medically beneficial" amendment was apparently aimed at reassuring physicians that they need not abuse infants with useless overtreatment. Of course, what "medically beneficial" treatment is begs the question of what criteria are used to judge such treatment, including the extent to which quality of life judgments can be used by parents and physicians in determining "medical benefit."[14] The changes involving sign size and location were entirely cosmetic. The only meaningful novelty in the January 1984 regulation was the suggestion of Infant Care Review Committees (ICRCs), a suggestion discussed later in this chapter.

These regulations took effect on February 13, 1984. In the meantime, a case destined to join the Johns Hopkins and Bloomington, Indiana, cases, the case of Baby Jane Doe, was being played out in the New York courts. It involved the other major category of handicapped infants, in addition to infants with Down syndrome, that seem especially vulnerable to nontreatment decisions: infants with spina bifida.

The Case of Baby Jane Doe

Baby Jane Doe was born on October 11, 1983, suffering from spina bifida, hydrocephaly, and microcephaly. She was the first child of young parents who had been married for approximately one year. Her physicians recommended immediate surgery to place a ventricular shunt to reduce cerebrospinal fluid pressure within the ventricles of her brain and to close her meningomyelocele. Her physicians believed this could increase her life expectancy from a matter of weeks to 20 years or more. But it was alleged she would likely be severely retarded, epileptic, paralyzed, bedridden, and subject to constant urinary tract infections. After lengthy consultations, the parents refused to consent to the surgery, opting instead for antibiotics and bandages to prevent infection. Her attending physicians did not disagree with the reasonableness or appropriateness of this decision, and even though the child had already been transferred to State University Hospital at Stony Brook, it is likely that had the decision been made even a year earlier, or in another part of the country, none of us would ever have heard of Baby Jane Doe.

In the "Baby Doe" regulation era, however, it was predictable that at least one child like Baby Jane Doe would be chosen as a test case to deter-mine the proper role of the state in decisions to withhold surgery from handicapped newborns.[16] In this case, a self-styled "right to life" Vermont lawyer, Lawrence Washburn, received a confidential tip about Baby Jane Doe and brought suit in New York to obtain an order to have the surgery performed. The trial judge appointed Attorney William E. Weber as guardian *ad litem* to represent the child and held a hearing on October 20. Weber, who the night before the hearing had told the parents he agreed with their decision, reversed himself at the hearing. He argued for immediate treatment on the basis that the medical records disagreed with what the physicians had told him and the parents about the child's prognosis. The trial judge ruled the infant in need of immediate surgery to preserve her life, and authorized Weber to consent to it. The parents appealed.[17]

The Appellate Division reversed the decision the following day, ruling that the parents' decision was consistent with the best interests of the child, and therefore there was no basis for judicial intervention. The court found both that the child was not "in imminent danger of death," and that the recommended shunt and spinal closure carried their own risks, including loss "of what little function remains in her legs."[18] Seven days later New York's highest court, the Court of Appeals, ruled that the trial judge had abused his discretion in hearing the case in the first place, because Attorney Washburn had "no disclosed relationship with the child, her parents, her family, or those treating her illness."* The court ruled that allegations of child abuse or neglect must be made to the state's Department of Social Services for appropriate investigation, and dismissed the suit on these procedural grounds.[20]

---

*Although most commentators have been favorably inclined to this ruling, which seems to preclude strangers from "interfering" with decision making concerning handicapped new-borns, Professor Robert Burt of Yale Law School thinks that we were too quick to accept this conclusion. He notes that the Baby Jane Doe case occurred just about the time of the 20th anniversary of the Kitty Genovese case. Ms. Genovese, it will be recalled, was killed early one morning on a public street following an hour and a half pursuit by her killer, during which she frequently and loudly called for help. Some 38 neighbors heard her cries, but none did anything to help her, not even by calling the police. The case has become symbolic of our anonymous society and the disappearance of any communal caretaking ethos. Burt asks, recalling this case, "Was [Washburn] an officious meddler? Or was he a good citizen prepared to seek protection for a fellow citizen who, though a stranger to him, appeared to be in need of help?" Burt raises this question because he believes "that the question of whether any communal caretaking bonds exist among strangers is raised with special symbolic and emotional force in social policy toward handicapped people generally and anomalous infants, who are mentally retarded or physically disabled, specifically.[19] We think he is generally correct; although in the case of Baby Jane Doe, Washburn should have contented himself with notifying New York's Department of Social Services.

The Federal Government and Baby Jane Doe

Meanwhile, HHS received a "hotline" complaint from an unidentified private citizen that Baby Jane Doe was being discriminatorily denied indicated medical treatment. The complaint was referred to the New York State Child Protective Services, which, on November 7, 1983, concluded that there was no cause for state intervention. Prior to this, however, HHS had obtained the record of the state court proceedings, which contained the child's medical records through October 19. After personally reviewing them, Surgeon General Koop concluded that he could not determine the basis for denial of treatment, including whether it was based solely on handicap, without "immediate access to, and careful review of, current medical records. . . ." Therefore, beginning on October 22, HHS repeatedly asked University Hospital to make Baby Jane Doe's medical records (after October 19) available to it so it could conduct an investigation under section 504 of the Rehabilitation Act of 1973.

The hospital refused, and in early November HHS brought suit in US District Court to obtain the child's medical records so it could conduct its section 504 investigation. The District Court focused the issue on whether or not it could be "clearly determined" from the record that the hospital was not in violation of section 504. The court concluded that the hospital failed to perform the surgery not because of the child's handicap, *but because of parental refusal*; therefore, the hospital was not in violation of the act. The court also found the decision of the parents "reasonable" based on "the medical options available and on a genuine concern for the best interests of the child."[21] Arguing that the hospital had a duty under section 504 to seek judicial review of a parental refusal under certain circumstances, HHS appealed. The parents and hospital, on the other hand, argued that section 504 was never intended to serve as a basis for governmental intervention in medical decision making.

Stated simply, the government's position was that examination of the child's medical record was necessary to determine if she was denied surgery *because* of her microcephaly. It argued this would be as unlawfully discriminatory as refusing to perform surgery on an individual because the person was black, because it would not be based on medical criteria, and thus would not be a "*bona fide* medical judgment."

In reviewing HEW's and HHS's regulatory history with respect to the issue of what authority section 504 gave the government to investigate, the Court of Appeals noted that in 1976 HEW adopted the position that section 504 did *not* give the government authority to establish new patients' rights to "receive or refuse treatment." Rather HEW's authority was to make services "accessible" or available to the handicapped, so as to provide them with "an equal opportunity to receive benefits." In May 1977, HEW explained the difference in this way:

> A burn center need not provide other types of medical treatment to handicapped persons unless it provides such medical services to nonhandicapped persons. It could not, however, refuse to treat the burns of a deaf person because of his or her deafness.

In fact, it was not until the May 1982 letter to hospitals that HHS ever suggested that section 504 might apply to actual medical treatment decisions. After reviewing the development of the Baby Doe regulations, the court found that "the regulatory history of 504 is inconclusive," and HHS's current position on the scope of the enabling statute is "flatly at odds with the position originally taken by HEW."[22]

This left the court with the task of interpreting the statute based on its language and legislative history. Section 504 provides:

> *No otherwise qualified handicapped individual* in the United States. . .shall, solely by reason of his handicap, be excluded from the participation in, or be denied the benefits of, or be subjected to discrimination under any program or activity receiving Federal financial assistance [emphasis added].

The Court of Appeals concluded that Baby Jane Doe fit the definition of a "handicapped individual," but determined she was not "otherwise qualified" because this phrase referred to handicapped individuals who could benefit from services *in spite of* their handicap rather than cases, like Baby Jane Doe's, in which the handicap itself was the subject of the services. The court also noted that nothing in the legislative history of the Rehabilitation Act of 1973, which had to do primarily with employment and vocational education, envisioned any governmental role in medical treatment decisions. The court therefore concluded that the Rehabilitation Act did not give HHS any authority to interfere with "treatment decisions involving defective newborn infants." Accordingly, HHS's request to continue its investigation by obtaining access to Baby Jane Doe's medical records was denied.[22] Prior to the decision, Baby Jane Doe's parents agreed to have the shunting procedure performed, and her myelomeningocele had closed naturally. On April 5, 1984, she went home with her parents.

The decision devastated HHS's Baby Doe regulations, cutting their legislative foundation out from under them. On the basis of the decision, the American Medical Association (AMA), the American Hospital Association (AHA), and others brought suit in federal district court to enjoin the mandatory provisions of the regulations. In the meantime, attention shifted to Congress.

Federal Legislation

The Second Circuit Court's opinion was based on its interpretation of Congressional intent. Therefore, Congress was free to explicitly legislate in this area. And it did. Instead of acting indirectly by amending the Rehabilitation Act of 1973, however, Congress concentrated on the more traditional legal role of the government, child abuse. It, accordingly, moved enforcement back to the traditional level, the states. On October 9, 1984, President Ronald Reagan signed the Child Abuse Amendments of 1984 into law. This statute, among other things, explicitly brands the withholding and withdrawal of medically indicated treatment and nutrition from disabled infants as a type of child abuse. It requires the individual states, as a condition for continued federal funding of their child abuse programs, to establish special procedures to deal with this form of child abuse.

On April 15, 1985, HHS issued final regulations to implement the new law.[23] The most controversial provision of the statute, and one that prevented the AMA from supporting it, is the wording of the exceptions to the rule against withholding or withdrawing "medically indicated treatment" in the face of a "life-threatening condition." Treatment may be withheld if:

1. The infant is chronically and *irreversibly comatose;*

2. The provision of such *treatment would merely prolong dying;* not be effective in ameliorating or correcting all of the infant's life-threatening conditions; *or otherwise be futile* in terms of survival of the infant; or

3. The provision of such *treatment would be virtually futile* in terms of the survival of the infant and the treatment itself under such circumstances would be *inhumane* [emphasis added].

The "virtually futile" exception was seen by most involved in drafting the statute as providing sufficient latitude for physicians to make reasonable medical judgments regarding most treatments. In its original December 1984 proposed regulations, HHS took the extreme position that "virtually futile" referred exclusively to situations in which "the treatment is highly unlikely to prevent imminent death." This seemed to many to be simply an attempt to restrict physician judgment by regulation in a way that Congress had refused to do by legislation. In the final rule, however, medical judgment is again given central authority, and specifically includes the withholding of "other than appropriate nutrition, hydration, or medication" to an infant when any of the above-listed exceptions apply. Whether or not one of the exceptions applies is determined solely on the basis of "reasonable medical judgment," which the regulation defines as a "medical judgment that would be made by a reasonably prudent physician, knowledgeable about the case and the treatment possibilities with respect to the medical conditions involved."[23] These regulations answer one question that was prominent during the debate and compromise: Can nutrition and hydration ever be withheld from an infant? The answer is yes, when fluids and nutrition are not "appropriate" in the attending physician's "reasonable medical judgment." The Department's use of the word "imminent" was eliminated altogether in the final regulations. "Merely prolong dying" was expanded from "imminent" to "in the near future" (but something less than "many years of life"). All this, again, is left up to "reasonable medical judgment." Since such a decision can be extremely problematic, the development of Infant Care Review Committees, discussed later in this chapter, was also recommended.[23]

The Child Abuse Amendments of 1984 thus leave us legally in almost precisely the same situation we have been in for the past two decades. In its introduction to the proposed regulations, HHS seemed to concede as much: "The protection of children from abuse and neglect, including medical neglect, has always been a state and local responsibility."

While superficially appealing, the thrust of the 1984 Amendments is to require state child protection agencies to spend much more time and effort on potential abuse and neglect in neonatal care. Although some abuses have been noted in the literature, the Amendments appear more a solution to a political problem than to a real world medical one. For example, HHS was not able to uncover even one case of discriminatory child abuse or neglect in more than a year of operating its "hotline." Furthermore, current state laws already permit state child protection agencies to investigate cases of alleged abuse and neglect of infants. Encouraging the devotion of further resources to this area, while other much more prevalent forms of child abuse go underinvestigated, seems unwarranted.

The Supreme Court's Decision on the Baby Doe Regulations

It was primarily for the reasons already discussed that the Supreme Court struck down the Baby Doe regulations when it finally reviewed them in June 1986. As previously noted, following the case of Baby Jane Doe, the AHA and others asked a US District Court to enjoin the four mandatory sections of the Baby Doe regulations (notice posting, mandatory reporting, access to medical records, and expedited action to effect compliance). The lower court invalidated the regulations, and the Second Circuit Court summarily affirmed the lower court's decision based on its own previous Baby Jane Doe opinion. Accordingly, it is fair to say that the original Baby Jane Doe case was the subject of this appeal to the Supreme Court.

Somewhat inexplicably, Justice John Paul Stevens, writing for the Court did not examine the reasoning of the Second Circuit in any detail, although he seemed to agree with it. In a footnote, for example, he stated, "The legislative history of the Rehabilitation Act does not support the notion that Congress intended intervention by federal officials into treatment decisions traditionally left by state law to concerned parents and the attending physicians or, in exceptional cases, to state agencies charged with protecting the welfare of the infant."[24]

Instead, the centerpiece of the Court's analysis was that *it is parents, not hospitals, who are refusing to treat handicapped newborns.* State laws regarding child neglect apply to parental refusals, but section 504 does not, since in the absence of parental consent the infant is neither "otherwise qualified" for treatment nor has the infant been denied care "solely by reason of his handicap." The plurality noted that HHS's original position, based on the case in Bloomington, Indiana, was that section 504 did apply to parental refusals and that the hospitals violated 504 by even allowing such infants to remain in their care. But HHS abandoned this position in its final rules, noting that section 504 did *not* authorize HHS to override parental refusals. Instead HHS relied on two possible categories of 504 violations to justify the rules: (1) a hospital's refusal to furnish a handicapped infant with medically beneficial treatment "solely by reason of handicap"; and (2) a hospital's failure to report cases of suspected medical neglect of handicapped newborns to a state child protective services agency.

Justice Stevens concentrated almost all of his analysis on the "axiom of administrative law" that an agency's basis for a regulation must include "a rational connection between the facts found and the choice made; and that an agency's action "must be upheld, if at all, on the basis articulated by the agency itself." Stevens argued that no such "rational connection" exists for the first rationale because HHS could find *no* case in which a hospital denied treatment to a handicapped infant "solely by reason of handicap." This was true in the original Baby Doe case from Bloomington, Indiana, and in the case of Baby Jane Doe. Moreover, in the 49 cases HHS investigated in 1983 and used as a basis for the final rule, none involved a finding that a hospital had refused to provide care to which the infant's parents had consented. Physician surveys that indicated attitudes supportive of nontreatment[25] were found irrelevant because HHS had not used them as a basis for the regulation, and HHS did not contend that physicians (rather than parents) were making the nontreatment decision.

Regarding the second rationale, the one for the reporting regulations,

Stevens says three things: (1) the record reveals *no* case where a hospital failed or was accused of failing to make such report; (2) much more evidence of Congressional intent is needed when the federal government commands a state to do something; and (3) the way the states discharge their child abuse and neglect protection functions is "wholly outside the nondiscrimination mandate of section 504." Section 504 *could* apply if the hospital refuses to treat a handicapped child because of the handicap when parents want the treatment. But mandatory reporting does not seem needed here, since it is reasonable to assume that the parents themselves would bring such a case to the attention of the authorities.

The plurality's decision not only invalidated the four mandatory rules, but also affirmed the lower court's much broader injunction. That injunction forbids "federal continuation or initiation of regulatory and investigative activity directed at instances in which parents have refused to consent to treatment. . .and efforts to seek compliance with affirmative requirements imposed on state child protective service agencies."

The opinion is a strong affirmation of federalism. In this area federal authority stems primarily from funding, and if the federal government wants to improve the lot of the handicapped, it can do so by making a much wider range of services available to them. On the other hand, areas of child abuse and neglect are traditionally areas of state authority, and the Court sees no reason to suppose that Congress meant to change this traditional division of governmental authority when it enacted section 504.

Justice Byron White, joined by two others, dissented. In his view, HHS could properly take attitudinal surveys of physicians into account in promulgating regulations whose purpose was to "foster an awareness by health care professionals of their responsibility not to act in a discriminatory manner with respect to medical treatment decisions for handicapped infants." He reached this conclusion because he differed with the plurality on the centrality of parental consent in treatment decisions. In his view the survey literature made clear that the "parental consent decision does not occur in a vacuum. In fact, the doctors (directly) and the hospital (indirectly) in most cases participate in the formulation of the final parental decision and in many cases substantially influence that decision."[24]

Unfortunately, like its progenitors, the case itself is "checkered." Justice Stevens objects to Justice White's dissent on the grounds that, "like bishops of opposite colors, the opinions of Justice White and the Court of Appeals do not even touch one another," because Justice White limited his discussion to cases in which treatment is not directly related to the handicap (like treatment of an esophageal obstruction in a child with Down syndrome), whereas the Court of Appeals was concerned only with cases, like

Baby Jane Doe, in which the handicap was itself the condition needing treatment. This oversimplifies the disagreement, but the bishop analogy seems appropriate to much of the 1982–1986 discussion about the "Baby Doe" regulations.

From the start, for example, the Reagan Administration was concerned primarily with playing "right to life" politics, and not with enforcing section 504. So close was the Administration's political agenda in pursuing the Baby Doe regulations to its view on abortion, that when the President was asked about the US Supreme Court's recent abortion decision* at his mid-1986 news conference, he responded by talking about the Baby Doe decision instead. Noting correctly that the Court had ruled that the federal government was "getting into something that properly was the province of the states," he went on to say, "I feel very strongly that we're talking about human life. And the case that prompted this entire act was one in which the determination is made that this life is to be taken away and yet it isn't done as you would with an animal, it isn't done with a merciful putting to sleep or—they just let it starve to death."

Child neglect by parental treatment refusal has *always* been a matter of state law. It still is. The Court did *not* hold that parents have a right to refuse treatment for their handicapped children. The law of the case is that review of such decisions is a matter for the states. Since there is *no* evidence that the states are doing an inadequate job, and since Congress did not authorize HHS to get directly involved when it enacted 504, there is no reason why the status quo concerning the respective powers of the federal and state governments should be changed in this area. The 1984 Child Abuse Amendments explicitly recognize the respective roles of federal (funding) and state (child neglect enforcement) governments. Finally, section 504 was never explicitly or implicitly meant to apply to individual medical treatment decisions in which the handicap itself influences the possible benefit that can be derived from the treatment. Unfortunately, while this point is acknowledged by the plurality, it is not discussed, so what application, if any, HHS could make of section 504 *if* it developed a sufficient factual record for rule-making is not determined by this case.†

The proper legacy of the Baby Doe regulations is twofold: it highlights the inherent powers of the states in the area of child neglect, and it demonstrates that the most effective way the federal government can help the handicapped is not simply to enforce section 504, but also to fund service programs that directly benefit the handicapped.

*See Chapter 6.

†An excellent history of sec. 504 is Scotch RK: *From Good Will to Civil Rights: Transforming Federal Disability Policy*. Philadelphia, Temple University Press, 1984.

Standards of Care

The focus on child abuse, rather than on section 504 of the Rehabilitation Act of 1973, is proper. But this does leave the entire legal field precisely as it was before the Administration's May 1982 letter to hospitals: withholding customary medical treatment can be child abuse under certain circumstances.[12] The originally perceived problem was that the child abuse standards were vague and somehow permitted Down syndrome children with treatable esophageal or intestinal atresia to die untreated. This, however, was never lawful, and conflicting perceptions of the reasonableness of parental refusals, rather than purposeful maliciousness, probably accounted for the hospital's failure to act in the few reported cases relied upon by HHS in adopting its original proposals.

On the other hand, the child abuse standard of requiring "customary medical care" does not state a useful or precise legal standard in many areas of infant care simply because there is no such thing as "customary medical care" in many difficult and problematic cases. This is precisely what makes these cases so difficult for physicians. In its January 1984 regulations, HHS believed it was being helpful by requiring that only "medically beneficial treatment" be used; but, of course, this is no better since physicians "customarily" use only treatment they consider "beneficial."[15] Nor did the four examples HHS recited in the Appendix to the regulations provide more useful guidance. The first three dealt with Down syndrome, spina bifida, and anencephaly, respectively. The fourth is more general:

> Withholding of *certain potential treatments* from a *severely premature* and low birth weight *infant* on the grounds of *reasonable medical judgments* concerning the improbability of success or risks of potential harm to the infant would not violate section 504 [emphasis added].

This simply substitutes another vague phrase, "reasonable medical judgment," for "medically beneficial care." It also further complicates the issue by adding the terms "success" and "risks" without identifying their limits. In fact, in the context of example 3, which immediately precedes it and approves withholding of all medical treatment from an infant with anencephaly "who will inevitably die within a short period of time," the HHS examples seem to permit physicians to utilize quality of life criteria in making "medical" judgments—precisely the opposite of what Dr. Koop has stated he intended the regulations to do.[2] The Department of Health and Human Services attempted to justify its position by stating that in such cases treatment would be "futile" since it would "merely temporarily prolong the process of dying."

The problem, of course, is that if we have the medical technology to prolong the life of an anencephalic child and yet opt not to use it, this is *not* a medical judgment, but an ethical one based primarily on the desirability of prolonging the anencephalic child's life.* The real answer seems to be that it is not "beneficial"—medically, ethically, or any other way—to prolong the life of infants who will never experience anything.[2] This is, however, a nonmedical judgment based entirely on the consequences of living without cerebral function. The point is not necessarily that these HHS guidelines permit quality of life factors to be taken into account. It is that without taking such factors into consideration, we would be left with a technologically driven rule that would require the use of all treatments that prolonged life under all conditions.

The new statute's "medically indicated treatment" standard is, of course, no better, and its "clarifying" definition only creates more confusion. That is why we are where we were when we started: call it "customary," " indicated," "beneficial," or "appropriate," what must be provided is that care necessary to avoid violation of the state's child abuse and neglect laws. The idea that more specific standards are likely to be developed in any other way than through articulation by national professional associations and individual court decisions seems fanciful. Certainly randomly assigned Baby Doe squads dispatched from Washington were not the answer; nor do vaguely worded notices provide helpful guidance for would-be child protectors.[14]

A more fruitful way to think of the issue would be to concentrate not on the role of governmental enforcement mechanisms, nor on the role of "medical custom," but on the infant. We began our analysis of the child neglect laws with the observation that these laws require that medical care always be provided when it was in the child's "best interests." This term has a seductiveness about it that suggests we can always do something "best" for the child. With the typical Down syndrome child, this is probably true, because the child can experience life. In many cases, however, all choices are "tragic"; there is no "best" or even good outcome possible. It may, therefore, be more useful to rephrase our standard. One that has been suggested is to search for the "least detrimental" or the "least worst" alternative for the child. In the context of withholding life-sustaining treatment from an infant, however, we think the standard that should be explicitly stated and examined in the particular case is what we term the "better off dead" standard, i.e., the physician and family should not be permitted to withhold life-sustaining treatment from an infant unless there is objective evidence,

---

*It has been suggested that anencephalic infants should be used as a source of organs for transplant. Under current law this is not permissible, since these infants do not meet any currently acceptable definition of death because they have sufficient brain stem function to breathe on their own. Society (rather than medicine) would have to redefine such infants as nonhuman or subhuman before their use as an organ source could be acceptable.

from the infant's "point of view," that the infant would be better off dead than alive. This is a very high standard and will mean that almost all infants will be treated; but it is flexible enough to permit withholding of treatment when the burdens of the treatment in terms of factors like pain, discomfort, and degrading conditions outweigh any potential benefits in terms of increased length of life.

We purposefully include "degrading conditions" to encompass individuals who although they feel no pain also experience nothing (or will never be able to experience any meaningful thoughts), such as children born with trisomy 13.* A very strict best interests standard might require their treatment (on the theory that if they can possibly experience anything at all, from their own perspective this would be better than nothingness). However, if it can never result in the child experiencing a meaningful thought, we believe such treatment is properly labeled futile from the child's perspective, even if the child's "nothingness" existence causes it no conscious pain or discomfort. We recognize that this makes the "best interest" test at times imprecise, but without some room for consideration of the child's circumstances for living, we degrade and dehumanize the child by requiring it to exist like a plant or pet, much more for our own "good" than for its own. In this regard philosopher John Arras seems correct: "Ethical ambiguity pervades the issue." He argues, and we agree, that "we can either attempt to sustain the lives [of all handicapped infants] or we can engage in the risky business of designating a threshold of meaningful human life. The latter alternative might well be dangerous, but the former is pointless. . . ."[26] Our proposed "better off dead" standard, taking into account demeaning conditions of nonconscious existence in extreme cases, does not answer all of the difficult questions in the neonatal intensive care unit. It does, however, provide a somewhat more realistic basis for addressing the treatment decision than a simpler resort to the best interests test.

Work in three areas is required: enunciating substantive principles, ensuring proper facts are available to the decision makers, and developing reasonable procedures to apply the substantive principles to the facts of the case. In this regard the landmark "Principles of Treatment of Disabled Infants," developed by a broad coalition of medical and advocacy groups for the disabled in 1983, provides a reasonable beginning:

> When medical care is clearly beneficial, it should always be provided. When appropriate medical care is not available, arrangements should be made to transfer the infant to an appropriate medical facility. Considerations such as anticipated or actual potential of an individual and present or future lack of available community resources are irrelevant and must not determine the deci-

*See Chapter 1.

sions concerning medical care. The individual's medical condition should be the sole focus of the decision. These are very strict standards.

It is ethically and legally justified to withhold medical or surgical procedures which are clearly futile and will only prolong the act of dying. However, supportive care should be provided, including sustenance as medically indicated, and relief of pain and suffering. The needs of the dying person should be respected. The family should also be supported in its grieving.

In cases where it is uncertain whether medical treatment will be beneficial, a person's disability must not be the basis for a decision to withhold treatment. At all times during the process when decisions are being made about the benefit or futility of medical treatment, the person should be cared for in the medically most appropriate way. When doubt exists at any time about whether to treat, a presumption always should be in favor of treatment.[27]

These "Principles" should be periodically reassessed by the groups involved. We suggest, for example, that it seems unnecessarily narrow and unrealistic to ignore "present and future community resources," to focus exclusively (primarily is probably more realistic) on the individual's medical condition, and to resolve doubt always in favor of treatment, apparently no matter what its dimensions.

Those guilty of abusing the handicapped by denying them appropriate treatment should be prosecuted, and questionable cases should be referred to courts and child abuse agencies by hospitals. In court, the relevant facts can be examined by a politically appointed and accountable decision maker, in a neutral, public forum, on the basis of clearly articulated principles. There is no simple solution to this complex problem, but the combination of carefully crafted professional standards, an adequate development of medical facts, and public review of individual problematic cases in court, provides the most likely method by which the best interests of the child will remain central in decision making.

A More Radical Proposal

Some commentators, including Australians Helga Kuhse and Peter Singer, have argued that there should be a period of time after birth, perhaps 28 days, during which the child can be legally killed if it is severely handicapped. The decision would be made by the parents and physician, perhaps with the oversight of a hospital review committee.[2] There are a number of rationales for this proposal, but the primary ones are: (1) there is no moral justification for distinguishing between killing and letting die; and (2) focusing just on the best interests of the child neglects other important interests, such as those of the parents, the other children, potential future children, and society.[2] We agree that treatment decisions involving severely handicapped newborns are intrinsically difficult, but we believe that they should remain difficult and that they should be made in an atmosphere that mandates very serious reflection in the face of possible legal consequences for terminating the life of a handicapped child. We take this position primarily because of the devastating effect that an explicit social policy permitting the killing of certain handicapped newborns would be likely to have on all living handicapped individuals.* Moreover, if parents have the right to end the lives of their retarded or severely defective newborns, it is easy to conclude that if they do not exercise this right, then they alone should be responsible for caring for the child.[28] The argument would be that the community need not bear any responsibility for this act of "family privacy." This would strongly skew the decision making in favor of terminating treatment. Thus, Professor Robert Burt argues persuasively, "claims for parental privacy rights in withholding care have an inevitable public significance . . . formal social legitimation of these actions transforms private conduct into public performance, approves and invites imitation." Such formal legitimation could erode the "fragile public connection between an impaired child, and his parents and their community, upon which any child's welfare, upon which his very life, inevitably depends."[28]

Kuhse and Singer argue that their planned change in the law "would do no more than allow parents to make a decision, shortly after birth, to end life which has started out with difficulties so great that it is best that it not be prolonged."[2] This both understates and overstates the case. As we have seen, it greatly overstates the case with regard to the parents' right to choose abortion prior to birth; the proper demarcation is prior to viability.† Moving the boundary from viability to 28 days after birth makes the decision one that is different in kind, not just degree. Viability may be just as arbitrary a "bright line" for protection of life as birth, but it is much less arbitrary than 28 days (or any number of hours or days) *after* birth. Abortion may be justified primarily on the basis of reproductive liberty in terms of choosing whether or not to continue to permit one's body to be used for the gestation of the fetus. But it need not be justified on the basis of reproductive liberty extended to permit the destruction of one's viable fetus, newborn, or 6-year-old child. This is the difference between permitting a woman to have the fetus removed from her body and permitting a woman to destroy her viable child after it has been removed.

Perhaps even more astonishing than the overstatement of a woman's right to abortion is the understatement of the current law. The proposal

---

*The primary proponents of this proposal recognize the problems, but think that the proposal's impact on living handicapped individuals can be limited by assuring them that it will not be applied to anyone who could appreciate their own future (and thus worry about it being applied to them).[2]

†See Chapter 6.

assumes that parents cannot now make a decision to withhold treatment, even though it is clear from all the cases both we and the proponents can muster that they *can*. The law permits parents and their physicians great latitude in deciding not to treat severely handicapped newborns. As we have noted, there is only one case of an attempted prosecution in the United States, and only a handful of attempted (and equally unsuccessful) prosecutions elsewhere in the common law world.[4, 5, 29] This means that the law is extremely tolerant of parental and physician discretion in the newborn nursery. The Massachusetts Supreme Judicial Court accurately stated US law when it noted that a physician will not be criminally responsible for withholding life-sustaining treatment as long as the physician acts on a "good faith judgment that is *not grievously unreasonable by medical standards.*"[30]

Kuhse and Singer might retort in either of two ways: (1) yes, but we should change the "black letter" law to reflect practice so that decisions will not be made out of fear (even if irrational) of the law; and/or (2) yes, but the law requires that infants, like Baby Doe, be passively starved to death, rather than actively and mercifully put to death. The answer to both of these objections, it seems to us, is that we as a society want the decision for death to be difficult and made with at least some chance for accountability. The current child abuse laws provide this. Starving the child to death also makes the decision more difficult. Sufficient drugs can certainly be given to prevent pain and suffering (even if this hastens death),[31] but we do not believe that any useful social purpose will be served by making it easier for parents, doctors, and nurses to terminate treatment of severely defective newborns. This comes close to Professor Robert Burt's position:

> The true enormity of these actions to withhold life from newborns, viewed from our contemporary perspective, will remain in high visibility only if advance social authorization is withheld, and only if the parents and physicians who wish to take action are willing to accept some significant risk that they will suffer by such action. Their suffering will come in increasing intensity if criminal prosecution is instituted, if a jury finds them guilty of unconscionable conduct, and if a judge imposes sanctions on them accordingly.[32]

Burt argues that while this scheme (basically the present law) gives no guarantee that every newborn will be kept alive, it at least acts as a "powerful incentive to favor the child's continuing life."[32] Faced with even the remote possibility of criminal sanctions, however, physicians might choose to prolong the agony of defective newborns even when all reasonable hope of a cure or survival is gone.[33] One potential way to help ameliorate this fear, protect newborns and their parents, and perhaps improve on the decision-making process itself would be to utilize "ethics committees" as consultants in particularly difficult cases.

INSTITUTIONAL ETHICS COMMITTEES

In terms of procedures, HHS continues to recommend, but not require, that hospitals establish Infant Care Review Committees to help police child abuse and neglect policies. Since ethics committees are viewed by many as a procedural "way out" of the ethical dilemmas presented in the neonatal field, it is appropriate to examine their history and potential in this area. The concept remains ill-defined, the committee's mission and structure vague, and the impact on patient care uncertain. To exert a positive influence in patient care the committee's goals must be clearly defined, their substantive principles clearly articulated, and their procedures fair.

In late April 1984, the American Academy of Pediatrics (AAP) released their "Guidelines for Infant Bioethics Committees," and urged all hospitals to establish such committees. The guidelines were developed by the Academy as a response to the Administration's "Baby Doe" regulations and as an alternative to them. The President's Commission for the Study of Ethical Problems in Medicine also suggested that in difficult cases "an 'ethics committee' or similar body might be designated to review the decision making process."[34]

Types of "Ethics Committees"

The concept of ethics committees is not new; in one variation or another such committees have been used in the hospital setting whenever there has been a value conflict that has been explicitly identified and cannot be ignored. For example, prior to *Roe v. Wade*,[35] some state statutes prohibited abortions unless an abortion review committee found that the pregnant woman's life was in danger.[36] And in the human experimentation setting, Institutional Review Boards (IRBs), designed to approve research proposals and consent processes, have existed in most hospitals since the early 1970s.[37] Committees were mandated in Oregon and California to review the cases of individuals for whom psychosurgery was recommended.[38] When Dr. Barney Clark received his artificial heart, a multidisciplinary committee, which included the surgeon, a member of the IRB, a social worker, and another individual, reviewed his medical history and suitability prior to approving him as a candidate.[39] All of these committees differ from one another, however, and the term "ethics committee" itself is contentless.

The use of such committees has had neither universal appeal nor consistent success. In Seattle, in the late 1960s, patient selection committees were used to decide which of the candidates for kidney dialysis should have access to this life-saving procedure. The decision was based not on some general theory of justice or fairness, but on the notions that some individuals may be more worthy than others, and that a "worthiness" decision should not be made by a physician alone. As one physician member put it, "it's a lot more reassuring to play one-fifth God—to share the decision with other people."[40] As laudable as the notion of community decision making may be, the public perception that social worth was used as a criterion for living or dying was repulsive and led to the abandonment of the committee. Likewise, the New Jersey Supreme Court in the Karen Ann Quinlan case envisioned a multidisciplinary committee to review decisions to remove individuals from mechanical life support systems if they were in a persistent vegetative state in order to "diffuse the responsibility"[41] for the decision. This was soon seen as an improper use of such a committee; the court found medical prognosis the determining factor, and only qualified physicians could make this determination. Thus, New Jersey "ethics committees" have been replaced by "prognosis committees" made up entirely of consulting physicians.[42, 43]

Committee Functions

Ethics committees for complex treatment decisions have thus arisen for a variety of reasons, from confirming a medical diagnosis or prognosis, to selecting among candidates for a medical procedure, to reviewing research protocols. There is no obvious way to classify such committees, but they can be usefully viewed from the perspective of public policy if they are classified functionally. Such committees have two primary functions: protecting the health care institution and providers, and protecting the patient.

Institutions and their staffs often see the primary function of ethics committees as protecting them against potential legal liability for treating or not treating particular patients. This is, for example, the primary function of the early abortion review committees, the dialysis patient selection committees, and the Karen Quinlan "prognosis committees."[42, 43] By using committee review, legal liability can be either drastically minimized or eliminated altogether. This is a legitimate institutional goal, but such committees should probably be termed "risk-management" or "liability-control" committees instead of ethics committees.

The much more important potential function of ethics committees is the protection of the autonomy and dignity of individual patients. This is, for example, the primary function of IRBs, psychosurgery, and artificial heart committees, although their use also protects the institution. The notion is that, because of their unique vulnerability, some categories of patients merit special protection to ensure that their human rights are not violated. Some settings, such as institutions for the mentally ill and mentally retarded, also lend themselves to the "Human Rights" committee approach. Handicapped newborns are patients meriting protection, and a properly structured committee to protect infants (instead of institutions) may be desirable.

Infant Review Committees

The President's Commission concluded that "seriously erroneous decisions about the treatment of newborns" in this country "appear to be very rare." Those that do occur tend to happen because of one or more shortcomings in the current system:

1. Failure to communicate appropriate information to all involved in the decision;

2. Failure of all involved to understand the basis of a decision to treat or not to treat;

3. Taking actions without the informed approval of the parents or other surrogates.[34]

These concerns can probably be most directly and constructively addressed by requiring an expert consultant in the child's condition to explain the child's prognosis and treatment alternatives to both the attending physician and the child's parents. In cases in which treatment would be beneficial to the child, it should, of course, be rendered. In cases in which the benefits of therapy are "less clear," the President's Commission opined that an ethics committee "might be designated to review the decision making process."[34] The purpose of this review would include verification of the information used to make the decision, confirmation of the propriety of the decision, resolution of disputes concerning the decision, and, where necessary and appropriate, referral of the case to public agencies, including child protection services.

In the April 1985 regulations promulgated under authority of the 1984 Child Abuse Amendments[23] (like the January 1984 Baby Doe Regulations[15] on which they are based), the Administration took a step beyond the Presidential Commission's cautious suggestions about the potential usefulness of ethics committees and encouraged each recipient of federal funds that cares for infants to establish an Infant Care Review Committee (ICRC).*

---

*This part of the "Baby Doe" regulation was never challenged, since such ICRCs are not mandatory under the Baby Doe regulations (or under the Child Abuse regulations).[15, 23]

The proposed committee is composed of at least eight members, including a practicing physician, a practicing nurse, a hospital administrator, a social worker, a lawyer, a representative of a disability group, a lay community member, and a member of the facility's medical staff who shall be chairman.[23] The committee's function is twofold: (1) to assist the facility in developing standards, policies, and procedures for treating handicapped infants; and (2) to assist in making decisions concerning medically beneficial treatment in specific cases. When specific cases are decided, the ICRC is required to designate one member to act as a special advocate for the infant to ensure that "all considerations in favor of the provision of additional treatment are fully evaluated and considered by the ICRC." The ICRC must also engage in retrospective review of "all records involving the withholding or termination of medical or surgical treatment to infants."[23]

The proposal by the American Academy of Pediatrics (AAP) is similar in spirit to the Administration's, but it tilts more in the direction of protecting the institution by keeping difficult cases out of court than protecting the infant. The core committee itself is identical to the Administration's, with a pediatrician knowledgeable about the nursery taking the place of a staff physician, and two additions: a member of the clergy, and a "person trained in ethics or philosophy." This composition enhances the likelihood that "ethics" rather than medical issues will be discussed. The requirement for a "special advocate" for the infant has been eliminated, however, making it unclear whose function—if anyone's—it is to present the arguments in favor of treatment. This is troublesome given the ability of the committee to exclude even the infant's parents from "the deliberative portions of the meeting." Also, unlike the Administration's model, the AAP's proposal contains no substantive rules for the ethics committee to apply, not even the "Principles of Treatment of Disabled Infants," which the AAP itself helped draft.[23]

What Role for Ethics Committees?

Four basic roles have been suggested for ethics committees: education, consultation, policy making, and decision making. Ethics education is a laudable mission, but it generally requires an expert in the field to be effective. A group of nonexperts is unqualified to teach much of substance to other nonexperts, and thus the diverse ethics committee is unlikely to be an effective medical ethics educator (at least until the committee members themselves have mastered some of the aspects of the subject matter). Similarly, consultation is crucial, but almost always demands the knowledge or experience of an expert. If consultation concerning the patient's prognosis is indicated, for example, a medical expert in the particular condition the patient has should be consulted, not a committee of generalists. Nonetheless, consultation may be procedurally useful just to slow down the decision-making process so all relevant facts can be gathered and properly considered.

This leaves two realistic roles for ethics committees: policy making and individual case decision making. These are the two functions of one of the primary legal institutions in our country: the administrative or regulatory agency. Specifically, administrative agencies develop and promulgate agency policies through regulations and rule-making procedures (the procedures followed, for example, in developing the Baby Doe regulations). These regulations have *general applicability* to all persons who are subject to the agency's authority. In performing this function, the agency acts like a legislature. The second function these agencies perform is deciding in individual cases, through an adjudicatory process, if a *specific person* has violated its regulations. In performing this function, the agency acts like a court. Agencies are set up to regulate certain areas because of their expertise and because their procedures are less formal and more efficient than either legislatures or courts. This is, of course, the stated rationale for ethics committees: they have the expertise and closeness to the hospitals that legislatures lack, and they may be able to make quicker, less public, and more efficient decisions than courts.

Policy Making

Ethics committees have neither the authority nor the jurisdiction to make policy. And even if the hospital trustees delegate such authority to them, they are likely to succeed in formulating policy only in the short run. Ultimately it will be seen as illogical and unfair to have fundamentally different policies regarding the treatment of handicapped newborns at different hospitals, or even in different areas of the country. Policy in this area will have to be nationally based and consistent from one hospital to another. In the meantime, however, while there is no national consensus on the appropriate treatment of certain categories of handicapped newborns, some diversity may be both tolerable and desirable as a method to help shape a more universal policy. But, as soon as a national consensus does develop, it will not be fair or feasible for individual hospitals to ignore it and set their own idiosyncratic policies. For example, a brain death definition must be universal and socially acceptable.[44] Hospitals cannot alter the definition to suit their own purposes, even if it relates solely to using anencephalic infants as organ donors.

Individual Case Adjudication '

Individual case adjudication is the only function ethics committees might be uniquely suited to perform in the long run. Such adjudication should have three characteristics: (1) an impartial and competent tribunal; (2) the right of affected parties to participate through special procedural devices such as notice, opportunity to produce evidence, and the right to cross-examine opposing witnesses; and (3) a requirement that the decision be based on the record established before the tribunal and that it be consistent with accepted principles and rationally explained.[45] In the ethics committee context some modifications might be appropriate, but fairness to the parents and the child demands that each should be represented, in person or by someone of their choice, throughout the proceedings, with the opportunity to present and cross-examine witnesses. Whatever decision is reached should be on the basis of the evidence presented to the committee, and the evidence should be reviewed in a written document that contains a reasoned and principled basis for the decision. This implies two things: (1) a set of substantive principles upon which to base decisions must be developed before this procedure can be used in a nonarbitrary manner; and (2) since "due process" must be the primary concern of adjudication, a lawyer should be the chairman of the committee.

New decision-making procedures will ultimately be judged on the basis of three criteria: accuracy, efficiency, and acceptability.[45] Ethics committees will probably be as accurate as the current physician-patient, physician-parent model (and more accurate if they can gather relevant information that might not otherwise be considered), less efficient in terms of time and effort, and worthy of public acceptability only if their primary function is the protection of the infant. If their primary function is protection of the institution, such committees will serve only to postpone the day of infant-centered reform by temporarily creating the illusion that something is being done to protect handicapped newborns. Experimentation with such committees seems in order; however, it is premature to pretend that ethics committees can solve the very difficult substantive issues raised by neonatal rescue medicine by simply adding a procedural layer to the decision-making process. The development of substantive standards for decision making must remain our first priority.

Even though we strongly support the development of professional standards (with broad public input), attention to accurate factual development, and more procedural fairness in neonatal decision making, we are under no illusions that any completely acceptable standards or scheme will ever be developed. The area of treatment decisions for severely handicapped newborns is one of "tragic choices."[46] Basic to a tragic choice is "the inevitability of paradox, of unresolved tensions and ambiguities, of opposites in precarious balance. Like an arch, tragedy never rests."[47] True tragic choices have no happy outcomes, only better accommodations.

This conclusion will be unsatisfying to many because it implies that no easy answer will ever be found, but rather that we must continue to ponder what it means to be human in a technological age that sometimes permits "life" to be sustained long after any of the attributes we usually associate with humanness have disappeared. We think that it is worthwhile not only in itself to contemplate what it means to be human and attempt to identify the minimal attributes an infant should possess to merit treatment, but also because it forces physicians and others to concentrate on more than just medical technology and how it can be used. While the goal of defining "humanness" may be ultimately unreachable, it is a goal worthy of our efforts. Without such a goal, we are left to wander aimlessly, like the cowboys in Sam Shepard's play, *True West*. One of the cowboys chases the other; as we now pursue medical technology:

> They take off after each other straight into an endless black prairie. . .What they don't know is that each one of 'em is afraid, see. Each one separately thinks he's the only one that's afraid. And they keep ridin' like that straight into the night. Not knowing. And the one who's chasin' doesn't know where the other one is taking him. And the one who's being chased doesn't know where he's going.

Chapter 8 _____

Teratology

_____

Literally translated from Latin, "teratology" means the study of "monsters," the study of abnormal development and congenital malformations. By current convention, it denotes the study of abnormal embryonic and fetal* development as it is influenced by environmental agents (teratogens) such as drugs, chemicals, viruses, and radiation. Animal studies may help establish the teratogenic potential of an agent and define teratologic mechanisms, but the final proof that an agent is teratogenic in humans must be demonstrated in humans.

It is important to distinguish between a teratogen and mutagen. A teratogen acts on the somatic (nonreproductive) cells or tissues of the developing organism, causing structural or functional defects. Its effects are limited only to the individual fetus whose mother was exposed to the agent while pregnant. A mutagen acts on the germ cells and alters the genetic material, thereby affecting future generations.[1] Some agents, such as radiation, may have both teratogenic and mutagenic effects.

Until relatively recently, it was generally assumed that the mammalian embryo and fetus developed in a shielded environment, the maternal uterus, and that external factors did not have a significant influence on development.[2] With increasing use of x-ray film studies for obstetric management in the 1920s and 1930s, it was discovered that the fetus could be functionally and morphologically damaged by such extrinsic factors.[3]

*In this chapter we use the term embryo to identify the conceptus from implantation (end of second week of development) to the end of the eighth week of development, and fetus to identify the conceptus from the ninth week of development until birth.

Experimental teratology in the modern sense began in the 1940s when it was demonstrated that environmental factors such as maternal dietary deficiency and x-ray exposure could adversely affect intrauterine mammalian development,[4, 5] and the association between rubella infection and abnormal fetal development was recognized.[6] However, it was not until the thalidomide tragedy of the early 1960s, in which thousands of severely malformed infants were born as a consequence of the maternal use of this drug during early pregnancy, that the significance of teratology to clinical medicine came into sharp focus.[7] Today there is a growing recognition of the potential hazards to reproduction resulting from our increasingly toxic environment, whether formed by medicine, agriculture, or industry. As a leading commentator has noted:

> Morbid curiosity, mixed with a modicum of human sympathy, has from ancient times focused attention upon errors in development and abnormalities in the newborn, but it is only in this century that their acceptance as inescapable hazards of procreation has yielded to scientific inquiry into root causes and that a hope has been engendered of significantly reducing the risk. Ironically, . . . it was man's capacity for making things worse that did most to direct inquiry into causes and thus spark the hope of prevention.[3]

SCOPE OF THE PROBLEM

Drug utilization among pregnant women is surprisingly high. In summarizing drug exposures during more than 50,000 pregnancies, the National Institutes of Health (NIH) Collaborative Perinatal Study[8] determined that the average consumption was about four drugs per pregnant woman, excluding vitamins and iron. Twenty percent of the pregnant women avoided all medications, but 40% took drugs during the first trimester. The most common drugs included analgesics, sedatives, antiemetics, antibiotics, antihistamines, and diuretics. More than 1.2 billion drug prescriptions are written each year, there is unlimited self-administration of "over-the-counter" drugs, and approximately 500 new pharmaceutical products are introduced annually.[9] The potential for drug teratogenicity is thus truly remarkable. The risks for teratogenicity are escalated even further if environmental chemicals (e.g., industrial pollutants, food additives), physical agents (e.g., ionizing radiation, ultrasound), and infectious agents are added.

The most notable observation is that despite the numerous potential teratogenic hazards to which the human conceptus is invariably exposed, the vast majority of infants are born healthy. This may be attributed to homeostatic and adaptive protective processes of both the mother and the conceptus. Since absolute security from teratogenicity is unattainable, recognition and understanding of the causes and mechanisms of teratogenicity are likely to be most helpful in taking preventative measures.

GENERAL PRINCIPLES OF TERATOLOGY

Knowledge of the principles of teratology is basic to understanding the cause-and-effect relationships of any agent and its potential to cause a defect.[10] The most important determinant factors that govern teratogenicity are the specificity of the agent, the exposure time during embryonic or fetal development, the genotype of the mother and the conceptus, the dosage, and concurrent exposure to other agents.

Specificity of the Agent

Certain embryonic tissues have a relatively greater sensitivity to specific teratogenic agents, an effect termed organotropism. The primary action of teratogens may be variable:

(i) a teratogen may exert a direct action by itself or its metabolite(s) on the primordial embryonic organ which is to be malformed later or (ii) it may cause, first, some disturbance in certain embryonic tissues other than the respective primordium, and this newly formed condition could secondarily induce defective development of the primordium or (iii) the primary target of the action of a teratogen is not developing embryonic cells but certain maternal tissues or the placenta. Some disturbances caused in the latter secondarily lead to malformation in the embryo.[11]

Teratogenic agents may impinge upon developing cells to change their prescribed course in embryogenesis through various mechanisms including: (1) mutation; (2) chromosomal nondisjunction and breaks; (3) mitotic interference; (4) alteration of nucleic acid integrity of function; (5) depletion of precursors and/or substrates needed for biosynthesis; (6) alteration of energy sources; (7) enzyme inhibition; (8) osmolar imbalances; and (9) alteration of cellular membrane characteristics.[12] These mechanisms are believed to occupy a pivotal position in the series of events between the causative agent and the end result.

Exposure Time

Susceptibility to teratogenic agents varies with the developmental stage at the time of exposure.[10] Teratogenic susceptibility can be represented as a

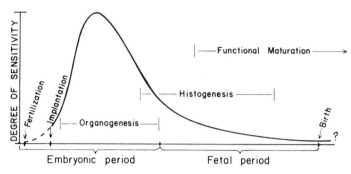

FIG 8–1.
Curve approximating teratogenic sensitivity at different periods in mammalian develop-ment. Although the curve does not apply specifically to any one species, it is more directly applicable to higher primates and man in which the fetal period is prolonged and post-natal development relatively insignificant except for nervous system functions. (From Wil-son JG: Environmental effects on development-delay, in Assali NS (ed): *Pathophysiology of Gestation.* New York, Academic Press, 1972, p 17. Used by permission.)

hypothetical curve in relation to various developmental processes (Fig 8–1). Knowledge of human embryonic differentiation can suggest the stages of susceptibility in humans for a given organ system. During approximately the first two weeks of embryogenesis, a teratogen can be lethal; however, if the embryo survives, no demonstrable adverse effects occur other than per-haps a slight delay in the overall developmental schedule.[10] Presumably, early embryonic cells have not achieved specific developmental roles. Thus, if one cell is destroyed, a surviving cell normally can assume its function unless the insult produced chromosomal or genetic abnormalities that inter-fere with the cell's metabolic processes. This is not, however, an absolute phenomenon but a general rule. Exceptions have been reported, at least in animal experimentation in which malformations were caused by chemical insults at the predifferentiation stage.[13, 14]

The period of organogenesis, characterized by the segregation of cell groups into primordia that will form future organs, is a time of particular vulnerability for induction of structural defects in organs and systems, and typically occurs before the woman knows she is pregnant.[10] Teratogens also act in an organ-specific fashion. A teratogen may affect one organ system at one stage of development and another system at another stage. The pre-cise time at which the insult occurs determines not only whether a malfor-mation will occur, but also the specific spectrum of anomalies. For example, in the rat, 100 rads of radiation produces no anomalies on days 8 to 11, but causes numerous anomalies on day 9 (eye, brain, spinal cord, heart, aortic arch, and urinary system) and day 10 (eye, brain, and urinary system).[12]

Following organogenesis (for most human organ systems, this is over by the fourth month), embryonic development is characterized primarily by increasing organ size and differentiation for specialized tissue needs. A teratogenic exposure at this time can affect the overall growth of the embryo or the size of a specific organ but usually will not produce a visible malformation.* For example, after the 12th week, administration of androgens to a pregnant woman may produce clitoral enlargement of her female fetus, but it will not cause displacement of the urethral orifice or labioscrotal fusion. Anomalies can also result from secondary effects. For example, hypertrophy of the intima of an artery could lead to vascular occlusion, causing secondary atrophy of a distal organ.

Finally, fetal enzyme development follows a well-defined sequence of maturation: different enzyme forms, with different substrate activities and specificities, appear at detectable stages. This ontogenic development is regulated by biologic signals (triggers), particularly hormones. However, stimulation by exogenous inducing agents may interfere and may possibly modify the normal arrangement. Because potential hazards to the fetus from transplacentally acquired drugs or other environmental toxins may derive from abnormally produced metabolites formed within the fetus, induction of fetal metabolic activity may be a determinant mechanism of teratogenicity.[15]

Genotype

Susceptibility to teratogens depends on the genotype of the embryo or fetus and the manner in which this interacts with environmental factors and the maternal phenotype (Fig 8–2).[10, 16] Genetic determinants give individuals, strains, and species their distinctive similarities and dissimilarities in normal structure and function. Analogously, variation in susceptibility to a potential teratogenic drug or toxic chemical depends on complex processes, which are at least partially under genetic control, including: (1) absorption; (2) biotransformation; (3) distribution; (4) exertion; and (5) interaction with receptor sites. Each of these five processes is controlled by different genes, hence by different proteins.[17] Twin studies on the half-life of various drugs have emphasized the importance of genetic factors in drug metabolism. Whenever a drug is given to identical twins and nonidentical twins, much more similarity in half-life has been observed for the identical twins.[17, 18]

---

*Brain and gonadal tissue, which continue to differentiate, are possible exceptions.

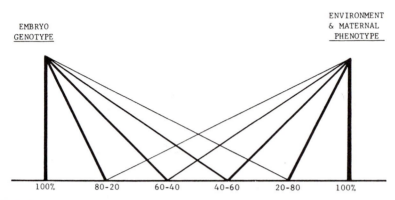

FIG 8–2.
Chart suggesting that relatively few developmental defects are caused by either genetic or environmental influences alone, and, instead, that most teratologic manifestations are caused by some ratio of interaction between the two. The maternal body (phenotype) is an important part of the embryo's environment, and as such it is able to influence both normal and abnormal development. (From Wilson JG: Environmental effects on development-delay, in Assali NS (ed): *Pathophysiology of Gestation*. New York, Academic Press, 1972, p 289. Used by permission.)

Pharmacogenetics

Pharmacogenetics may broadly be defined as the area of genetics that deals with variation among individuals (including embryos and fetuses) in response to drugs and toxic chemicals. Two categories of genetic influences may be recognized: (1) polygenic/multifactorial pharmacogenetic conditions, and (2) monogenic pharmacogenetic conditions.

Polygenic/Multifactorial Pharmacogenetic Conditions
For genetic traits, continuous variation is usually best explained on the basis of polygenic inheritance. This assumes that there are a large number of genes at different loci, each having a small individual effect, which cumulatively determine the phenotype of an individual with regard to a specific trait.† The usual model assumes that this continuation results in a normal distribution (the bell-shaped curve). These genes, of presumably minor individual effect, determine most ordinarily inherited differences (stature, skin color, blood pressure) between apparently normal people. When environmental factors are also involved, the term multifactorial is applied.

Assuming that past a given threshold (in the normal distribution of genes within the population), an abnormal phenotype can occur, then the

†See Chapter 1.

heritable nature of most common birth defects that are not known to result from chromosome abnormalities or single genetic mutation is explained. Most common anomalies are associated with normal chromosome complements and have too low a proportion of affected siblings (after one affected child the risk for any subsequent progeny is usually 2% to 5%, depending upon the anomaly) to reasonably support a hypothesis of simple Mendelian inheritance. The genetic aspect of several such conditions (cleft palate, pyloric stenosis, congenital hip dislocation) can be explained most satisfactorily by assuming polygenic inheritance with a threshold past which an abnormal phenotype would result. In a similar fashion, the susceptibility of an embryo or fetus to a teratogen may be described in terms of the polygenic/multifactorial inheritance model.‡

Monogenic Pharmacogenetic Conditions

Monogenic (Mendelian) factors can also be responsible for differences in teratogenic susceptibility. That is, a few individuals, embryos, and fetuses may be unusually sensitive or resistant to certain drugs or toxic chemicals because of a single mutant gene. Insight into genetically determined enzyme deficiencies have identified these conditions as special forms of "inborn errors of metabolism" in which the substrate is a drug or toxic chemical.[17] An important example is that of pseudocholinesterase deficiency, an autosomal recessive condition. The muscle relaxant succinylcholine chloride is a routinely used drug before the administration of general anesthesia to allow the easy insertion of an endotracheal tube. It is also used for patients undergoing electric shock treatment to help prevent muscle spasm injuries. Normally, the relaxing effect of succinylcholine chloride lasts only two to three minutes, because an enzyme known as pseudocholinesterase very quickly inactivates the drug. About 1 in 2,500 individuals is homozygous for an autosomal recessive mutation of the gene for pseudocholinesterase, however. Since the variant enzyme is ineffective at inactivating the drug, paralysis lasts much longer—hours, or even days—and may even be fatal unless respiration is artificially maintained. The difficulty can be reversed by transfusion of either normal plasma or a highly purified preparation of human enzyme.*

‡One of the first lines of evidence that demonstrated the importance of genetic influences on teratogenicity was that of cleft palate induced by cortisone in the mouse. The same dose administered under identical conditions produced a frequency of 100% in the A/J inbred strain and only 20% in the C57BL6 inbred strain.[19] In humans a similar example of susceptibility to norethindrone exists, in that only 18% of female offspring developed clitoral hypertrophy following administration of this drug to their mothers during a specific time and with a specific dose.[20]

*Other examples of monogenic pharmacogenetic abnormalities include warfarin resistance, heparin resistance, or inability to catabolize (decarboxylate) drugs like isoniazid or hydralazine.

Dose-Response

Manifestations of abnormal development increase in frequency and degree as dosage increases.[12] At any given time an embryo or fetus can respond to a teratogen in one of three ways, depending on the dose level: at a low dose there is no effect; at an intermediate dose a pattern of organ-specific malformations can result; at a high dose the embryo or fetus may be killed, causing the organ-specific teratogenic action to go unrecognized. Further increase in dosage eventually reaches the maternal lethal range. Although there is no standard ratio between maternal-effect levels and the embryotoxic ranges of dosage, animal data indicate that teratogens exert their action within a relatively narrow range, usually between one half to one fourth of the average dose (LD50)† that would kill the mother. The effect also depends upon the developmental stage during which the drug is administered. That is, an agent may be teratogenic at a given dose during one state of embryonic or fetal development, but teratogenic only at a higher or lower dose at a different stage. Similarly, at one dose level an agent might be lethal yet not teratogenic, whereas at another level it could be either lethal or teratogenic. In general, the preimplanted embryo has a lower LD50 than the fetus during organogenesis.[21]

The four basic processes that determine the actions of drugs are absorption, distribution, biotransformation, and excretion. During pregnancy, these processes and the multitudinous factors that can affect their rates must be considered, not only with respect to the physiologically transformed pregnant female, but also with respect to the embryo or fetus and the placenta.[22] The route of administration must also be considered, because some agents appear teratogenic only if administered in a particular fashion. This is probably related to absorption phenomena.

Finally, small doses administered over several days may produce a different effect than an equal total amount administered at one time. Sequential administration of small doses may induce an enzyme system that can degrade the teratogen, thus possibly causing less damage than if the entire dose were administered at one time. Conversely, a drug administered sequentially might destroy those cells that catabolize the drug, leading to more deleterious consequences than might otherwise be expected.

Concurrent Exposure

The teratogenic potential of one agent may be altered by exposure of the embryo or fetus to other agents, as well as to normal metabolites, and

---

†LD50 is the median lethal dose; a dose that is lethal to 50% of test subjects.

altered physiologic states. This is clinically important because drugs are frequently given to patients in combination. Examples of drug interactions include *p*-aminosalicylic acid, causing decreased gastrointestinal absorption of rifampin or isoniazid; compounds containing cations such as calcium, magnesium, aluminum, or iron, reducing the absorption of tetracyclines; and cholestyramine, delaying absorption of thyroxin, warfarin, and other acidic drugs.[17]

PROOF OF TERATOGENICITY

The most reliable test for teratologic risk in humans is one carried out in humans.[12] However, recognition of a teratogenic agent in humans is often difficult. Many isolated case reports and retrospective studies have suggested a strong association between particular environmental factors and the occurrence of congenital malformations. But such reports must be cautiously interpreted because they may represent mere association and are often based on tenuous data.

There are two major epidemiologic methods of examining a relationship between exposure and outcome. One method is to observe groups of individuals who differ in exposure and determine if they differ in the occurrence of the outcome of interest. This is most commonly referred to as a prospective or cohort study. The other approach is to select groups that differ in the presence of the outcome variable (cases and controls) and determine if they differ in terms of past exposure. This is referred to as a retrospective or case-control method. Statistical analysis is required in both instances to determine if an association between exposure and outcome differs from what would be expected by chance alone.*

Observations that may implicate a particular agent as a teratogen include:

1. The agent was associated more often with cases having a particular anomaly than with appropriate controls.

2. An anomaly or pattern of anomalies is consistently associated with the suspected teratogen.

3. The agent was present during the stage of organogenesis when the anomaly would have been likely to occur.

---

*There are, of course, many important considerations that enter into decisions of appropriate design for use in a specific study. The specific advantages and limitations of these epidemiologic methods are discussed in detail elsewhere.[23, 24] Terminology in the epidemiologic literature is not always consistently used; it is the method, not the label applied to it, that is important.

4. The anomaly was less common prior to the time the potential teratogen was available (e.g., phocomelia was almost unreported prior to the time thalidomide was introduced).

5. The anomaly can be produced in experimental animals by administration of the agent during a stage of organogenesis comparable to that believed to be involved in causing the anomaly in humans.†

It was not until the thalidomide catastrophe that regulatory agencies began to request the inclusion of teratogenicity studies as part of the toxicologic studies required prior to the release of chemicals as drugs, food additives, or pesticides. Through such monitoring it was hoped that the public's health could be safeguarded. No method of teratogenicity testing is universally applicable to all agents. The following recommendations have been made:

1. At least two species, one preferably nonrodent, should be utilized to determine potential teratogenic hazards of chemicals.

2. Rodent species that can be recommended are the mouse, the rat, and the hamster.

3. The nonrodent species currently recommended is the rabbit.

4. Research is required into the usefulness of additional nonrodent species in teratologic assessment.

5. Retrospective and prospective studies should be initiated when possible in human populations.

6. Additional data should be collected to permit accurate assessment of the effects of variables such as maternal age and ethnic origin on the normal incidence of malformations in the human population.[26]

TERATOGENIC AGENTS

Drugs and Chemicals

Table 8–1 lists those drugs with documented teratogenic effects that most often concern patients and frequently lead to questions in clinical practice. A detailed discussion of these agents is beyond the scope of this chapter.‡ The omission of certain agents from this list does not imply their safety has been proved.

†However, negative animal data do not prove that a drug is innocuous to humans.[25]
‡The reader is referred to other sources for additional information.[10, 27–29]

TABLE 8–1.
Documented Drug Teratogens in Humans

AGENT	EFFECTS	COMMENTS
Alcohol	Fetal growth retardation, microcephaly, mental retardation, short palpebral fissures, unusual dysmorphic facies, ± cardiac defects, occasional other major and minor malformations	30%–45% of infants born to women who drink 3 oz of pure alcohol daily (6 drinks) will have major signs of fetal alcohol syndrome. "Safe" amounts of alcohol consumption are uncertain. Ingestion of smaller amounts (1–2 oz) (2 drinks) may cause a small reduction in average birth weight and may or may not be associated with an increased risk of malformations.
Aminoglycosides (neomycin, kanamycin, gentamycin)	Eighth cranial nerve damage; hearing deficits	Risks primarily with prolonged exposures
Androgens (testosterone, ethinyl testosterone norethindrone, norethindrone acetate)	Masculinization of the external genitalia in female offspring; advanced genital development in male offspring	Labioscrotal fusion only prior to 12 weeks; after 12 weeks clitoral enlargement, but not labioscrotal fusion; minimal, if any, risks from oral contraceptives
Anticoagulants (warfarin [Coumadin], dicumarol).	Intrauterine growth retardation; nasal hypoplasia; stippled epiphyses; broad short hands; short distal phalanges; eye anomalies (optic atrophy, cataracts, microphthalmia); hypertelorism; mental retardation	Risk of full syndrome possibly as high as 25% when exposure in first trimester; later exposure associated with spontaneous abortions, stillbirths, abruptio placentae, and fetal or neonatal bleeding; anticoagulant of choice during pregnancy is heparin
Antithyroid drugs (e.g., iodine, propylthiouracil, methimazole)	Hypothyroidism, cretinism, hypertrophic fetal goiter	Goiter may result in hyperextension of the fetal head causing positional dystocia during labor; adverse effects usually avoidable by keeping mother on minimal maintenance dose *Continued.*

TABLE 8–1. *Continued*

AGENT	EFFECTS	COMMENTS
Chemotherapeutic drugs: folic acid antagonists (methotrexate, aminopterin); alkylating agents (busulfan, chlorambucil, cyclophosphamide)	Increased frequency of spontaneous abortions; variety of structural functional defects	Folic acid antagonists contraindicated for treatment of psoriasis during pregnancy; if used for the treatment of neoplastic diseases, patients should be counseled regarding uncertain (but probably high) teratogenic risks
Diethylstilbestrol (DES)	Females: vaginal adenosis and clear cell adenocarcinoma; cervicovaginal structure defects (e.g., transverse ridges, septa, cervical stenosis, cervical incompetence); upper müllerian duct system anomalies (e.g., "T"-shaped endometrial cavity, hypoplastic uterus, fallopian tube structural defects) Males: epididymal cysts, hypotrophic testis, microphallus, varicocele, capsular induration, altered semen analysis	Vaginal adenosis in about 50% of women whose mothers took DES in first trimester; risk of adenocarcinoma about 1/1000 in exposed women
Isotretinoin (Accutane)	Increased abortion rate, nervous system defects, microtia, cardiovascular defects, microphthalmos, cleft palate, and craniofacial defects	Used in treatment for severe cystic acne, first trimester exposure results in approximately 25% frequency of anomaly
Lithium	Congenital heart defects, most commonly Ebstein anomaly	Drug used in manic-depressive psychosis; risk of cardiac malformation as high as 8% if exposure in first trimester; late pregnancy exposure associated with toxic effects on the neuromuscular system, thyroid, and kidneys
Phenytoin (Dilantin, hydantoin, diphenylhydantoin)	Fetal growth retardation, microcephaly, developmental delays, and mental	Full spectrum of anomalies may occur in 5% to 10% of exposed infants;

Drug	Anomalies/Effects	Comments
	retardation; dysmorphic craniofacial features, including a short nose with depressed nasal bridge, hypertelorism, ptosis of the eyelids, strabismus, and a wide mouth; hypoplastic nails and distal phalanges; occasional cleft lip, cleft palate, cardiac anomalies, and genitourinary anomalies	additional number may show some features of the syndrome
Streptomycin (dihydrostreptomycin)	Eighth cranial nerve damage; hearing deficits	Risks primarily with prolonged exposures
Tetracycline	Hypoplasia and discoloration (yellow, gray, brown) of tooth enamel; tetracycline incorporated into bone	Tetracycline has no proved adverse effect in the first trimester; adverse effects occur in second or third trimester exposures
Thalidomide	Bilateral limb anomalies (amelia, phocomelia, radial reductions); absence of the external and internal ears; cardiac anomalies; various other anomalies	The most vulnerable period for teratogenicity between days 35 and 48 after the last menstrual period, with 20% of exposed infants showing effects; no teratogenic effects seen in rodents
Trimethadione (paramethadione)	Cleft lip and/or palate; cardiac anomalies; microcephaly; mental retardation and developmental delay; "V"-shaped eyebrows; low-set ears with anteriorly folded helix; irregular teeth	Previously used for treatment of petit mal seizures; 80%–90% of first trimester exposures resulted either in spontaneous abortion or infant with congenital anomalies
Valproic acid (Depakene)	Neural tube defects; risk for other anomalies not yet well assessed	Commonly used drug for seizure disorders; incidence of neural tube defects (NTDs) in exposed fetuses is 1%–2%. Women exposed during the first trimester should be offered prenatal diagnosis for NTDs (amniotic fluid measurement of α-fetoprotein and ultrasonographic studies).

Alcohol Consumption

Concern regarding alcohol consumption during pregnancy dates back to biblical times: "Behold, thou shalt conceive, and bear a son; and now drink no wine or no strong drink. . ." (Judges 13:7). However, it was not until recently that a specific dysmorphic condition, the so-called fetal alcohol syndrome (FAS) characteristic of offspring of chronic alcoholic mothers was described.[30, 31] The Fetal Alcohol Study Group of the Research Society on Alcoholism has recommended that the diagnosis of FAS be made only when the patient has signs in each of these three categories:

> *Prenatal and/or postnatal retardation* (weight, length, and/or head circumference below the tenth percentile when corrected for gestational age).
> *Central nervous system damage* (signs of neurological abnormality, developmental delay, or intellectual impairment).
> Characteristic *facial dysmorphology* with at least two of these three signs: (1) microcephaly (head circumference below the third percentile); (2) microphthalmia and/or short palpebral fissures; (3) poorly developed philtrum, thin upper lip, and/or flattening of the maxillary area.[32]

This syndrome may not be due to alcohol per se; other factors such as poor protein intake, pyridoxine or other B-vitamin deficiency, alcohol contaminants like lead, or genetic predisposition may play important etiologic roles.

The incidence of FAS is difficult to specify because of variabilities in study populations and differences in research methodologies. Several investigators have estimated that there are one to three cases of FAS per 1,000 live births.[33–35] However, much higher frequencies have been reported for certain populations, for example, for American Indians on some reservations.[36, 37] There will be an estimated 1,800 to 2,400 new cases of FAS each year in the United States.[38] Some children do not show the full FAS but exhibit some manifestations of the syndrome. The term "possible fetal alcohol effects" (FAE) has been applied in such cases. The most commonly observed anomaly in FAE has been growth retardation. Possible fetal alcohol effects occur far more frequently than FAS, with an estimated incidence of 36,000 cases per year in the United States.[38]

There is no consensus as to the dose-response relationship with respect to the amount and/or pattern of alcohol consumption by a pregnant woman and the likelihood of adverse effects on her fetus. It even remains unknown whether there exists a minimum "safe" level of alcohol consumption or whether any consumption of alcohol produces some risk to the fetus.[39] Naturally, the most pronounced fetal effects have been found to occur with the heaviest and most prolonged maternal drinking. In terms of amount, the smallest reported quantity associated with full-blown FAS was six bottles of beer (about 2.5 ounces of ethanol) taken daily throughout pregnancy; the shortest duration of drinking related to FAS was the first eight weeks of pregnancy only. *When* drinking occurs is probably also an important factor. In one recent study, an average daily consumption of as little as 10 gm of ethanol (about one drink) in the week prior to recognition of pregnancy was related to a decrease in infant birth weight of 225 gm (after adjustment for gestational age, sex of child, and maternal age, weight, height, pregnancy weight gain, social class, gravidity, and parity).[40] Another study showed that women who reduced their drinking early in their pregnancies had infants with less growth retardation than women who continued to drink heavily.[41] There is no good information from human studies on the effects of "binge" drinking as compared to regular drinking by pregnant women, but animal work has indicated that acute ethanol doses of critical amounts can have detrimental consequences.[42]

A review of both animal and clinical research data concluded that a clear relationship between alcohol use and adverse pregnancy outcome has been demonstrated only for heavy and prolonged maternal alcohol abuse of at least 5.0 oz of absolute alcohol per day.[39, 43] However, other effects are clearly induced with lesser alcohol intake. Although a numerical value for a safe pattern of alcohol consumption during pregnancy cannot be specified, these studies conclude that there is currently no evidence for adverse effects associated with "light" alcohol consumption, such as one glass of wine each day (0.5 oz of absolute alcohol per day).[39, 43]

What, then, are the current recommendations regarding alcohol consumption during pregnancy? The American Council of Science and Health concluded in 1981 that the intake of large amounts of alcohol is clearly hazardous to fetal development.[44] The Council further stated that although no safe levels of alcohol ingestion have been defined (or ever would be), the health risks associated with small amounts are low, if they exist at all. They recommended that women should be cautious about alcohol consumption during pregnancy. Those who choose to drink should limit alcohol consumption to two drinks or less a day. While recognizing that total abstinence was the safest course, the Council expressed concern that excessive health warnings might confuse perceptions of hypothetical risks and thereby desensitize some women to all warnings.[44]

Based upon their own review of the scientific literature, the American Medical Association Council on Scientific Affairs issued a report in 1983 on the effects of maternal alcohol use.[45] The Council concluded that pregnant women who drink heavily place their fetuses at risk, and that there is a possibility of a dose-response phenomenon through which different levels of alcohol intake may be approximately associated with differing degrees and types of adverse effects. Fetal risks from moderate or minimal alcohol consumption have not been established. The Council made the following recommendations: (1) physicians should be alert to signs of alcohol abuse among women of child-bearing age and take appropriate diagnostic and therapeutic measures; (2) until more definitive information is available, physicians should inform patients what research does and does not show and encourage them to decide about drinking in light of the evidence and their own situations; and (3) although there is no definitive research support of statements linking low amounts of alcohol consumption with adverse fetal effects, physicians should advise their patients that abstinence is the safest course.[45]

Cigarette Smoking

Cigarette smoking is probably the most common addiction among women in our society. Smoking during pregnancy may result in a wide spectrum of biochemical and physiologic alterations in both the mother and the fetus including the following: (1) interference with the fetal oxygen supply due to carbon monoxide and its functional inactivation of fetal and maternal hemoglobin; (2) vasoconstrictive action of nicotine causing reduced perfusion of the placenta; (3) reduced appetite and, in turn, reduced caloric intake by women who smoke; (4) decreased maternal plasma volume; (5) reduction in maternal blood levels of vitamin B_{12}, vitamin C, folate, and other substances essential for tissue growth, collagen formation, and integrity of blood vessel linings; (6) reduction in leukocyte RNA synthesis, phosphokinase activity, and in the plasma levels of 14 amino acids (eight essential ones) and carotene; and (7) increased maternal plasma norepinephrine and epinephrine and serum cortisol concentrations.[46, 47]

Possible interference with placentation or implantation has been suggested by the observed increased rate of spontaneous abortions among women who smoke. A prospective Swedish study showed that smokers had a 20% increase in the spontaneous abortion rate among wanted pregnancies and a 34% increase if the pregnancy was unwanted.[48] In another retrospective, case-controlled study, which took into account a number of variables such as age, number of previous spontaneous abortions, induced abortions, and live births, the spontaneous abortion rate was 41% among smokers compared to 28% for controls (odds ratio of 1.8).[49] A 1975 study of a large group of spontaneous abortions found a significant *reduction* in chromosome aberrations in the abortuses of women who inhaled cigarettes.[50] This rate was 50% as compared to the noninhalers' rate of 62%. This increase in abortuses with normal karyotypes was explained by an increase of spontaneous abortions (of chromosomally normal embryos) as a result of cigarette smoking.* Smoking during pregnancy has also been implicated in causing an increased risk for the offspring having mental developmental abnormalities (hyperactivity, short attention span, lower scores on spelling and reading tests), congenital malformations, sudden infant death syndrome, and cancer.[52, 56–58]

The best documented adverse effect of smoking during pregnancy is fetal growth retardation. A review of five studies, comprising nearly 113,000 births in the United States, Canada, and Wales, found that from 21% to 39% of the incidence of low birth weight was attributable to maternal cigarette smoking.[59] Infants of smokers weighed 100 to 300 gm less at birth than babies of comparable nonsmokers, and the proportion of babies weighing less than 2,500 gm usually doubles with maternal smoking.[47, 55] The term, "fetal tobacco syndrome," has recently been proposed to apply to an infant when the following four conditions are met:

1. The mother smoked five or more cigarettes a day throughout the pregnancy.

2. The mother had no evidence of hypertension during pregnancy (specifically, no history of preeclampsia and documentation of normal blood pressure at least once the first trimester).

3. The newborn has symmetrical growth retardation at term (>37 weeks), defined as: a birth weight less than 2,500 gm, and a ponderal index [(weight in gm)/(length in cm)] greater than 2.32.

4. There is no other obvious cause of intrauterine growth retardation (e.g., congenital infection or anomaly).[60]

The American College of Obstetricians and Gynecologists (ACOG) has recommended that, "Ideally, the patient should plan to stop smoking entirely and permanently."[61] ACOG, however, recognizes that it may be more realistic to attempt to eliminate or reduce smoking during pregnancy. Specific recommendations are:

---

*Data from the Ontario Perinatal Mortality Study showed that perinatal mortality increased directly with the level of maternal smoking during pregnancy.[51] Increases in smoking levels were also associated with increases in the frequency of early fetal death and of neonatal deaths due to premature delivery. These deaths were, in turn, linked to smoking-related increases in the incidence of bleeding during pregnancy, abruptio placentae (premature separation of the placenta), placenta previa (a placenta which develops in the lower uterine segment, in the zone of dilation), and the premature and prolonged rupture of the membranes. These findings have also been observed by others.[52–55]

1. Identify the smoker at the first prenatal visit and then begin an intensive education program about the dangers of smoking.

2. Consider obtaining a baseline carboxyhemoglobin level at the first visit and then repeating these at intervals throughout pregnancy . . . [to use] as objective evidence to the patient that smoking has resulted in abnormal change.

3. Education by example is important. Smoking should be prohibited within the clinic and hospital setting.[61]

Possible legal approaches to both alcohol and cigarette consumption during pregnancy include outlawing the sale of alcohol or cigarettes to pregnant women, placing warning labels on containers, and posting warning notices in bars and taverns.[62, 63] Prohibition of sales to pregnant women is unlikely to be effective (since other individuals can purchase these items for them) and seems excessively draconian and discriminatory.[64] Posting warnings at public places also seems excessive and may also be counterproductive, as women may react to such "warnings" by assuming the notices are just silly and overly cautious. Warning labels are reasonable, as long as they convey scientifically sound information. Even though education's history of changing health habits is "rather bleak,"[65] attempting to do more than educate by sound information and example will likely lead to coercive measures to force unwilling adults to change their life-styles. Such force will not be successful unless it is excessive and involves measures such as fines and imprisonment for disobedience and surveillance that is debasing and demeaning in a free society.† While we believe women should drink only moderately, if not at all, during pregnancy and should cease smoking altogether, we do not believe we should adopt criminal laws to foster this behavior.‡ Almost all women take every reasonable step to protect their fetuses from harm, and it is the responsibility of society and the medical profession to let women know what these steps are and to give them the opportunity and resources to make them realistic.

---

†Horror specialist Stephen King gives us one example of effective coercion in his short story "Quitters, Inc." Quitters promises its clients that they *will* stop smoking, without drugs or sermons. The company was set up by a Mafia chief, who shortly thereafter died of lung cancer. The company's "pragmatic" approach was simple. The first time an individual smoked another cigarette, their spouse was subjected to a series of electric shocks while the client was forced to watch; this was repeated, with increasing voltage, eight times; the ninth time, the arms of the client's child were broken. If an unusual client slipped a tenth time, he was killed and became part of the company's 2% failure rate.

‡For a more detailed rationale against the use of force in pregnancy see the discussion on maternal-fetal conflicts in Chapter 10.

Chemical Teratogens in the Workplace

There has been an increasing awareness over recent decades of the potential hazards to the embryo-fetus of chemical agents encountered in the workplace. Since World War II the number of women of childbearing age in the work force has increased dramatically, and equal rights to work have put women who may be pregnant in contact with agents and stresses previously not commonly encountered. As early as 1942, the US Department of Labor recommended that pregnant women avoid occupational exposure to certain known toxic substances. However, epidemiologists within industry have been concerned with the dearth of refined methods and lack of a discernible overall scientific approach to assessing reproductive hazards in humans.[66] Many chemicals have been tested for teratogenic potential in laboratory animals. Chemicals have been identified that are consistently positive in multiple species; others, consistently negative; and the rest, between extremes. But animal teratology cannot provide definitive answers to problems of human reproductive health. The ability to detect developmental toxicity in human populations depends on the frequency of the event as well as the uniqueness of the alteration compared with the background level. The background level in human spontaneous abortion, stillbirths, mental retardation, and malformation is high enough to make it difficult to detect an agent contributing slightly to the occurrence of such abnormalities.

As with nearly all other potential adverse effects of exposure to toxic amounts of chemicals, protection to concepti is generally directed through "management" of exposure, often by removing women from the workplace.[67] Available experimental and epidemiologic data characterizing adverse effects of chemicals have been used to formulate guidelines to protect workers such as those established by the US Occupational Safety and Health Administration (OSHA), or the Threshold Limit Value (TLVs) set by the American Conference of Governmental Industrial Hygienists (ACGIH), or the Maximal Allowable Concentrations (MACs) by the Federal Republic of Germany, which fixed upper limits of exposure as a function of chemical concentration and duration of exposure. These levels are selected on the basis of the most sensitive findings and appropriate margins of safety, depending on the nature of the toxic effects that are the limiting factors. To date, however, no OSHA standard, TLV, or MAC has been imposed in which teratologic effects have been the most sensitive parameter to select limits of exposure. Instead, other toxicologic effects have been the determining factors in selection of guidelines.

The American College of Obstetricians and Gynecologists has recommended that evaluation of the pregnant worker "include information on the work activity, including physical stress and chemical exposure." Contact with occupational physicians and nurses at the woman's work site is suggested for specific exposure information and assisting in observation between visits. "Synergistic effects of existing medical problems, self-medication, or physical stresses or toxic chemicals in the home" must also be taken into account.[68]

In an effort to make physicians more aware of the hazards of the workplace to pregnant workers, the Council on Scientific Affairs' Advisory Panel on Reproductive Hazards in the Workplace recently prepared a report reviewing the exposure effects of 120 chemicals.[69] These agents were considered for review based on an estimation of their imminent hazard, i.e., widespread use and/or inherent toxicity.* Just a few of the many areas of concern are presented in Table 8–2. Omission of any chemical from Table 8–2 does not mean that its safety has been proved, and much more research is needed.

Radiation

It is now well recognized that x-rays adversely affect human prenatal development as well as that of all laboratory species tested. In humans an increased incidence of fetal and neonatal death, central nervous system defects, and growth retardation has been associated with in utero exposure to therapeutic pelvic irradiation, and exposure to atomic bomb radiation in Hiroshima and Nagasaki.[72–76]

Maternal exposure to radiation usually occurs, however, because of medical indication on a selective basis (e.g., pelvimetry) or unknowingly, as in a chest x-ray film, gastrointestinal series or intravenous pyelogram. Such prenatal exposures produce more emotional responses by lay persons and physicians alike than any other agent to which women are exposed during pregnancy. There is good evidence to indicate that exposures in the range of diagnostic x-ray films (200 to 5,000 millirads) present an extremely low risk to the embryo. Both animal and human data support the conclusion that there is no increased risk in the incidence of congenital malformations as compared to the general population risk.[77] This does not mean, however, that there is a categorical "zero" risk to the embryo exposed to lower doses of radiation. Whether there exists a linear or exponential dose-response relationship or a threshold exposure for genetic, carcinogenic, cell-depleting, and life-shortening effects has not been determined. A recent review concluded, "Medically indicated diagnostic roentgenograms are appropriate for

---

*It is beyond the scope of this chapter to provide a detailed discussion of the numerous potentially teratogenic chemicals found in the workplace. Excellent reviews are available.[70, 71]

pregnant women, and there is no justification for terminating a wanted pregnancy in women exposed to 5 rads or less because of a radiation hazard."[77]

Diagnostic radiation rarely exceeds exposure doses of greater than 5 rads. For example, a chest x-ray film, cholecystogram, upper gastrointestinal

TABLE 8–2.
Selected Environmental Chemicals That May Be Potentially Teratogenic in Humans

CHEMICAL AGENT	EFFECTS	COMMENTS
Carbon disulfide	Increased frequency of spontaneous abortions and premature births	Menstrual disorders in exposed females; oligospermia and libido and erection failure in exposed males
Carbon monoxide	Increased frequency of spontaneous abortions and stillbirths; low birth weight; brain damage (microcephaly, spasticity, retarded psychomotor development)	
Dichloro-diphenyl-trichloro-ethane (DDT)	Increased frequency of premature deliveries	
Inhalation anesthetics	Increased frequency of spontaneous abortions in women chronically exposed; no evidence for increased risk of malformations in offspring	Suggested increased risk of spontaneous abortions in wives of chronically exposed males
Lead	Increased frequency of spontaneous abortions and stillbirths, neurologic defects, intrauterine growth retardation, and postnatal failure to thrive	Risk probably increased with lead concentrations in maternal blood of greater than 400 mg/L
Methyl mercury	Cerebral palsy, chorea, ataxia, tremors, seizures, mental retardation, polyneuritis, and blindness	Teratogenic effects can occur even in third-trimester exposure; methyl mercury selectively concentrated in the fetal brain, resulting in atrophy of the granular layer of the cerebellum and a spongiose softening in the visual cortex and other cortical areas
Polychlorinated biphenyls (PCBs)	Dark ("cola" colored) skin, eye defects, premature tooth eruption, gingival hypertrophy, hypotonia, and severe acne	Widely used as plasticizers and heat exchange fluids, PCBs break down slowly under natural conditions and accumulate in the food chain. These chemicals are preferentially stored in tissues with high fat content.
Smoking	Increased frequency of abortions, stillbirths, and neonatal deaths; intrauterine growth retardation	Maternal cigarette smoking associated with increased frequencies of abruptio placentae and placenta previa; decidual necrosis at the margin of the placenta significantly more frequent in smokers than in nonsmokers
Vinyl chloride	Increased frequency of spontaneous abortions, central nervous system defects, craniofacial anomalies, genital organ defects	

series, intravenous pyelogram, and barium enema deliver 5, 300, 330, 585, and 485 millirads, in that order.[78] Concern has been expressed over a dose of 5 to 10 rads. But from a practical standpoint serious risk to the fetus does not occur until a dose of 10 rads or more has been absorbed. If the fetus absorbs 50 rads or more at any time during gestation, there is a significant possibility that the fetus might be damaged, with growth retardation, microcephaly, and mental retardation being the predominant observable effects.[77] No report of a bona fide radiation-induced congenital malformation has been made in a human being that has not exhibited growth retardation or a central nervous system abnormality. Finally, if the dose absorbed by the embryo during the early stages of organogenesis amounts to several hundred rads, there is a reasonable possibility that the embryo might abort. Later in pregnancy such exposures are less likely to result in spontaneous abortion, but irreparable injury to the central nervous system can occur.[77]

In 1977, the American College of Obstetricians and Gynecologists, in cooperation with the American College of Radiology, issued a statement of policy on diagnostic x-ray film use in fertile women.[78] The recommended guidelines are:

> The use of x-ray examination should be considered on an individual basis. Concern over harmful effects should not prevent the proper use of radiation exposure when significant diagnostic information can be obtained . . .
> There is no measurable advantage to scheduling diagnostic x-ray examinations at any particular time during a normal menstrual cycle [since the developing ovum is at risk prior to ovulation as well as subsequently].
> The degree of risk involved in an x-ray examination if the person is pregnant, or may become pregnant, should be explained to the patient and documented in her record.

TERATOGEN COUNSELING

In our current environment, pregnant women, and those contemplating pregnancy, are inevitably exposed to scores of agents that are potential teratogens. A major problem is determining the level of risk or safety of such exposures. As detailed earlier, any statement about human teratogenesis must, by definition, be incomplete. Only a few agents have undergone scientific scrutiny well enough to define hazards or safety and thereby provide clinically relevant information. Unfortunately, the vast majority of agents have been inadequately studied for their teratogenic potential.[79]

How then should the physician approach counseling patients about possible teratogenicity? The first step is gathering information that is as current and complete as possible through a careful literature search.* The physician may also wish to consult with or refer such a patient to a health professional with special education or experience in teratology and birth defects.

The counseling session should be performed in a sympathetic manner so that the patient is not unduly alarmed or burdened by guilt.† Most questions will involve agents of either low-level risk or unknown risk. Couples must be provided with a careful explanation of general principles of teratology, the 2% to 3% background level of birth defects in the general population, and the possibility of individual susceptibility of a given fetus to any specific agent. The period of development during which the conceptus is exposed to an agent should be taken into account. Although a categorical "zero" risk can never be given, cautious general reassurance can usually be provided. When faced with a situation in which a drug is deemed necessary for the health of the woman or her embryo or fetus, we suggest a course of therapeutic nihilism. That is, only the most necessary therapeutic agent with the least known teratogenic potential should be given for the shortest period of time possible to achieve the therapeutic result. The risk-benefit ratio must always be carefully weighed, and the pregnant woman should give her informed consent.

Certain patients, however, will have been exposed to agents that are recognized as associated with a significant teratogenic potential. They must be counseled regarding the known risks to the conceptus and the spectrum of abnormalities that might occur. These couples frequently inquire about prenatal diagnosis and should be informed that amniocentesis for chromosomal analysis is not specifically informative for this category of birth defects. Amniocentesis to determine the level of α-fetoprotein may be diagnostically useful in certain exposures. For example, the incidence of neural tube defects is in the order of 1% to 2% in fetuses exposed to valproic acid during the first trimester.[80] Ultrasonography may detect some anatomical defects; however, a negative study does not necessarily mean that the fetus has not been affected. Given the choice between giving birth to a child with a significant risk of having a serious defect and that of aborting, many couples choose the latter. Psychological support for the couple's decision should be provided. In particular, follow-up counseling is advised for after

---

*Additional information may be available through the following resources: Center for Disease Control, Office of Public Inquiries, Birth Defects Branch, 1600 Clifton Road, N.E., Atlanta, Georgia 30333, (404) 329–3534; and Environmental Teratology Information Center, P.O. Box 12233, Mail Drop 1801, Research Triangle Park, NC 27709, (919) 541–3418.

†See Chapter 2 on counseling.

the abortion or after the birth of an affected baby. Technical multispecialty support for the handicapped infant is essential.‡

PUBLIC POLICY ISSUES IN THE WORKPLACE

The premier public policy issue in the workplace is expressed in the question, how can the fetus be protected from harm without discriminating against fertile and pregnant women workers? This is an especially critical issue since more than half of all women over 18 are in the work force, and their proportionate share for financing child rearing is growing. We are nowhere near achieving equality in the work force. Pay differentials between men and women have narrowed, but the average man continues to earn "almost 50 percent more per hour than does the average woman of the same race, age, and education."[81] Motherhood is the major factor responsible for this differential, and as long as women remain primarily responsible for child rearing, these sex differences in the labor market are likely to persist. While fair fetal protection policies will not ensure equality, they can at least ensure that an unfair situation is not made worse. The long-term goal, of course, must be to clean up the workplace so that neither women nor men are exposed to harmful chemicals and other mutagens and teratogens simply as a consequence of working.

Without losing sight of this goal, it is useful to understand the significant limitations current law and regulatory agencies have in this area. The primary regulatory agencies are the Occupational Safety and Health Administration (OSHA), the Environmental Protection Agency (EPA), and the Nuclear Regulatory Commission (NRC). The primary regulator of hazardous occupational exposures for over 75 million US workers, OSHA is charged with ensuring that employers provide their workers a work environment free from "recognized hazards" likely to cause death or serious physical harm. Although OSHA can promulgate permanent health standards for a single hazardous substance or group or class of substances, it has been persuasively argued that its rules can apply only to employees directly (and not to fetuses), and thus that OSHA has no direct jurisdiction over fetal protection policies.[81]

The EPA has authority to regulate certain exposures to reproductive health hazards and has concentrated its efforts on pesticide manufacturers (who are required to submit information on the potential reproductive effects of their products) and farmworkers (who are often exposed to pesticides and herbicides). No single agency regulates radiation exposure. The

‡See Chapter 7.

EPA is revising the 1980 federal radiation protection guidelines for workers. The regulations of the Nuclear Regulatory Commission provide for maximum exposure levels, including limitations on exposure to gonads and lifetime cumulative dose, and protection of minors.[81]

At least 15 of the Fortune 500 companies have policies that exclude fertile and/or pregnant women from some jobs. Exclusionary policies vary greatly, and are subject to Title VII of the Civil Rights Act of 1964 that prohibits employment discrimination on the basis of sex. The Pregnancy Discrimination Act of 1978, an amendment to Title VII, specifically forbids discrimination on the basis of pregnancy, childbirth, or related medical conditions. There are two basic exceptions that permit discrimination. The first is if a "bona fide occupational qualification" exists that is reasonably necessary to the normal operation of the business (e.g., actress, sperm donor, guard at violent male prison). Courts have also concluded that a "business necessity" can be used to set standards for employment even though these will exclude most women from consideration. Three tests must be met: the reason for the rule must be compelling; it must carry out a business purpose effectively; and there must be no acceptable alternative. Examples include educational qualifications, strength and agility tests, height and weight requirements, and previous experience.

Federal court rulings on Title VII suggest a fetal protection policy that applies only to women is presumptively discriminatory. To overcome the presumption, the employer must produce scientific evidence that the exposure level in the workplace involves a significant risk of harm to unborn children of female but not male employees, and that the policy significantly reduces the risk. However, even if the employer proves this, discrimination may still be proved by demonstrating that an acceptable alternative policy would protect unborn children with a less adverse impact on women.[82–85]

While these agencies and federal laws offer some assistance to some women, in general it seems fair to conclude that companies can get away with very restrictive fetal protection policies and that women will seldom be able to challenge them effectively in court. Nor are state worker compensation laws helpful. Compensation is not available for loss of reproductive function because this is not a *job* disability. Nor is compensation available for loss of a fetus or damage to a fetus because the injury must be *personal*, and not one suffered by someone other than the worker. Thus, workers have no remedies under workers' compensation systems in most states for adverse reproductive effects suffered on the job.[82]

This leaves workers who suffer reproductive injuries with the tort system. Workers will not be permitted to sue their employers in most cases, because workers' compensation is their exclusive (albeit inadequate) remedy for injury on the job. They *may*, however, be able to sue the product's manufacturer in certain cases (e.g., the asbestos cases)[86] in which exposure was from a product the employer purchased from another manufacturer. On the other hand, the fetus is not an employee, and so may be able to sue its mother's employer if it is injured by a negligent or intentional exposure to a teratogen. It is primarily because of this *potential* liability that companies are adopting "fetal protection policies." The label notwithstanding, their real purpose seems to be "company asset protection." All states now recognize the right to bring a lawsuit for prenatal injuries, although many jurisdictions deny recovery unless the fetus has reached the stage of viability at the time of the injury. Although a theoretical possibility, there are two strong reasons why such an action might fail. The first is that the injury occurred prior to viability in a state that required it to occur after viability for recovery. Since most teratogens are likely to act on previable fetuses, this is a major drawback. In addition, even when the fetus has standing to sue, causation will be an extremely difficult issue to prove given the high background rate of handicaps, and the confounding factors such as nonemployment exposure to various teratogens. Thus it should come as no surprise that there is no record of any successful lawsuit by a damaged child against its mother's employer for prenatal injury.[82]

All this, of course, begs the question: what policy should employers and employees adopt regarding fetal protection? The first option, as previously noted, should be to eliminate the hazardous exposure to all workers. If this is not possible, because of prohibitive cost or lack of knowledge of a safe level, a fetal protection policy that optimizes worker privacy and autonomy while providing reasonable protection to the fetus should be the general goal. A sound starting assumption is that women employees will do everything reasonable to protect their fetuses, including taking whatever steps are necessary, if given the opportunity to do so, in an atmosphere that does not penalize them (by demotion, firing, or mandatory leave without pay). This mandates that all workers be informed of all hazardous exposures, including teratogens. Unions must insist on this as a minimum. Men and women working with teratogens must understand the risks to their fetuses and every effort should be made to provide them with the *option* to work at another job for a period of time during which they begin to attempt pregnancy, until after they give birth, without loss of seniority. Monitoring women for pregnancy would be a terrible invasion of their privacy and would likely be only minimally effective since damage to the fetus may have already occurred by the time the pregnancy is confirmed.

In the end, pregnant women must be responsible for their fetuses. We believe this responsibility should be primarily ethical and moral, and not legally enforced.* The state can, however, foster responsible parenthood by

---

*See discussion of maternal-fetal conflicts in Chapter 10.

funding research on mutagens and teratogens, encouraging employers to clean up their workplaces, enforcing the provisions of Title VII to prohibit discrimination on the basis of sex, and requiring employers to notify workers of all hazardous substances they are likely to come into contact with on the job, and what hazards exposure to these substances might have on their offspring. Given reasonable governmental and employer policies, prospective parents are likely to act in the best interests of their future children.

Chapter 9 _____

Noncoital Reproduction

_____

Now that 1984 has come and gone, Huxley's vision of our future in *Brave New World* looms larger than Orwell's. Huxley envisioned the abolition of parenthood and the family that would take place with the full cooperation of society as it attempted to improve on natural reproduction.* We are on our way. The last few years have witnessed scientific and societal developments in noncoital human reproduction and corresponding steps to redefine parenthood and family relationships. On the scientific side, we witnessed the first birth from surrogate embryo transfer (SET)[1] and the first birth from a frozen embryo. On the societal side, there have been major reports by government-appointed panels on noncoital reproduction in the United Kingdom (the Warnock Report),[2] Australia (the Waller Report from Vic-

_____

*In Orwell's world of *1984*, AID (artificial insemination by donor) was mandatory, and sexual pleasure and the family were destroyed to help maintain the tension necessary in a society dedicated to perpetual warfare. In Aldous Huxley's *Brave New World*, the family was also destroyed; but he portrayed a society controlled not by fear but by gratification and reinforcement. Abolition of the family was followed by complete sexual freedom; but reproduction was handled by the state, in "hatcheries" in which embryos were produced and monitored in an artificial environment: "[Of] course, they didn't content themselves with merely hatching out embryos: any cow could do that. 'We also predestine and condition. We decant our babies as socialized human beings, as Alphas or Epsilons, as future sewage workers or. . .' He was going to say 'future World controllers,' but correcting himself, said 'future Directors of Hatcheries,' instead." In both futuristic scenarios, the critical elements of governmental success were the separation of sex from reproduction, and the abolition of the family. In Margaret Atwood's futuristic *The Handmaid's Tale,* the role of sex is reduced to stylized ritual, with forced surrogacy; insemination is done coitally while the surrogate lies between the legs of the infertile wife. One surrogate describes her station: "We are two-legged wombs, that's all; sacred vessels, ambulatory chalices."

toria),[3] and Canada (Ontario),[4] and Congressional hearings on the subject in the United States.[5]

Techniques for noncoital reproduction close a circle opened with the introduction of effective contraception that made sex without reproduction dependable. Society seems as supportive of the new techniques for reproduction without sex as it was of contraception, but we seem more anxious about the implications these techniques raise and consequently more interested in public regulation of them. As with in vitro fertilization (IVF) and surrogate motherhood, the major justification offered for using these new techniques has been the resulting infants. Their pictures have appeared in newspapers and magazines around the world, and *People* magazine even named the world's first IVF child, Louise Brown, one of the ten most prominent people of the decade, one who dominated it "by simply being."[6]

Ambivalence is nonetheless apparent in the language used to describe the new techniques in various countries. In Australia, they are sometimes referred to as methods of "abnormal" reproduction; in England as "unnatural" reproduction, and in the United States the preferred term is "artificial" reproduction. We use the term "noncoital" since it is the most descriptive and the least value-laden. With developments occurring rapidly in noncoital reproduction, especially in North America, Australia, and Europe, it seems prudent to reflect on the societal issues raised by these techniques and to assess their future. The policy problem is how to deal effectively "with a series of sequential challenges" to current clinical practices.[7] It will often be critical to make distinctions, usually previously irrelevant, between the genetic, gestational, and rearing parents when sorting out individual rights and responsibilities.[8] Indeed, it is now possible for a child to have five "parents": a genetic and rearing father, and a genetic, gestational, and rearing mother.[9]

We believe it is more fruitful to explore the generic issues posed by methods of noncoital reproduction than to examine the methods themselves separately. While it would be possible to explore all of the potential methods of noncoital reproduction, including artificial insemination by husband (AIH), ovum donation, and the various possible combinations, such as IVF, SET, and frozen embryos with implantation in a surrogate mother (so-called "full surrogacy"), in this chapter we concentrate on the methods that present society with the most difficult generic problems. For example, AIH poses no problems of identifying the rearing parents or any issues regarding the sperm donor and so is *much* less problematic than artificial insemination by donor (AID) itself. Fifty years ago, about the time of the publication of *Brave New World*, AIH children were commonly referred to as "Test Tube Babies."[10] At that time, the notion of asking a physician to inject "strange semen" (AID) was described as "outlandish" and lacking in "tact, decency, and moral feeling."[10] Society has obviously come a long way attitudinally in the past half-century. Similarly, the problems in ovum donation are so analogous to those involved in AID that a separate consideration would be redundant. Issues involved in the myriad of possible combinations can likewise be addressed by looking at the individual methods themselves. Issues raised by cloning and ectogenesis, which are not so remote as to be relegated to science fiction, are analogous to those involving use of frozen embryos.

None of these technologies and techniques are neutral. Their very existence forces us to decide to use them or not, and also creates a new potential burden for the infertile, "the burden of not trying hard enough."[11] Noncoital reproduction forces us to confront issues of lineage, legitimacy, parenthood, family, and identity. These techniques not only change how humans can reproduce, but they also threaten to change how we think about human reproduction, and perhaps how we think about humanness itself.

In reviewing the social policy issues raised by these methods, we have found it useful to construct Table 9–1 in which we list the most important policy issues raised by these techniques, and in the cells we assign values to their importance. The values assigned represent our view of the normative importance of each issue in the context of a specific noncoital method of reproduction. We do not contend that these values are unambiguous or incontrovertible, but we believe the attempt to quantify provides a useful impressionistic model to compare and contrast the relative societal importance of the issues raised by each technique. Even a cursory examination of Table 9–1 explains, for example, why we begin our discussion with IVF rather than AID: IVF poses far fewer societal issues. As the President's Commission properly cautioned, the state of the law regarding AID is "chaotic" and by using it as the paradigm for other methods of noncoital reproduction, like IVF and embryo transfer (ET), we risk repeating "the chaos surrounding artificial insemination . . . with egg donors and borrowed wombs."[12]

OVERVIEW OF SOCIETAL ISSUES

In Vitro Fertilization (IVF)

In vitro fertilization followed by embryo transfer requires highly sophisticated biomedical technology to obtain one or more ovum, fertilize them in a Petri dish, and transfer the embryo to the woman's uterus. Nonetheless, when confined to married couples (using an ovum of the wife and the sperm of the husband), IVF actually presents far fewer societal problems than AID, because the genetic, gestational, and rearing parents are identical.

TABLE 9–1.

Index of Relative Importance of Societal Issues in Noncoital Reproduction*†

ISSUES‡	AID§	SURROGATE MOTHER	IVF§	SET§	FROZEN EMBRYO
Potential for noninfertility use	2	2	2	2	3
Protection of embryo	0	0	3	3	3
Identification of mother	0	3	0	3	3
Identification of father	2	2	0	2	3
Donor screening	2	2	0	2	2
Donor anonymity	2	2	0	2	2
Opportunities for commercialization	1	3	0	3	3
Total	**9**	**14**	**5**	**17**	**19**

*(From Elias S, Annas GJ: Social policy considerations in noncoital reproduction. *JAMA* 1986; 255:62. Courtesy of *JAMA;* copyright 1986, American Medical Association.)

†1 indicates of societal concern, but not sufficient to require uniform guidelines; 2, of sufficient societal concern to require uniform guidelines; and 3, of sufficient societal concern to justify discouraging or perhaps prohibiting the procedure altogether if reasonable uniform guidelines cannot be agreed on and enforced.

‡Definitions: *Potential for noninfertility use:* Use of the technology to gain access to the embryo for research or genetic manipulation; avoidance of pregnancy for "convenience" of the genetic mother; use of technique for eugenic purposes. *Protection of the embryo:* Exposure of the embryo to the potentially hostile laboratory environment; research that would not directly benefit that embryo; use that would devalue the embryo and human life. *Identification of mother:* Difficulty in distinguishing between the genetic mother and gestational mother and determining who will be legally identified as the presumptive rearing mother. *Identification of father:* Difficulty in distinguishing between the genetic father and the rearing father and determining who has legal responsibility for rearing the child. *Donor screening:* Requirements for gamete donors and method of ensuring compliance. *Donor anonymity:* What records should be kept, by whom, and how access can be gained to them by the child. *Opportunities for commercialization:* Buying and selling gametes, embryos, or children and the implications for society.

§AID indicates artificial insemination by donor; IVF, in vitro fertilization; and SET, surrogate embryo transfer.

Accordingly, IVF rather than AID should be used as the starting point for any analysis of the policy implications of noncoital reproduction. As noted in Table 9–1, IVF raises two major societal issues: indications and protection of the embryo.*

Medically, IVF has been developed primarily to permit married couples with infertility due to the wife's irreparable fallopian tube disease to have children. In vitro fertilization may also prove useful in cases in which the husband has a low sperm motility. A more controversial indication is "idiopathic infertility" in which evaluation of the couple (i.e., history, physical examination, laparoscopy, testing of fallopian tube patency, endocrine profiles, semen analysis, etc.) reveals no cause for infertility. An estimated 10% to 15% of infertile couples fall into this category. Possible explanations in-

*In vitro fertilization also raises the more universal issues of resource allocation and informed consent. Is the procedure worth offering at all if its success rate cannot be dramatically increased from its current level of less than 20%, and how should candidates for the procedure be counseled concerning its extremely high probability of failure?

clude immunologic factors, undiagnosed abnormalities of oocyte or sperm transport, undefined physical or chemical barriers preventing sperm penetration of the ovum, genetic abnormalities, and unrecognized uterine abnormalities. Virtually all cases of infertility, exclusive of intractable anovulation and those women without a uterus, are potential medical candidates for IVF.[13]

Legally and ethically, who should be considered a candidate for IVF? For example, should single women with fallopian tube disease be considered candidates for the procedure? This question should probably be answered the same as, "Should single women be considered candidates for AID," i.e., should medical technology be used to assist in the creation of single-parent families? The US Ethics Advisory Board (EAB) recommended that IVF be restricted to married couples.[14] In Australia, it has been recommended (even more restrictively) that, while it is acceptable to favor married couples who have had children during the experimentation phase, after IVF becomes established procedure, priority should be given to those married couples who have not had any children. This issue must be resolved on a broader base then medical practice because the family issues involved are not medical. In addition to life-style and marital status, financial status plays a large role. Is infertility a disease, and should its treatment be covered by medical insurance?

Because of the extracorporeal fertilization of the ovum and temporary in vitro development of the embryo, even more controversial new issues are presented: defining the steps that should be taken to protect the embryo and determining the extent to which experimental protocols are applicable to clinical use of IVF. All members of the US Ethics Advisory Board,[14] the Warnock Commission,[3] and the Waller Commission[4] agreed that the human embryo is worthy of respect and legal protection and cannot be treated like a hamster or other experimental animal.* The groups also agreed that

---

*The Waller Commission approved embryo research "in order that the success rate of the clinical IVF program be improved . . ." It also permitted embryos to develop no more than 14 days because this is the end of the stage of implantation, and "after this stage the primitive streak is formed, and differentiation of the embryo is clearly evident." The committee approved this by a 7–2 vote; but by the same 7–2 margin voted that no human embryo be brought into existence solely to be used in research because it was morally unacceptable to use a "genetically unique human entity" solely as a "means to an end." The United Kingdom's Warnock committee was split. All agreed with the US EAB's approach that the "embryo of the human species should be afforded some protection in law." The 14-day limit was also adopted, but on the basis that "day 15 marks the time of the formation of the primitive streak, and the beginning of individual development of the embryo." The committee did recommend that it be permissible to create embryos for research purposes alone, but the vote was very close (9–7). Even so, the Warnock committee unanimously condemned the routine testing of drugs on human embryos because of the large numbers of embryos this would require. The Ontario Commission adopted the 14-day limitation, recognizing that it is "arbitrary" but "could easily be amended" if "the state of medical knowledge at some future date indicates that it is inappropriate."

no research should be permitted after 14 days following laboratory fertilization, but the reasons for this cutoff date varied, including that 14 days is the time normally associated with implantation, when individual development of the embryo begins, and marks the beginning of the formation of the primitive streak. Until the basis of the 14-day limit is more clearly articulated and publicly accepted, it cannot serve as a legitimate regulatory boundary. Are we concerned with what the embryo *is,* what it looks like, or what it feels? Or are we concerned with what it *will be,* or what it will never have a chance to be, or with what it will look like or feel? Or is the focus of our concern something else entirely?

Artificial Insemination by Donor (AID)

Artificial insemination by donor has become widely accepted, with an estimated 250,000 AID children in the United States alone.[15] But familiarity has not resolved the societal problems raised by this technique. About half the states have enacted laws making the consenting husband of the woman inseminated the lawful father of the resulting legitimate child, but half have not. Controversy continues regarding the methods of selecting and screening donors, the use of single women as recipients, the types of records kept, and what information about their genetic father, if any, the children should be able to obtain. Nonetheless, AID is the accepted paradigm for all other methods of noncoital reproduction as evidenced by Commissions like Warnock and Waller.[3, 4] It may be an unworkable paradigm, however, because it potentially places the private contractual agreement among the participants regarding parental rights and responsibilities above the best interests of the child, and because it raises a series of societal issues that remain unresolved.[15] Indeed, by beginning one's analysis with AID and assuming that deciding about parenthood by contract is socially accepted as currently practiced, we ignore the relevance of legitimacy, lineage, and individual identity tied up in kinship, and thus bypass fundamental questions about the definition of fatherhood and its role in the family and the life of the child.[16] If, on the other hand, legitimacy is no longer a major social issue in the United States, and lineage is much more important in a country like England where hereditary titles might be at stake,† Alexander Pope's question, "To Whom Related, and By Whom Begot?" may be less relevant today.

Probably the most interesting and problematic societal issue still unre-

---

†In England, the issue of hereditary titles is very much alive, as the Royal College of Obstetricians and Gynaecologists noted in their IVF Report.[34] The RCOG quoted with apparent approval a December 20, 1982, publication of the Law Commission on Family Law and Illegitimacy: "The Commission was advised that children born following AID should not succeed to a title of honor, either that of the husband of the inseminated woman or that of the donor of the sperm."

solved in AID is donor screening. In AID, this is a two-step process: a general pool of candidates is selected (e.g., medical students), and then some additional screening is done to ensure that the potential donor does not have specific conditions, such as sexually transmissible diseases. Neither of the two steps in the process has been either well thought out or standardized. As to the initial screen, two points should be made. The first is that the term "donor" is descriptive only from a biologic perspective. From a legal and ethical perspective, virtually all sperm suppliers are actually "sperm vendors," since they sell their sperm for money.[15] While this distinction may seem one without a difference, it has practical consequences for both physicians and sperm suppliers. Primarily, the sperm vendor should not sign a consent form (since he is *not* a patient, and is not consenting to the physician treating him), but a contract in which he agrees to deliver his sperm for pay. The elements of the agreement can be tailor-made to the setting and should spell out the vendor's obligations in terms of his own physical and genetic health, including accurate family history, the quality of the semen he has agreed to produce, and a waiver of any rights to any child resulting from the insemination.

Second, far too little attention has been devoted to identifying the pool from which sperm vendors are drawn. The vast majority of physicians use medical students and house officers. It is often alleged that these individuals are the most convenient because they are always around. But the janitorial staff or the hospital security staff would qualify equally well on convenience grounds. What is really occurring is that physicians are making eugenic decisions, selecting what they consider "superior" genes for AID. In general, they have chosen to reproduce themselves, as sociobiologists would probably predict. Although physicians may believe that society needs more individuals with the attributes of physicians, it is unlikely that society as a whole does. Lawyers would likely select law students; geneticists, graduate students in genetics; military officers, students in military academies, and so forth.[15] The point is not trivial. Selecting donors in this manner is in the best interests of physicians, not infertile couples. Since the couple is not usually permitted to select the donor, physicians should develop guidelines that permit donation by a random sample of the population.

Actual screening of the donor and the donor's sperm demands the development of uniform professional standards that do not exist, and a reasonable enforcement mechanism to ensure that they are followed. For example, in the case of human immune virus (HIV), it seems reasonable to exclude men who engage in high risk activities from participation as sperm donors. It may also be reasonable to test the donors for HIV antibodies, freeze the sperm, and retest the donor 6 to 12 months later. Only if both tests are negative can one conclude that the sperm cannot transmit HIV to the potential child.[17]

Surrogate Mothers

Relying not on new medical technology but on lawyers as brokers, surrogate motherhood has received increased media attention in the past few years. This method employs a fertile woman who is artificially inseminated with the sperm of the husband of an infertile woman. The surrogate agrees to bear a child for the infertile couple and turn it over to them upon birth, either by giving the child up for adoption or by relinquishing her parental rights and obligations.

This is a much more socially problematic practice than either AID or IVF because it raises new issues of maternity (identity of rearing mother) and the commercialization of motherhood, as well as the older AID question of paternity, donor screening, and donor anonymity. The maternity issue, i.e., identifying the woman with the legal right and obligation to rear the child, involves the surrogate's ability to change her mind and keep the child, and perhaps even successfully sue the sperm donor for child support, as well as the child's interest in knowing its genetic lineage and having its gestational mother care for it. The commercialism issue involves paying the surrogate mother for her "services," and whether or not such payment is properly seen as compensation for gestational services, or as "baby buying," an activity prohibited in almost all states.[13] The Ontario Law Reform Commission has recommended that surrogate contracts should be specifically enforceable and argues persuasively that this is required to protect the parties.[4] Nevertheless, because of the trauma of removing a newborn from its gestational mother against her will, we do not believe contracts with surrogates should be specifically enforceable against the surrogate.* A suit against her for money damages for the emotional harm suffered by the contracting couple should she change her mind and keep her child might, however, be successful. The lack of legislative or judicial recognition of the surrogate mother contract has been one of the major obstacles to increasing the popularity of this method. We believe that the potential problems, as

---

*Following an almost five-year battle between the Attorney General and a surrogating parenting corporation, the Kentucky Supreme Court ruled in 1986 that Kentucky's baby-selling statute did *not* prohibit surrogate motherhood arrangements so long as the price was agreed upon *before* conception, and the surrogate mother retained the right to cancel the contract up to the point of relinquishing her parental rights after the birth of the child (*Surrogate Parenting Associates v. Kentucky*, 704 S.W.2d 209 [1986]). We think this case was wrongly decided since we believe that the essence of surrogate motherhood is not new science, as the majority of the court argued, but old commercialism.[18] On the other hand, treating the gestational mother's right to rear the child as inalienable prior to birth seems reasonable because of her greater physical and psychological bonding to the child. Because of the lack of data, the Ethics Committee of the American Fertility Society has recommended that surrogate motherhood only be pursued as a "clinical experiment."[19] This however, seems to place too much emphasis on surrogacy as a "medical solution for infertility,"[19] rather than on surrogacy as a contractual, commercial enterprise.

illustrated in the 1987 case of Mary Beth Whitehead, are so critical that this inhibition should remain. Our guess is that commercial surrogacy will wither if legislation to regulate and legitimate it is not enacted. Such legislation would amount to a societal approval of this method and likely encourage imitation.

The arguments in favor of commercial surrogacy are that it promotes reproductive autonomy for those who could not otherwise reproduce, is "womb rental" rather than baby selling, and is unlike payment for adoption because the deal is made prior to pregnancy, and the resulting child is genetically linked to one of the adopting (contracting) parents (the father). We believe, nonetheless, that only women desperate for money would produce children for pay, and that commercialism in babies degrades both mother and child. Although we generally do not believe in outlawing specific methods of human reproduction, we oppose positive societal encouragement of commercial surrogacy.

SURROGATE EMBRYO TRANSFER: A SOCIAL POLICY CASE STUDY

The most recent development in noncoital reproduction is surrogate embryo transfer (SET), and even though it has not proved popular, this technique provides a useful model to examine the major policy implications of all forms of noncoital reproduction. Sometimes described as "uterine lavage for preembryo transfer,"[19] SET involves the nonsurgical recovery of an embryo by uterine lavage from a surrogate who has been artificially fertilized with the sperm of an infertile woman's husband, and the subsequent transfer of that embryo into the uterus of the infertile woman.[1] Almost all of the issues of IVF and surrogate mother combined are raised by SET. We say "almost all" because the bonding and likelihood of the embryo donor refusing to undergo the lavage procedure and retaining the pregnancy (should one result) is much less likely than the risk that a surrogate mother who carries the child to term will opt to keep it.[20] Surrogate embryo transfer directly presents all of the other issues: indications, protection of the embryo, maternity, paternity, donor screening and anonymity, and commercialization (see Table 9–1, p. 225).

Indications

Surrogate embryo transfer has been introduced using the same indication as that used for the initial IVF trials: infertility in married couples due to irreparable fallopian tube disease.* This raises at least two questions: in what sense is infertility a disease, and in what sense is use of SET (or any other method of noncoital reproduction) a therapeutic treatment for infertility? A similar question can, of course, be asked of the most popular form of birth control, sterilization; is sterilization a treatment for fertility? Diseases are, to a large extent, social constructs, and it seems fair to conclude that both physicians and society have defined involuntary infertility as a disease. Although it is a condition from which individuals suffer, it has generally been treated only in the context of a marital relationship. The "treatment" may be more accurately described as a "service," since the disease or disability is not treated or cured (as it would be in a fallopian tube transplant), but the condition is technologically bypassed. The indications for such noncoital reproduction services must be defined on a broader base than medical practice, since the value of the traditional family unit and the relationship of childbearing to child rearing are not medical issues. Proponents of using new reproductive techniques based on contracts among adults rather than on marriage and family relationships have argued that the traditional family unit is giving way to multiple models and that our practices should mirror reality. They in effect justify noncoital reproduction outside the traditional family on the basis that the traditional family unit is breaking up. But, is this move to multiple family models to be fostered, or should society attempt to reverse it? We currently have no social policy on "families." Nonetheless, it seems disingenuous to argue on the one hand that the primary justification for noncoital reproduction is the anguish an infertile married couple suffers because of the inability to have a "traditional family," and then use the breakup of the traditional family unit itself as the primary justification for unmarried individuals to have access to these techniques.

Protecting the Embryo: Parental Rights and Duties

We can assume that the embryo, once transferred into an otherwise infertile woman, is highly regarded by both the woman and her husband. In IVF there would be no embryo without the in vitro beginnings and development. But SET actually jeopardizes the well-being or survival of an existing embryo by removing it from its "safe harbor," the donor's uterus. The justification is that the embryo donor had no intention of having the child herself, and the removal is just part of a larger procedure to attempt a pregnancy that otherwise would not have occurred. This simply restates the argument that "all we are doing is making babies," a laudable objective, but

---

*In addition, SET could be used when the woman has no ovaries (i.e., after surgical removal) or abnormal ovaries (e.g., streak gonads in 45,X individuals).

not an end that justifies any means. For example, the desire to have a child does not justify kidnapping another's child, or forcibly removing an embryo from a "donor" who has changed her mind. It may also not justify putting a healthy embryo at risk, any more than we would be justified in exposing the embryo to teratogens prior to implantation.

Who should have the authority to make decisions concerning the extra-corporeal embryo in SET? The understanding is that the embryo, once removed from the donor, will be transferred to the infertile wife. However, even with such a contract, the "donor" maintains the ability to continue the pregnancy. Once the embryo is transferred, the recipient contributes the gestational site and assumes the risks of pregnancy, and she should therefore have the final decision-making authority over the embryo. Because of her greater contribution and risk and to provide certainty of identity and responsibility necessary to protect both mother and child at the time of birth, the gestational mother (rather than the genetic mother) should be deemed the child's legal mother for all purposes.[13, 18] Her husband should likewise be deemed the child's legal father.

The period of embryonic life that has received the greatest attention has been its brief extracorporeal existence. This in vitro period exposes the embryo to an artificial and potentially teratogenic or lethal environment and provides an opportunity for genetic engineering. Both authority and responsibility during this period are undefined. Although ethically bound to follow through with transfer, the physician could destroy the embryo or transfer it to a woman other than the sperm donor's wife. Legal control over the extracorporeal embryo should be vested in the sperm donor who has contributed genetically to it and who has the most interest in seeing it successfully implanted as his future child. The ovum donor relinquishes all rights and responsibilities to the embryo when it is voluntarily flushed from her uterus. Furthermore, since the *only* justification for SET is to enable the married woman to bear a child that was genetically her husband's, the sperm donor and the physician with custody of the embryo should have authority only to do those things that would reasonably promote this objective. Consequently neither would have the authority to "volunteer" the embryo for research or donate it to another woman.

Donor Selection

Donor selection has always been the most discussed issue in AID, and remains a central issue in all forms of noncoital reproduction (except IVF with married couples). When donors are selected on the basis of some particular desirable trait or set of traits, eugenic decisions are being made. The question is how such decisions should be made. A Nobel Prize sperm bank has already been established, and a counterpart panel of ovum donors can be envisioned, as can catalogs of frozen embryos. Since most desirable genetic traits are polygenic/multifactorial, however, such banks are unlikely to ever be very popular or effective in producing individual traits in offspring, at least until the technology exists to clone specific embryos.

How should the women who will be used as donors in SET be selected? Fertility is obviously important, but should they already have had children? Should they be married, single, or divorced? What should their economic and social status be? What medical and genetic characteristics should rule them out as donors? What types of genetic and psychological screening tests should be performed and who should perform them? What kinds of agreements regarding preinsemination intercourse retained pregnancies and abortion should they be asked to make prior to the procedure? What relationship, if any, should the donor have with the child? None of these questions have self-evident answers, and all should be resolved before SET (or any similar technique) is made widely available.

Donor Anonymity and Record Keeping

The basic thrust of current AID policy is to protect the sperm donor from any claims the resulting child might have on him.[15] This protection has been almost obsessional, and in the process the interests of the child are usually given a lower priority. In both AID and SET, two basic issues are raised from the child's perspective: (1) Does a child have a significant interest in having only two unambiguously identified parents? and (2) Does the child have a significant interest in knowing how it was conceived, implanted, and gestated? If the answer to the first is yes, we may wish to devise a system in which at least one, but only one, mother and one father can possibly be identified for each child. If we cannot ensure such unique identification, it would seem that the child should have access to identifiable information about his genetic mother in the SET setting, and his genetic father in the AID setting. We admit that this is a difficult issue; however, since such information could be kept secret only by purposeful deception, since the child has no voice in the matter, and since it may be an extremely important psychological (and possibly medical or genetic) issue to the child seeking information about his genetic heritage, records should be kept of all births in a way that they can be matched with donors.[15] We think medical professionals should maintain these records. But if they refuse, legislation may be needed to require their deposit with a court of relevant jurisdiction. The donor can effectively waive any right to access to such records, but no one should be able to effectively waive the child's future access to genetic, medical, and perhaps even personal information about the donor.

These records could have two "levels": level one would be medical and genetic history that did not identify the donor; level two would contain the donor's actual identity. Access to level one information should be guaranteed. Access to level two should be possible if the child can demonstrate a "need to know." The objection that such a practice might make AID impossible because donors would not be willing to be identified seems misplaced. The only survey of donors we have been able to locate found that 60% would donate even if their identity was made known to the resulting children,[21] and a 1985 Swedish law requiring that children be able to learn the identity of their AID father at the age of 18 only temporarily discouraged sperm "donation."[21]

FROZEN EMBRYOS

It seems reasonable to freeze the embryo in SET if the planned recipient becomes ill or has an accident immediately prior to the planned transfer; or in IVF to preserve multiple embryos for use in subsequent cycles. In IVF this eliminates the need for repeated ovum retrievals should the initial pregnancy attempt fail, allows greater convenience in determining time of transfer, and may even increase the efficacy of the procedure.[23] Freezing embryos, however, forces us to reexamine all of the issues raised by noncoital reproduction (see Table 9–1). This is not because of freezing *per se* (assuming it can be accomplished without damage to the embryo) but because freezing raises the possibility of transferring the embryo to a multitude of potential donees over an extended period of time.

The recent case of a wealthy US couple who died leaving two frozen embryos in Australia caused an international debate about their legal status and what should be done with them, including their possible implantation in a surrogate.[3] Other potential problems include confusion of parental identity because the embryo may not be genetically related to either of its rearing parents; frozen embryos could be implanted in surrogates for convenience; embryos could be maintained for generations (raising the possibility of a woman giving birth to her genetic aunt or uncle); siblings could be born from different sets of parents; embryos could be removed using the SET embryo removal procedure from any woman, and (when the technology is available) karyotyped, examined for nonchromosomal genetic defects, and discarded, treated, frozen for reimplantation during the woman's next cycle or at some future time, donated to another woman, or sold.

The possibility of frozen embryo banks, in which embryos are produced to order by matching the sperm and ovum of "ideal" types and then sold to parents for genetic or eugenic purposes, also raises concerns of commercialism. Even if we accept paying a surrogate mother for the "work" of pregnancy, we could still reject traffic in embryos since in this case there is absolutely no ambiguity about what is being bought or sold. We may even wish to go further and require procedures similar to adoption when frozen embryos are used. This amounts to "prenatal adoption" when neither prospective parent has contributed genetically to the embryo, although such a procedural requirement seems extreme and confuses notions of "what will be" with those of "what is."

Before launching any regulatory initiative in the United States, it is useful to review recent action in the United Kingdom, Australia, and Canada on these issues.

COMMISSION REPORTS

United Kingdom

In July of 1984, the government-sponsored Warnock Commission, named after its chairperson, Dame Mary Warnock, issued a report that made 63 specific recommendations: 33 involving a proposed licensing board to regulate clinical services and research; 7 involving the National Health Service's infertility program; and 23 involving new British laws, including naming of 7 new crimes.[2] The Warnock Commission, for example, proposed outlawing all aspects of surrogate motherhood, including both for profit and nonprofit organizations, and professional activities designed to "knowingly assist in the establishment of a surrogate pregnancy." The British Government has already legislated to ban commercial surrogacy, and the other proposals are under debate.

The commission also expressed concern about payment to sperm donors, ovum donors, and embryo donors, but adopted a much more cautious approach to this problem. It recommended legislation be "enacted to ensure there is no right of ownership in a human embryo," but stopped short of suggesting that the purchase and sale of gametes be outlawed, apparently because it believed such a move would threaten the sperm supply for AID. Accordingly, its official recommendation was that "*Unauthorized* [by the state licensing authority] sale or purchase of human gametes or embryos should be made a criminal offence."[2] The Commission did not suggest what guidelines the licensing commission should adopt, or if it should become involved in price-setting for gametes and embryos. This matter awaits resolution.

Australia

The Australian Commission for the State of Victoria was, if anything, more aggressive than its British counterpart. Under the direction of Law

Professor Louis Waller, the Commission issued reports in August 1983 and August 1984.[3] These reports made a total of 54 recommendations, many of which were written into laws dealing with the Status of Children (passed May 15, 1984), and Infertility (passed Nov 2, 1984). These laws continue the Australian ban on sales of human tissues, including sperm, ova, and embryos; and outlaw cloning, fertilization of a human ovum with an animal gamete, use of children's gametes, mixing of sperm in AID, and all commercial forms of surrogate motherhood.

The infertility legislation also sets up a system of state regulation for AID, IVF, freezing and experimenting on embryos, counseling of participants, and required record keeping. In addition, a standing committee is created to study and report to the government about new developments in this field. One of the issues not yet considered in Australia by either the government or the Waller Commission, for example, is SET (the Warnock Commission recommended that SET "not be used at the present time"). The Status of Children legislation creates an irrebuttable presumption that the woman in whose womb a child gestates is the mother of that child.

On the issue that has received the most press coverage, the disposition of frozen embryos, the Warnock and Waller Commissions diverged considerably. The Waller Commission recommended that in the absence of specific instructions from the gamete donors, frozen embryos in storage should be destroyed upon the death of the gamete donors. The Warnock Commission, on the other hand, recommended that their fate be determined by the storage facility, in effect treating them like unclaimed baggage. While there are problems with both "solutions," the Waller approach seems more reasonable, since the interests of the gamete donors are superior to those of the storage facility.

Canada

The Ontario Law Reform Commission's Report was prepared following Warnock and Waller and relies heavily on both of them. The Commission came up with 67 specific recommendations, generally favoring artificial reproduction "where medically necessary to circumvent the effects of infertility and genetic impairment."[4] As this statement implies, the Commission recommended that these procedures be legislatively defined as the "practice of medicine." Access to them should be restricted to "stable single women and to stable men and stable women in stable marital or nonmarital unions." Gamete banks that buy and sell sperm, ova, and embryos were permitted to operate under state license and to extract payment by users "to defray reasonable costs, and perhaps, to provide a reasonable profit."[4]

The most notable divergence is in the area of surrogate motherhood.

The Commission recommended a legislatively established regulatory scheme to govern surrogate mother arrangements. All agreements must be in writing and have the prior approval of the Family Court, which will "assess the suitability of the prospective parents for participation in such an arrangement," including the couple's medical need for using it. The court would also assess the "suitability of a prospective surrogate mother," including her physical and mental health, marital status, and likely impact on her children of the arrangement. The most controversial recommendation is:

> A child born pursuant to an approved surrogate motherhood arrangement should be surrendered immediately upon birth to the social parents. Where a surrogate mother refuses to transfer the child, the court should order that the child be delivered to the social parents. In addition, where the court is satisfied that the surrogate mother intends to refuse to surrender the child upon birth, it should be empowered, prior to the birth of the child, to make an order for transfer of custody upon birth.[4]

While payment is permitted, no payment shall be made without prior court approval. Finally, the Commission recommends that five years after its regulatory scheme has been implemented, "a review of all aspects should be undertaken by an appropriate governmental body." The surrogate motherhood enforcement provision, which makes a gestational mother's rearing rights alienable before birth, could face serious constitutional problems relating to violation of privacy and personhood in the United States.

The United States

The United States had a National Commission to examine fetal experimentation in the mid-1970s, an Ethics Advisory Board (EAB) in the Department of Health, Education and Welfare (now the Department of Health and Human Services), and most recently, a Presidential Commission on Bioethics. The first Commission proposed strict regulations on fetal experimentation,[24] the EAB recommended that research on IVF go forward under similarly regulated conditions,[14] and the President's Commission endorsed the views of the EAB on IVF, and spent little time on other methods of noncoital reproduction. The Commission did, however, recommend that AID donors should be screened for their "genetic history," that records of source and sample should be kept, and that steps should be taken to ensure that the confidentiality of the donor is protected to the "greatest extent possible."[25] Federal law requires EAB approval for any federally funded embryo research, so the demise of the EAB in 1979 has meant no federal funding, and a de facto moratorium on open embryo research in the United States since then. We currently have a Working Group on Gene

Therapy (a subcommittee of NIH's Recombinant DNA Advisory Committee), but no national commission comparable to Warnock, Waller, or Ontario to develop public policy.[26] One should be established.[5, 22, 27] Like Australia, but unlike the United Kingdom, our laws relating to parenthood and reproduction are primarily state laws. Accordingly, the debate about the appropriate legislative responses to the challenges of these noncoital methods of reproduction is already under way in many state capitals.

PROPOSED LEGISLATIVE ACTION

Since they have not been adequately debated in public, it is premature to attempt to answer all of the issues raised by these techniques, but it is foolish not to act on those that can be relatively easily resolved. Of the three issues that generate the most concern (see Table 9–1), two are capable of legislative solution now: identification of the mother and commercialization.

Identification of the Mother

Identification of the mother gets a higher "point value" in Table 9–1 than identifying the father because the mother plays a much more significant role in the gestation and birth of the child than the father. Unlike the father, for example, the gestational mother will always be present and easily identifiable at the moment of birth. The social policy issue is whether the genetic or gestational mother will be *legally* presumed to have the right and responsibility to rear the child. This situation will arise in SET, in the use of surrogate mothers generally, and in the use of donor (usually frozen) embryos. We believe that it is critical for the protection of both the mother and child that the legal mother (i.e., the woman with rearing rights and responsibilities) be identifiable at the time of birth. This confirms the child's maternal legitimacy and provides the child with a caretaker and a person legally responsible for the child's welfare, and able to consent to its treatment. It also protects the gestational mother from exploitation. Given the need for certainty and the greater biologic and psychological investment of the gestational mother in the child, we think the Victorian Parliament was correct in codifying the traditional legal presumption: the gestational mother should be irrebuttably presumed to be the child's legal mother for all purposes. She may later agree to give the child up for adoption or otherwise relinquish her parental rights and responsibilities, but that decision is one she will make as the child's legal mother, and the child's legal mother will *always* be readily identifiable. A state statute codifying this traditional legal presumption, and making it irrebuttable, would be protective of both mother and child.*

Commercialism

The social policy goal is to prevent children from being viewed as commodities that can be purchased, sold, returned, and exchanged, because this view will lead to attitudes and practices detrimental to the well-being of children as well as to a reconceptualization of human life and the value of human life. It would seem that surrogate motherhood has enough potential legal and personal problems surrounding it that it is unlikely to survive as a viable option unless laws are passed that encourage it by clarifying its legal status. Surrogacy can be viewed as a voluntary degradation of oneself because it treats one's body as a mere incubator, and degradation is no more acceptable because it is voluntary.[16] Money, of course, makes it worse, be-

---

*Only one case has reached even a lower court on this subject, and that case was dealt with extremely superficially and can hardly be termed "the law." The case (*Smith & Smith v. Jones & Jones,* 85-532014 DZ, Detroit, MI, 3d Dist. March 15, 1986) involved an infertile couple (because the wife lacked a uterus) who contracted to have her ovum fertilized with her husband's sperm, and the resulting embryo implanted in a married surrogate who would gestate it, and then present the child to its genetic parents. Thus we had a case of "full surrogacy." A few weeks prior to the birth, lawyers for the two couples went to court to ask Judge Marianne O. Battani to declare the genetic parents the legal parents so, among other things, their names would appear on the birth certificate. The judge agreed, mainly we think because no one was appointed to represent the child, and no legal arguments were presented in opposition to the petition. The judge based her ruling primarily on her view that the state's paternity statute should apply equally to maternity. Unfortunately, as the judge appears to have realized by describing the gestational or "birthing mother" as "a human incubator for this embryo to develop," the opinion demotes pregnant women to the status of incubators. The decision also makes identification of the child's legal mother *at birth impossible.* The judge dealt with this by ordering that HLA tissue-typing confirm "maternity," but understood that this would not be possible for at least a few days (perhaps more) after birth. While many will applaud the judge for putting contracts before biology, the judge was not faced with the case her opinion raises: what if *neither* the genetic nor the gestational mother contracted for the child, but rather a third party who had no ovaries had contracted for the baby? Does it make any sense at all to say that *neither* the genetic nor the gestational mother is the mother, i.e., that biology has nothing to do with motherhood, only rearing rights that are the subject of a contract and a monetary exchange?[18] In view of the dubiousness of this result, we also find it unprofessional and distasteful that on the basis of this opinion, the lawyer for the couple sent a solicitation letter to obstetricians which said, among other things, that this decision "could have an overwhelming impact on your medical practice . . . [because the legal drawbacks to full surrogacy] have been virtually eliminated by Judge Battani's exciting and far-reaching opinion . . . I have available surrogates ready for immediate selection for any couple you may refer to me. If your practice does not include all of the medical procedures described, I have qualified physicians willing to undertake such procedures" [undated form letter from Noel P. Keane].

cause the motivation becomes entirely material, and a price is put on the product, i.e., the child. Although we oppose commercial surrogacy, we do not believe the law should prohibit a friend or relative to act as a surrogate out of love or compassion. This gets the state too closely involved in human reproduction, and a reasonable argument can be made that although giving a "gift" still treats the child as a thing in some ways, in the absence of a monetary exchange, the child is not treated as a commodity but remains a "priceless gift," the giving of which, like the giving of blood, is a gesture of love and altruism.[28] On the other hand, new problems of multiple known parents will have to be dealt with by the participants. Similarly, it may be reasonable to permit embryo donation, but commerce in embryos seems wrong. There is an almost universal consensus that kidneys should not be bought and sold, and this has recently been codified in federal law.[29, 30] The arguments against the sale of human embryos are even more compelling. A commercial market in prefabricated, selected embryos would encourage us to view embryos as commodities that are simply means to the ends we design (with or without regulation), rather than as human entities without a market price. British law professor Ian Kennedy has argued that we know intuitively that a human embryo is more valuable than a hamster or other experimental animal, and that is why we have trouble permitting experiments on human embryos.[31] Likewise, we know intuitively that the human embryo is more valuable than a kidney and of much more symbolic importance regarding human life; that is why we believe embryos should not be the subject of commerce.

Embryos, like babies from surrogate mothers, will be bought or sold, if at all, on the belief that they will produce a healthy child, and possibly one of a certain physical type, IQ, stature, and so forth. When the child is not born as warranted or guaranteed, what remedies will the buyer have against the seller? Accept, reject, return for a refund or another "item"? The problem with commerce in human embryos is that the sale of human embryos can become confused with the sale of human children.[27] Accordingly, it seems reasonable to outlaw the sale of human embryos. Sale of sperm and ova does not present the same problem, but the Warnock and Waller Commissions may well be on the right track in discouraging commerce in gametes and in limiting payment to out-of-pocket and medical expenses. It may be time to experiment with other methods to recruit sperm donors in the United States besides money. For example, as in France, couples who use AID could be required or requested to find one or more of their friends to act as sperm donors for other couples.

Forbidding the sale of human embryos does not improperly interfere with an individual's constitutional right to procreate (assuming *arguendo* that this right includes the right to use noncoital techniques), any more than legally limiting an individual to one spouse, and making it illegal to purchase either another spouse or a license for polygamy.†

CONCLUSION

No commission (or any two authors) can solve all of the social policy issues raised by noncoital reproduction. Nonetheless, previous work and this discussion demonstrate both that noncoital reproduction decisions cannot survive solely in the private domain of infertility specialists, and that the private contract paradigm used in AID is outdated and inadequate to protect children, parents, the family, and social values. We will need new guidelines and even some new laws. These guidelines can and should be developed by professional associations with public participation, and a reasonable start has been made.[19, 33, 34] Both the courts and legislatures are likely to look with favor upon professional guidelines in this area that have been well thought-out, and private practitioners should welcome reasonable and responsible guidance. In formulating more comprehensive guidelines, we suggest the following as useful foundations:

1. To protect the interests of resulting children and the legitimacy of noncoital reproduction, primary consideration should always be given to the welfare and "best interests" of the potential child, rather than to the donors, the infertile couple, or the physician or clinic.[13–15, 35–39]

2. To protect the interests of resulting children, complete and accurate records should be kept of all participants, including donors, so that donors can be matched with offspring. These records should be kept confidential, but in a manner that makes future access by the child possible if this is determined to be in the child's best interests.[15, 25]

---

†It also seems wrong for medical professionals involved in developing new techniques of noncoital human reproduction to patent the *processes* they develop. This is because patenting places them in a conflict of interest position in regard to candidly reporting on their research and could also restrict independent, unbiased evaluation by other investigators. But since other motives, like pursuit of the Nobel prize or tenure, might as easily contaminate research as the profit motive, we must condemn patenting noncoital processes on other grounds. We think the most persuasive is the argument that the government should not be involved in controlling or supervising, directly through its police powers, or indirectly through its patenting powers, the process of human reproduction. This is because the subject matter of the patent does not lend itself to patent infringement enforcement without potentially unbearable privacy violations.[32] The American Fertility Society has reached the same conclusion, but for different reasons.[19]

3. To protect all participants, uniform and complete standards for donor selection and screening, including genetic screening, should be developed and made public.[14, 15, 19, 38, 40]

Action on three levels is warranted: (1) a model state law designed to clearly define the gestational mother as the irrebuttably presumed legal mother for all purposes, and to outlaw the sale of human embryos should be enacted;* (2) professional organizations, with significant public participation, should develop and promulgate guidelines for sound clinical practice; and (3) a national body of experts in law, public policy, science, medicine, and ethics should be established to debate and monitor developments in this area and report annually to Congress and the individual states on the desirability of regulation and legislation.

At all levels, the primary focus of social policy formation should be on protecting the best interests of the planned-for children, even if their protection sometimes comes at the expense of some infertile couples and some gamete donors or vendors. This general policy is one that helps protect basic societal values and can provide noncoital reproduction itself with societal legitimacy.

Twenty-five years after he wrote *Brave New World,* Aldous Huxley opined, "That we are being propelled in the direction of *Brave New World* is obvious. But no less obvious is the fact that we can, if we so desire, refuse to cooperate with the blind forces that are propelling us."[41] More than another quarter of a century later, we still enjoy the opportunity to participate in shaping our reproductive future, but the opportunity will not last forever.

---

*Florida has already enacted a statute that provides "no person shall knowingly advertise or offer to purchase or sell, or purchase, sell or otherwise transfer, any human embryo for valuable consideration" (Fla. Stat. Ann. sec. 873.05[1]).

Chapter 10

Fetal and Gene Therapy

Some fetal disorders can now be approached by various experimental treatments, and a few abnormalities can be substantially corrected if not cured.[1] Genetic therapy holds great therapeutic promise for the future.[2] As technology evolves in the direction of fetal and gene therapy, our ability to intervene in more positive ways than pregnancy termination will grow. Our enthusiasm, however, must be tempered by the realization that results to date have been generally disappointing and, although research continues, there is no longer a general expectation of immediate widespread therapeutic application of these new methodologies. Nonetheless, the stakes remain high and the implications for successful fetal and gene therapy for medicine, society, the pregnant woman, and the fetus and the child are profound. In this chapter we review the current status and future prospects for fetal therapy by surgical, medical, and gene transfer approaches, and the major ethical and legal issues that these technologies raise.

FETAL SURGERY

Ascertainment of Abnormal Fetuses

Only a small fraction of potential candidates for antenatal surgery are currently identified. Sometimes a family history of a heritable abnormality will lead the obstetrician to monitor the fetus to determine if it is similarly affected. Some cases will be ascertained because of clinical suspicion (for example, oligohydramnios, which may be associated with urinary tract obstruction). With the current trend toward the liberal use of antenatal ultrasonographic monitoring for a variety of obstetric indications, the majority of cases in which fetuses are recognized as candidates for antenatal surgery will likely be diagnosed serendipitously.

Prerequisites for Fetal Surgery

Prior to considering a fetus for in utero surgery, a number of prerequisites must be met.[3] First, the extent of the fetal malformation must be delineated, and a careful evaluation must be made for possible coexisting abnormalities through detailed ultrasonographic studies (so-called level II ultrasound scanning) by an experienced ultrasonographer knowledgeable in fetal anatomy and the natural history of fetal disease. Ancillary procedures should include amniocentesis for chromosomal analysis, determination of α-fetoprotein levels, and, in some cases, viral cultures. Amniography or fetoscopy might also be considered. Second, the abnormality should be compatible with a reasonable expectation for a healthy infant as a result of the procedure. For example, surgery to repair a urinary tract obstruction would, in general, be contraindicated in a trisomy 18 fetus. Third, surgical intervention is indicated only when the fetus would be better off because of the performance of surgery before delivery, rather than after birth. In certain situations, the gestational age of the fetus will dictate whether or not preterm delivery followed by neonatal surgery offers an overall safer approach than in utero surgery. The primary rationale for fetal surgery is that the fetal condition will progressively deteriorate to a point of irrevocable injury unless surgical intervention is undertaken.* Fetal surgery requires a multidisciplinary team that includes an experienced obstetrician, ultrasonographer, pediatric surgeon, geneticist, and neonatologist (who will be required to manage the infant after delivery). Preferably, additional members would include a bioethicist, psychiatrist or psychologist, and social worker. Infants should be delivered at a tertiary medical center with a high-risk obstetric unit and intensive care nursery. Fetal surgery should also be performed only with the prior approval of an Institutional Review Board (IRB) and with the informed consent of the parents.[4]

STATE OF THE ART

Erythroblastosis Fetalis

Surgical treatment of fetal disease is not in itself new. In 1963, the first successful intrauterine transfusion for severe erythroblastosis fetalis was reported.[5] This procedure involves the percutaneous insertion of a needle into

---

*See discussion in Chapter 5 regarding interventions in a multiple pregnancy.

the fetal peritoneal cavity either under roentgenographic or ultrasound guidance, followed by injection of group Rh-negative erythrocytes. More recently, in utero transfusions have been carried out by percutaneous needle insertion into the umbilical vein under ultrasound guidance.[6] Intrauterine transfusion has now become an integral part of modern obstetric therapy.

Hydrocephalus

Current methods of ultrasonography permit the antenatal detection of at least some cases of fetal hydrocephalus during the second trimester; however, sensitivity and specificity have not been established. After 22 weeks' gestation, the outer border of the lateral ventricle should be extended no farther than half the distance of the midline to the skull wall.[7] In fetal hydrocephalus, the lateral ventricles become abnormally dilated prior to any changes in the biparietal diameter of the fetal skull. In addition, ultrasonographic studies of fetuses with hydrocephalus will detect associated intracranial anomalies in 37% of cases and extracranial anomalies in 64% of cases.[8] Thus, a complete ultrasonographic evaluation of fetal anatomy is mandatory prior to any intrauterine surgical intervention.

The most widely used in utero treatment of fetal hydrocephalus has been the placement of a ventriculoamniotic shunt under ultrasound guidance. The first reported placement of a silicone rubber shunt with a one-way valve was in a 24-week fetus with hydrocephalus caused by X-linked aqueductal stenosis.[9] The function of the shunt was confirmed by an increased cortical mantle thickness, a decreased ventricular-to-hemisphere ratio, and a normal biparietal diameter at 32 weeks' gestation.†

The data to date indicate that there may be a small but important group of infants born with severe hydrocephalus that might benefit from in utero treatment. Considerable screening is required to distinguish those fetuses that may benefit from such procedures (i.e., those with true obstructive

---

†The International Fetal Surgery Registry[10] has reported a total of 41 instances in which fetuses with hydrocephalus were treated by surgical decompression. Of these 41 fetuses, 39 were treated by chronic placement of a ventriculoamniotic shunt; the remaining 2 fetuses were treated by serial ventriculocentesis. The mean gestational age at the time of treatment was 27 ± 2.6 weeks (range, 23–33). Thirty-four of 41 fetuses (83%) survived after treatment, and 7 fetuses died during treatment or shortly thereafter (3 with lethal anomalies, 3 due to prematurity, and 1 as a direct result of needle trauma to the brain stem). Of the 34 infants who survived, follow-up data was available for 8.2 ± 5.8 months (range, 1–18). Twelve infants were reported as normal at follow-up; all had aqueductal stenosis representing 29% of all treated fetuses and 35% of survivors. Of the remaining 22 survivors, 4 infants were classified as having mild to moderate impairment (developmental quotients < 80), and 18 infants were classified as having severe handicaps and gross delay in reaching developmental milestones (in infants tested, developmental quotients < 60). The report concluded that "the results of intervention in cases of obstructive hydrocephalus are not encouraging . . . since treatment did not produce any obvious decrease in morbidity among survivors."

hydrocephalus without associated malformations) from fetuses with non-obstructive ventriculomegaly associated with intrinsic brain malformations or extrinsic severe anomalies.[11, 12] In general, however, the outcomes following such shunt procedures have been very disappointing. Indeed, most centers in the United States have abandoned clinical trials of such ventriculoamniotic shunting procedures.

Urinary Tract Obstruction

Fetal urinary tract obstruction may be ultrasonographically recognized by oligohydramnios, a massively enlarged bladder, and hydronephrotic kidneys.[13] Unrelieved complete urinary-tract obstruction as a result of posterior urethral valves or strictures leads to (1) hydronephrosis; (2) cystic dysplasia of the kidneys: (3) oligohydramnios with secondary facial deformities (hypertelorism, malformed low-set ears, depressed nasal tip, and micrognathia), flexion contractures in the extremities, and pulmonary hypoplasia; and (4) abdominal-wall muscle deficiency or "prune belly." In theory, drainage of urine from the bladder into the amniotic cavity prior to the time of irreversible damage may allow normal kidney development, restore normal amniotic-fluid dynamics, and thus prevent oligohydramnios and its sequelae.*

*Harrison and coworkers reported a case of an 18-year-old primigravid patient who underwent ultrasonographic evaluation at 20 weeks' gestation because of an inappropriately small uterus.[14] There was oligohydramnios, and it was determined that the male fetus had bilateral hydronephrosis, dilated redundant ureters, and a large thick-walled bladder with a dilated bladder neck. The renal parenchyma did not appear to be cystic. Because of the fetal position and the oligohydramnios, the placement of a catheter shunt from the bladder to the amniotic cavity was deemed impossible. Therefore, it was believed that bilateral ureterostomies offered the only hope of saving the fetus. At 21 weeks' gestation, the lower part of the fetal body was lifted through a hysterotomy incision; the dilated ureters were exposed through bilateral flank incisions, opened in the midportion, and marsupialized to the skin (Fig 10–1).[15] The fetus was then replaced and the incision closed. At 35 weeks' gestation, a 2,300-gm infant was delivered by cesarean section. The infant had mild facial deformities, limb contractures, a small chest, a slightly protuberant abdomen, and bilateral undescended testes. After nine hours at maximum supportive measures, the infant was permitted to die. At autopsy, the lungs were found to be hypoplastic, and the kidneys showed cystic dysplasia (Potter-type IV). In a second case, Golbus and colleagues reported a 41-year-old woman who, by ultrasonography prior to genetic amniocentesis at 17 weeks' gestation, was found to have twins, one of which was a male with marked ascites. At 23 weeks' gestation, this twin showed a marked increase in ascites, associated with a slight dilation of the left renal pelvis and ureter. At 30 weeks' gestation, the abnormal twin was found to have a significant decrease in ascites and to have oligohydramnios. An attempt to place an indwelling catheter percutaneously into the fetal bladder under ultrasonographic guidance was unsuccessful. At 32 weeks' gestation, a polyethylene catheter was placed in the fetal bladder under ultrasonographic guidance so that the curled end was in the bladder and the other end drained into the amniotic cavity. At 34 weeks' gestation, the infants were spontaneously delivered vaginally. The affected infant had the features of the "prune-belly" syndrome. At 1 day of age, the infant underwent bilateral high-loop cutaneous ureterostomies, correction of an associated intestinal malrotation, and excision of a portion of the redundant abdominal wall. Renal biopsies showed mild dysplasia.

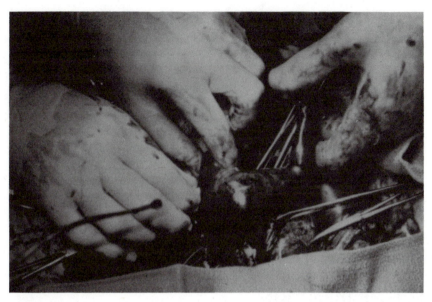

FIG 10–1.
Fetus undergoing bilateral ureterostomies at 22 weeks' gestation. From Harrison MR, Golbus MS, Filly RA: *The Unborn Patient: Prenatal Diagnosis and Treatment.* Orlando, Fla, Grune & Stratton Inc, 1984. Used by permission.)

The largest experience in the management of fetuses with congenital hydronephrosis is that obtained at the University of California, San Francisco.[12, 16] Among their first 26 fetuses, 8 had unilateral hydronephrosis and were followed up without intervention; all infants did well following post-delivery surgery. Three fetuses had bilateral hydronephrosis, which resolved spontaneously prior to delivery. Eight fetuses with bilateral hydronephrosis were shown to have poor renal function with the following results: three were not treated and died after birth with dysplastic kidneys and pulmonary hypoplasia; three women elected to terminate their pregnancies based on diagnostic studies showing irreversible disease; in two cases, a drainage procedure was successfully performed, but the infants subsequently died of irreversible renal damage. Seven fetuses had bilateral hydronephrosis and "equivocal" function. Four were delivered prematurely and subsequently underwent surgical correction; three did well and one had renal failure. In three fetuses, shunts were percutaneously placed in the bladder and drained into the amniotic fluid. Of these three, one infant died with multiple congenital anomalies, one developed severe renal failure, and one infant did well. The University of California, San Francisco group (Mitchel S. Golbus, M.D., personal communication) is currently evaluating a protocol on a limited number of cases in which the fetus is exteriorized at hysterotomy and operated upon for bladder outlet obstruction. Preliminary data suggest that such "direct" fetal surgery may offer the best outcome for such fetuses.

These investigators have also described a method (based on a combination of sonographic, biochemical, and physiologic criteria) of selecting those fetuses with bilateral urinary tract obstruction who they believe will be most likely to be aided by therapeutic intervention.[17] They have found that fetuses who later proved to have good function produced urine of hypotonic composition (suggesting intact glomerular and tubular function), whereas fetuses with poor function had isotonic urine.

From the very limited experience with surgery for fetal urinary tract obstruction, as well as the natural history of such anomalies, it appears that the chances of fetal salvage are optimized by decompression of the bladder and the restoration of amniotic fluid dynamics as early in gestation as possible.* However, the success rate measured by survival and ultimate prognosis remains to be established.

FUTURE DIRECTIONS

Diaphragmatic Hernia

Many infants with congenital diaphragmatic hernia cannot survive because of pulmonary hypoplasia caused by compression of the herniated viscera into the thoracic cavity. Using a fetal lamb model in which diaphragmatic hernias were created at about 100 days' gestation, Harrison and associates[12, 18] have developed a successful in utero surgical technique that

---

*A total of 73 cases of fetal obstructive uropathy, treated by placement of an in-utero long-term vesicoamniotic shunt, have been reported by 20 centers from around the world to the International Fetal Surgery Registry.[10] The number of cases in any one center ranged from 1 to 30, with 14 of the 20 centers reporting only 1 case. The mean (± 1 SD) gestational age at diagnosis of obstructive uropathy was 23 ± 4.6 weeks (range, 16–34). Eleven of these 73 fetuses (15%) were electively aborted on the basis of either a chromosomal abnormality (6 cases) or severe renal dysfunction (5 cases). Excluding these 11, the survival rate was 48.4% (30 of 62 cases). Of interest, only 5 of the 73 fetuses (6.8%) were female. Forty-three of the 73 treated fetuses (58.9%) died. Of these 43 fetal deaths, there were 14 stillbirths: 11 resulting from elective abortion, 2 occurring at the time of shunt placement (presumably the direct result of fetal trauma), and 1 occurring 6 weeks after placement of the shunt; in this last case, autopsy revealed previously unrecognized central nervous system abnormalities. Twenty-nine of the 73 cases (39.7%) resulted in neonatal deaths: 27 (all occurring within 6 hours of delivery) were due to pulmonary hypoplasia with respiratory insufficiency, 1 was due to chronic renal failure at two months of age, and 1 caused by respiratory distress syndrome (hyaline membrane disease). Of the 30 survivors, 2 had chronic illnesses: 1 boy had chronic renal failure, and the only surviving girl had persistent cloacal syndrome requiring surgery. The report concluded that "although the registry data do not provide proof, they suggest a possible benefit of prenatal therapy in selected cases of fetal obstructive hydronephrosis (e.g., in posterior urethral valve syndrome)."

involves reduction of the viscera from the thoracic cavity into the peritoneal cavity, repair of the diaphragmatic defect, and enlargement of the abdominal cavity by abdominoplasty using an oval silicone rubber patch sutured to the facial edges, followed by closure of the skin over this patch. They have concluded that the correction of congenital diaphragmatic hernia in utero appears physiologically sound and technically feasible. These investigators stress, however, that the in utero surgical repair of diaphragmatic hernias in human fetuses should be attempted only after considerable experimentation in laboratory animal models.[12, 17] The group at the University of California, San Francisco (Mitchel S. Golbus, M.D., personal communication) has attempted three such diaphragmatic hernia repairs. In two cases, the defects were considered irreparable at the time of surgery, and the pregnancies were terminated. In the third case, the repair was performed with the pregnancy continuing to 31 weeks' gestation. Unfortunately, the infant died shortly after birth from pulmonary hypoplasia.

Spina Bifida

Using fetal rhesus monkeys induced to develop neural tube defects by the administration of synthetic corticosteroids and thalidomide between day 18 and 28 of embryogenesis, a technique has been developed in which an agar-based medium, containing crushed bone particles, is used as a "bone paste" for sculpting overlays to enclose herniated nerve bundles.[19] Although such patching techniques may seal the spina bifida lesion, the effects on neurologic development and function are not yet established.

Gastroschisis

The morbidity and mortality rate in neonates with gastroschisis has been significantly reduced since the mid-1960s by improved surgical techniques; however, serious complications are not infrequent and include respiratory distress, matted viscera, and peel formation. Early in utero repair of gastroschisis may ultimately prove the method of therapeutic choice. Fetal gastroschisis models have been created in rabbits and lambs, which would allow such investigation to be undertaken.[20, 21]

Allogeneic Bone Transplants

Successful intrauterine allogeneic bone transplantations in the rhesus monkey at 120 to 135 days' gestation with use of either fetus-to-fetus bone transplants or particles of crushed bone mixed with an agar-enriched culture medium have been performed.[22] The investigators concluded that the immune surveillance system of fetal rhesus monkeys may be tolerant of such bone allografts, even when performed as late as the second trimester. Moreover, such transplants used in ablative long-bone surgery permit normal growth and development as compared with the contralateral unoperated extremity. Of particular interest was the fact that the "bone paste" had strong adhesive properties and could be sculpted into the desired conformation without forfeiting ultimate long-bone strength. These investigators suggest that this technique may offer potential for surgical repair of skeletal anomalies in utero.[22, 23]

HUMAN EXPERIMENTATION

Fetal research is one of the most controversial and complex areas in the entire field of human experimentation. The National Commission for the Protection of Human Subjects of Biomedical and Behavioral Research spent the first year of its existence (1974–1975) working on fetal experimentation under a Congressional mandate to make recommendations regarding fetal research before working on any other topic. This mandate itself was most influenced by *Roe v. Wade,* the 1973 decision of the US Supreme Court, which provided that the government could not interfere with the decision of a woman and her physician regarding abortion prior to fetal viability.[24] This decision invalidated criminal laws against abortion, increasing the number of fetuses aborted, and, therefore, the number of fetuses potentially available for research.†

As adopted by the US Department of Health and Human Services (HHS), federal regulations currently require that, prior to experimentation involving human fetuses, appropriate animal studies be done and that researchers have no role in any decision to terminate a pregnancy. The purpose of an in utero experiment must be to meet the health needs of the particular fetus, and the fetus can be placed at risk only to the "minimum extent necessary" to meet such needs. In the case of nontherapeutic research, the risk to the fetus must be "minimal" and the knowledge to be gained "important" and not obtainable by other means. The consent of both the mother and the father is required unless the father's identity is not known, he is not reasonably available, or the pregnancy resulted from rape.

The research protocol must be reviewed by an Institutional Review Board (IRB), which, in addition to its normal duties, must take special care to review the subject selection process and the methods by which informed consent is obtained. The consent process itself should probably be audited by a representative of the IRB as well. It has also been recommended by

†See Chapter 6.

some that a special advocate for the fetus be appointed to help caution the parents against consenting to an experimental procedure on their fetus that they may not understand or that they incorrectly may see as therapeutic. It appears, however, that by the time parents reach the major medical centers involved in this research, they have already made up their minds to go ahead with what they consider the last hope that their fetus may have. Thus, the advocate notion may be too little too late if its purpose is to beneficially influence the consent process.[25]

These federal human experimentation regulations technically apply only to those researchers who receive federal funds or are affiliated with institutions that have signed an agreement with HHS that all research in their institutions (and by their faculty and staff in other institutions) will be reviewed by their IRB. Nonetheless, these regulations are so fundamental to the protection of the integrity of the fetus, the potential parents, and the research enterprise itself, that they should be followed voluntarily in all institutions doing fetal research.

State Statutes

The states that have legislated in this area have used a much more rigid and punitive approach: fetal research in many states is a crime. Half the states now have statutes on fetal research; most of these (15) were passed soon after the US Supreme Court's abortion decision and in direct response to it.[24] In fact, more state legislation has been enacted regarding fetal research than regarding any other type of research, and this legislative activity, together with its poor quality, indicates the emotional nature of this research. Most state statutes prohibit or restrict both in utero and ex utero research, and the restrictions are generally more stringent than the federal regulations (only New Mexico's statute models itself on the federal regulations). In Massachusetts, for example, it is a crime to study the fetus in utero unless the study does not "substantially jeopardize" the life or health of the fetus and the fetus is not the subject of a planned abortion. Thus, therapeutic research (such as that on hydrocephalus) is permissible even in this restrictive state. Utah, the only state to deal exclusively with in utero fetuses, prohibits all research on "live unborn children." Eight states (Arkansas, California, Indiana, Kentucky, Montana, Nebraska, Ohio, and Wyoming) limit their prohibitions to the living abortus and so the prohibitions do not apply to fetal surgery at all. California, where much of the research to date has been done, restricts experimentation only on ex utero fetuses, outlawing "any type of scientific or laboratory research or any kind of experimentation or study, except to protect or preserve the life and health of the fetus."

State regulation is a hodgepodge of restrictions and prohibitions, with little consistency among states and no clear rationale. Nevertheless, researchers are bound by the law of the state in which they perform fetal experimentation, and knowledge of its provisions is obviously necessary in states that have such statutes.[24, 26]

Therapeutic Interventions

The line between therapy and experimentation has never been a completely clear one. Some argue for delineation of a transitional state called "pretherapeutic" or "investigational," and others contend that the distinction is usually intellectually pointless.[27] Therapy involves procedures done primarily for the benefit of the patient that are considered "good and accepted medical practice," whereas experimentation involves new or innovative procedures (not yet considered standard practice) for the primary purpose of testing a hypothesis or gaining new knowledge.[28] The courts have not always been consistent in applying these criteria and have even rejected, for example, the argument that the first artificial heart implant was done for other than therapeutic purposes.[29] Nevertheless, it seems fair and accurate to conclude that all of the procedures described in this chapter must currently be considered experimental and subject to the rules already summarized. Specifically, IRB review, detailed consent, and a consent auditor are all ethically and legally appropriate. An advocate for the fetus may also be appropriate in especially problematic cases.

Eventually, however, it is likely that at least some types of fetal surgery will become accepted medical practice. Then, the basic legal and ethical rules relating to therapy will apply. The most important issues will include informed consent, resource allocation, and potential maternal-fetal conflicts.

Consent

It is a fundamental premise of Anglo-American law that no one can touch or treat a competent adult without the adult's informed consent. This doctrine is based primarily on the value we place on autonomy or self-determination and, secondarily, on rational decision making. The first requires that individuals have the ultimate say concerning whether or not their bodies will be "invaded"; the latter requires disclosure of certain material information (a description of the proposed procedure, risks of death and serious disability, alternatives, success rates, and problems of recuperation) before one is asked to consent to an "invasion."[30]

All of this is relatively straightforward when one is dealing with an adult, but how does it apply when the therapy is aimed at the fetus? In the experimental setting, federal regulations call for the consent of the mother and the father prior to any permissible experimentation. In the therapeutic setting, the consent of either one of the parents is generally sufficient for beneficial procedures on children. In the case of the fetus, however, if the proposed procedure will place the mother at any risk of death or serious disability, only she would have the right to consent (and the corresponding right to withhold consent). Even after fetal viability, the US Constitution gives the woman and her physician the right to terminate the pregnancy if the mother's life or health is endangered.[24] In an analogous case, the US Supreme Court ruled that when conflict exists between a potential father and mother over the issue of an abortion, the mother's position should prevail because she has more at stake (that is, her own body and health) than the father.[31] The same logic applies here. The consent of the mother must be a necessary precondition for such surgery. Of course, her consent must be informed, and she should be told as clearly as possible about the proposed procedure and its risk to herself and her fetus, as well as about the alternatives, the success rates, and the likely problems of recuperation.

Resource Allocation

John Fletcher has raised resource allocation as one of the major ethical issues concerning fetal therapy.[32] Currently, the issue concerns how much funding the federal government and others should allocate to research in this area. This is fundamentally a political question, but it has ethical overtones. Is it acceptable, for example, to continue to place our most heavy emphasis on the extension of life for the elderly, rather than on providing fetuses and neonates with the best chance to live a healthy life? In an area in which early treatment can lead to the prevention of disease and misery, and, perhaps, can reduce significantly the cost of a lifetime of care, both research and treatment warrant a high priority. When fetal surgery becomes accepted medical practice, issues of screening, selection, and indications must also be addressed by insurance companies and other third-party payers. A liberal payment policy seems sensible.

MATERNAL-FETAL CONFLICTS

The emergence of fetal surgery brings the maternal-fetal conflict issue into sharp focus. This issue is, of course, at the heart of the continuing abortion debate, where the rights of the pregnant woman now take legal precedence. Putting the rights of the pregnant women first seems reasonable, but what if the woman "waives" her right to abortion? Does she then not take on a new duty to the fetus that she has decided will become a child, a duty to ensure that it will be born as healthy as she can reasonably make it?[33] This is a complex issue, but we believe that no pregnant woman should ever be legally forced to undergo medical procedures that threaten her with death or serious bodily harm for the sake of the life or health of her fetus. Much more difficult questions are raised when the intervention poses no physical threat to the woman (such as taking a vitamin pill), but she still objects to it on religious or personal grounds. Although this issue is not likely to arise very often, as most women will do almost anything to ensure the health of their fetuses, it is an issue of great symbolic importance because it determines what value and how much respect we accord to the autonomy of pregnant women. It has also been the most controversial issue touching fetal surgery. It therefore warrants careful review.

In 1979, four obstetricians suggested that when women in labor refuse surgical intervention recommended to save the life of their fetuses,

> It is probably that the patient hopes to be freed in this way of an undesired pregnancy . . . because it is an unplanned pregnancy, the woman is divorced or widowed, the pregnancy is an extramarital one, there are inheritance problems, etc.[34]

The view that women who refuse cesarean sections are willfully abusing their fetuses seems prevalent and deeply held (at least by some male obstetricians and judges) and is reflected in a number of cases in which judges have ordered women who refused surgical interventions during labor to undergo them. Almost all of the cases decided to date are lower court decisions and so are of dubious precedential value. The only state supreme court case (Georgia) was decided under emergency conditions, and the court misconstrued the law. Nonetheless, because these cases represent the only judicial pronouncements on this subject to date, they must be addressed.

The Georgia Case

Jessie Mae Jefferson was due to deliver her child in about four days when the hospital in which she would be attended sought a court order authorizing physicians to perform a cesarean section and any necessary blood transfusions should she enter the hospital and refuse.[35] She had previously notified the hospital that it was her religious belief that the Lord had healed her body and that whatever happened to the child was the Lord's will. At an emergency hearing conducted at the hospital, her examining physician testified that she had complete placenta previa, with a 99% certainty that her child would not survive vaginal delivery and a 50% chance that she herself would not survive it. On this basis, the court decided that the "unborn child" merited legal protection and authorized the administration of "all medical procedures deemed necessary by the attending physician to preserve the life of the defendant unborn child."

The next day, a public agency petitioned for temporary custody in the same court, alleging that the unborn child was "a deprived child without proper parental care" and seeking an order requiring the mother to submit to a cesarean section. The odds that the unborn child would die if a vaginal birth was attempted were put at 99% to 100% by the physician. The court granted the petition, on the basis that the

> state has an interest in the life of this unborn, living human being [and] the intrusion involved . . . is outweighed by the duty of the state to protect a living, unborn human being from meeting his or her death before being given the opportunity to live.

The parents immediately petitioned the Georgia State Court to stay the order. On the evening of the same day as the hearing, the court denied their motion, with a two-sentence conclusory opinion, citing *Roe v. Wade*[24] and *Raleigh Fitkin*[36] as authority. A few days later, Mrs. Jefferson uneventfully delivered a healthy baby without surgical intervention.

Court Decisions Regarding Surgery

Lower court decisions that were not appealed have been decided in courts in Colorado, Michigan, New York, and Illinois, and perhaps elsewhere as well. In the Illinois case, surgery was ordered and apparently thereafter the woman's consent was obtained.[37] In the Michigan case, which involved a woman who refused a cesarean section on the basis of religious objections, surgery was also ordered, but the woman fled the jurisdiction and reportedly had a normal vaginal delivery without complication to herself or her child.[38] In the New York case, Judge Margaret Taylor refused to order a cesarean section on the basis of a prolapsed cord after talking with the pregnant woman, a 35-year-old black woman who had borne ten children. The patient was competent and objected both on religious grounds and on the grounds that she had the right to control her own body. An hour after the judge's decision, the woman delivered a healthy baby without surgical intervention.[39] The best documented lower court case is one from Colorado.

The Colorado Case

The pregnant woman in the Colorado case was unmarried and had previously given birth to twins. She was described as obese, angry, and uncooperative. An internal fetal heart monitor suggested fetal hypoxia, and a cesarean section was recommended. Because of the patient's fear of surgery, she refused. Her mother, her sister, and the father of her child attempted unsuccessfully to change her mind. A psychiatric consultant concluded that she was neither delusional nor mentally incompetent.

The hospital administration was notified, and a decision was made to request court intervention. The hospital staff petitioned the juvenile court to find the unborn baby a dependent and a neglected child and to order a cesarean section to safeguard its life. An emergency hearing was convened in the patient's room, following which the court granted the petition and ordered the surgery. The cesarean section was performed, resulting in a healthy child and no complications for the mother. Because more than nine hours had elapsed between the tracings of the external fetal heart monitor that indicated distress (and six hours from internal tracings) and the delivery, the physician was surprised that the outcome was not poor. He indicated that the case "simply underscores the limitations of continuous fetal heart monitoring as a means of predicting neonatal outcome."[40]

These cases pose three questions: What is the state of the law? What should the role of the judiciary be in such disputes? And what position should physicians and hospitals take when confronted with a woman who refuses a cesarean section against medical advice?

State of the Law

The cases all lack an analysis of the precedents and place heavy and primary reliance on *Raleigh Fitkin*[36] and *Roe v. Wade.*[24] The courts should at least have considered the severe limitations of these two cases. *Raleigh Fitkin* involved a woman who was approximately eight months pregnant. Physicians believed that, at some time before giving birth, she would hemorrhage severely and that both she and her unborn child would die if she did not submit to blood transfusions. She refused blood transfusions because she was a Jehovah's Witness. The trial court upheld her refusal, and the hospital appealed to the New Jersey Supreme Court. In the meantime, the woman had left the hospital against medical advice, and the case was moot. Nevertheless, the court proceeded to determine that the unborn child was "entitled to the law's protection" and that blood transfusions could be administered to the woman "if necessary to save her life or the life of her child, as the physician in charge at the time may determine."[36]

This opinion is of limited value. First, no one was forced to do anything as a result of the opinion; that is, no transfusion was actually performed, and no police were dispatched to apprehend the woman and return her to the hospital. Second, it was a one-page opinion, with little policy discussion. Third, the extent of bodily invasion involved in a blood transfusion is much less than that involved in a cesarean section, which is major abdominal surgery. Fourth, the case was decided eight years before the US Supreme Court decision in *Roe v. Wade* and more than a decade before the same New Jersey court decided the case of Karen Ann Quinlan.

The second case, *Roe v. Wade*,[24] does stand for the proposition that the state has a compelling interest in preserving the life of viable fetuses. But it does *not* have such an interest if "the life or health of the mother" is endangered by carrying the child to term. The question that needs to be discussed is the relevance of the additional danger (physical or mental) to the mother of undergoing a cesarean section when its purpose is to protect the health of the fetus. In the Colorado case, for example, it was noted that excessively obese patients are "generally considered at increased risk of anesthetic and surgical complications." When do such increased risk factors outweigh the child's right to be born via cesarean section? The physician in the Colorado case cautioned that "had the patient steadfastly refused it might not have been either safe or possible to administer anesthesia to a struggling, resistant woman who weighed in excess of 157.5 kg."[40] Nothing in *Roe v. Wade*[24] gives either judges or physicians the right to favor the life or health of the fetus over that of the pregnant woman. No mother has ever been legally required to undergo surgery or general anesthesia (e.g., for bone marrow aspiration) to save the life of her dying child. It would be ironic if she could be forced to submit to more invasive surgical procedures for the sake of her fetus than for her child. For all these reasons, it is premature to label the conclusions of these quickly decided cases, which lack any meaningful analysis, "the law." The most that can be concluded is that the law in this area is very much in its infancy.

Judges in the Hospital

Judges are not terribly good at making emergency medical decisions. Perhaps the most famous example is the opinion of Judge Skelly Wright in the *Georgetown College* case.[41] The case involved an emergency petition to permit blood transfusions to a Jehovah's Witness patient to save her life. A lower court judge refused to issue such an order, but Judge Wright did, less than 1½ hours after he was approached by counsel for the hospital. He went to the hospital and interviewed the woman and her husband. The woman, a 25-year-old, who had a 7-month-old child, was "not in a mental condition to make a decision." Her husband refused but said if the judge ordered it, it would not be his responsibility. Because the judge believed that the woman's reasoning would be similar, he ordered the transfusion.

The full bench of the US Circuit Court of Appeals for the District of

Columbia refused to review the case, but some of its members dissented from this refusal and noted their concerns. Judge Miller, for example, noted that:

> [Judge Wright], impelled, I am sure, by humanitarian impulses doubtless was, himself, under considerable strain . . . In the interval of about an hour and twenty minutes between the appearance of the attorney in his chambers and the signing of the order at the hospital, the judge had no opportunity for research as to the substantive legal problems and procedural questions involved. He should not have been asked to act in these circumstances.[41]

Judge Warren Burger, former Chief Justice of the US Supreme Court, quoted Justice Benjamin Cardozo on judicial restraint:

> The judge, even when he is free, is still not wholly free. He is not to innovate at pleasure. He is not a knight-errant, roaming at will in pursuit of his own ideal of beauty or of goodness. He is to draw his inspiration from consecrated principles. He is not to yield to spasmodic sentiment, to vague and unregulated benevolence.

It is inappropriate for judges to act impulsively, without benefit of reflection on past precedent and the likely future impact of their opinions. The cesarean section cases discussed in this chapter suffer from a lack of reflection. Obviously, the delivery room is not conducive to such reflection, and judges probably do not belong there at all in such "emergency" circumstances.*

---

*A legally analogous situation occurs when a court authorizes a "search and seizure" of a substance that is inside the body of a criminal suspect. In the most famous case, the US Supreme Court ruled that having a physician take blood in a hospital to determine whether an individual was under the influence of alcohol was "reasonable" under the Fourth Amendment protection against unjustified searches and seizures because of the strong interest the community had in fairly and accurately determining guilt or innocence, the inability of determining intoxication by other means, and the very minor invasion of the body involved in drawing blood which, "for most people involves virtually no risk, trauma, or pain" (*Schmerber v. California*, 384 U.S. 757, 771 [1966]). In an earlier case the court had found a search unreasonable when police had broken into a suspect's room, attempted to extract narcotics capsules he had put in his mouth, and then rushed him to the hospital and insisted that an emetic be administered to induce vomiting. This was held to violate his interests in "human dignity" (*Rochin v. California,* 342, US 165 [1952]). Most analogous to the cesarean section cases, however, is the recent case in which the US Supreme Court upheld a lower court ruling that it would be unreasonable under the Fourth Amendment to order surgery to remove a bullet from an accused armed robber who shot his victim and was in turn shot by him. The court held, consistent with *Schmerber* and *Rochin,* that the interests of the accused had to be balanced against the interests of the state. The accused's primary interests were in maintaining "personal privacy and bodily integrity." Removal of the bullet would require, among other things, general anesthesia. In the court's words:

> When conducted with the consent of the patient, surgery requiring general anesthesia is not necessarily demeaning or intrusive. In such a case, the surgeon is carrying out the patient's own will concerning the patient's body and the patient's right to privacy is therefore

What Should the Law Be?

The law can take one of two paths, neither completely satisfactory. The first is to follow the lead of most cases and require the woman to submit to a cesarean section when her physician deems it necessary to protect her fetus. The problems with this approach are illustrated by these cases. First, the physician's prediction of fetal harm may not be accurate. Indeed, in most of these cases, serious errors were made. In Georgia, a 99% certainty turned out to be wrong; the supposed 1% reality occurred. In New York and Michigan, intervention also turned out to be unnecessary, and in Colorado the fetal heart monitor significantly overstated the amount of damage to the fetus from delayed delivery. So permitting physicians to judge when fetuses are in danger may simply be giving them a license to perform cesarean sections or fetal surgery whenever they want to, without regard to the pregnant woman's desires.[42]

But even supposing 100% accuracy, we should still permit pregnant women to refuse surgery, to protect their liberty as well as that of all competent adults. Practical considerations also support the rights of the woman over those of the fetus. Women may take matters into their own hands and not deliver in hospitals. Other interventions to which they might consent will be unavailable at home, and an opportunity to try to change their minds will be lost. The question of what to do with a woman who continues to refuse in the face of a court order remains. Do we really want to restrain, forcibly medicate, and operate on a competent, refusing adult? Such a procedure may be "legal," especially when viewed from the judicial perspective that the woman is irrational, hysterical, or evil-minded, but it is certainly brutish and not what one generally associates with medical care. It also encourages an adversarial relationship between the obstetrician and the patient, and it gives the obstetrician a weapon to bully into submission any pregnant women whom she or he views as irrational. Attempts at vaginal

preserved. In this case, however . . . the Commonwealth proposes to *take control of respondent's body,* to drug this citizen—not yet convicted of a criminal offense—with narcotics and barbiturates into a state of unconsciousness and then to search beneath his skin for evidence of a crime. *This kind of surgery involves a virtually total divestment of respondent's ordinary control over surgical probing beneath his skin* [emphasis supplied] (*Winston v. Lee,* 470 U.S. [1985]).

Not only was the burden on the citizen great, the state had other evidence available to make its case, so the search wasn't "reasonable." Analogously, a forced cesarean section is a much more intrusive and dangerous surgical procedure than the bullet removal and much more demeaning to the patient because it treats her simply as a container. On the other hand, the potential state interest in the life of the fetus (soon-to-be child) is very high. Nonetheless, we believe the reasonable balance must fall to the woman and her consent should be the sine qua non of surgery.

deliveries after one birth by cesarean section, for example, could fall victim to such a rule.

Could the case for forced cesarean sections be distinguished from fetal surgery when it becomes accepted medical procedure, or would pregnant women be forced to undergo fetal surgery as well? And if one can lawfully force surgery, one should certainly be able to restrain the liberty of a woman for the sake of her fetus, for example, by confining her during all or part of her pregnancy should she have an alcohol or drug problem that could adversely affect her fetus. It seems wrong to say that patients have the right to be wrong in all cases except pregnancy. In that case, why should only physicians have the right to be wrong?

The "waiver" argument that we opened this section with is not persuasive.[33] First, women never really do waive their right to an abortion; it is an inalienable right that they retain it up to the moment of childbirth if their life or health is endangered by continuing the pregnancy. Second, this argument takes a right designed as a shield to protect pregnant women and turns it into a sword to be used against them by individuals who "know better." Finally, women have a constitutional right to bear children if they are physically able. To have a legal rule that there are no restrictions on a women's decision to have an abortion, but if she elects childbirth instead, then the state will require her to surrender her basic rights of body integrity and privacy, creates a state-erected penalty on her exercise of her right to bear a child.[43] Such a penalty would (or at least should) be unconstitutional.

Nor does providing children the right to sue their mothers for not properly taking care of themselves and their future during pregnancy make policy sense. We may all agree that mothers should take care of themselves and their fetuses, but it is unlikely that the prospect of a damaged child suing its mother at some later date will be either an effective deterrent or a useful means of compensating the child. Indeed, it is more likely that this punitive approach will simply make it appear that we are doing something for fetuses when, in fact, we are not. Few children will ever find anyone to sue their mothers on their behalf, and, in any case even if they do, any funds gained would likely be those that would be used for the child's benefit.† Positive programs of education, the funding of maternal and child health programs, and medical research to help prevent the diseases that fetal surgery is designed to treat would be more effective. Extending notions of child abuse to "fetal abuse" brings the state into pregnancy without any likelihood of benefit and great potential for invasions of privacy and massive

---

†Such suits may, however, make sense if confined to cases in which the mother has given the child up for adoption or has relinquished her parental rights.

deprivations of liberty. Treating women as incubators while they are pregnant represses them and deprives them of their human dignity and autonomy, and so dehumanizes us all.

The arbitrariness and uselessness of after the fact criminal prosecutions of pregnant women who do not follow their doctor's "orders" is illustrated by an October 1986 California indictment against Mrs. Pamela Monson. The case had not been tried when this was written, but reportedly Mrs. Monson was, because of placenta previa, advised by her physician to refrain from taking drugs, stay off her feet, avoid intercourse, and seek immediate medical attention should she begin to hemorrhage. According to the police, she ignored this advice, staying at home after she first noticed some bleeding (having intercourse with her husband and taking some amphetamines), and not going to the hospital until many hours later. Her son was born with massive brain damage, and died six weeks later. Criminal charges were filed under California's child support statute, which includes "unborn children."*

The prosecution alleges that such "disobeying instructions" or "failure to follow through on medical advice" is grounds for criminal action. This strikes us as both silly and dangerous; silly because medical *advice* should remain *advice:* physicians are neither policemen nor seers; dangerous because medical advice is a vague term that can cover almost anything. To be effective in protecting fetuses, monitoring compliance would be necessary. This could require confining pregnant women to an environment in which eating, exercise, drug use, and sexual intercourse could be controlled. This could, of course, be a maximum security country club, but such massive invasions of privacy can only be justified by treating pregnant women during their pregnancy as fetal containers.†

Other quandaries arise if we apply child neglect statutes to fetuses. Unlike a child, the fetus is absolutely dependent upon its mother and cannot itself be "treated" without in some way invading the mother. The "fetal protection" policy enunciated by the prosecution seems to assume that, like mother and child, mother and fetus are two separate individuals, with separate rights. But treating them separately before birth can only be done by favoring one over the other in disputes. Favoring the fetus radically deval-

---

*If a parent of a minor child *willfully omits,* without lawful excuse, *to furnish* necessary clothing, food, shelter, or *medical attendance, or other remedial care* for his or her child, he or she is guilty of a misdemeanor punishable by a fine not exceeding $2,000.00, or by imprisonment [for one year] (emphasis added) (Cal. Penal Code, Sec. 270 [West, 1986]).

†Brain dead pregnant women can, however, properly be viewed as containers, and their respiration artificially maintained for the sake of their fetuses. Women in persistent vegetative states probably also have less interest in privacy than their fetuses have in life. See *University Health Services v. Piazzi,* CV86-RCCV-464. Richmond Co. Sup. Ct., Aug. 4, 1986, Fleming, J.

ues the pregnant woman and treats her like an inert incubator, or a culture medium for the fetus. This view makes women unequal citizens, since only they can have children, and relegates them to performing one main function: childbearing. It is one thing for the state to view the fetus as a patient; it is another to assume that the fetus's interests are in opposition to its mother, and to treat the fetus by requiring the mother to be its servant.

The alternative to using the power of the state to coerce pregnant women is to honor the unusual case of a woman's refusal. We assume that this is general practice at the vast majority of hospitals in the country regarding cesarean sections. We believe that it should apply to fetal surgery and other interventions during pregnancy as well and that it is the proper practice ethically and legally. This view may seem callous to the rights of the fetuses, as some fetuses that might be salvaged may die or may be born defective. This is tragic, but it is likely to be rare. It is the price that society pays for protecting the rights of all competent adults and for preventing forcible physical violations of pregnant women by coercive obstetricians and judges. The choice between fetal health and maternal liberty is laced with moral and ethical dilemmas. The force of law cannot magically make them disappear.

We reach this conclusion primarily because fetal surgery entails serious risks to the mother and requires her body to be "invaded" to reach and manipulate the fetus. If these considerations were not present (for example, if the fetus could be treated with a drug that the mother could take orally and that would not affect her own health), a much more difficult balancing test would be presented. In this latter case, we think that the woman would be morally wrong not to take the drug (assuming it is virtually 100% effective and had no adverse fetal or maternal effects). Nonetheless, we do not favor permitting police to forcibly administer such a drug under court order unless the woman has been judged mentally incompetent.[30] Education, counseling, and the provision of reasonable prenatal care seem a more positive and beneficial route in the long run.

MEDICAL THERAPIES

Many drugs have been utilized with the hope of improving the capacity for the fetus to adapt to postnatal life. Important examples include use of drugs to arrest preterm labor, prenatal administration of glucocorticoids to advance fetal lung maturity for the prevention of respiratory distress syndrome in premature infants, use of propylthiouracil to prevent intrauterine growth retardation and neonatal thyrotoxicosis in cases of maternal Graves disease, and pharmacologic cardioversion of fetal tachycardia to prevent fetal demise or severe congestive heart failure in the newborn.

The rationale for prenatal medical treatment of genetic disorders is that intervention will favorably influence conditions in which postnatal therapy is too late because the infant would be born already injured.

Metabolic Diseases

Methylmalonic Acidemia

Methylmalonic acidemia (MMA) is a rare disorder characterized clinically by recurrent vomiting, failure to thrive, developmental retardation, hepatomegaly (enlarged liver), intermittent neutropenia (abnormal decrease in the number of neutrophil cells in the blood) and thrombocytopenia (abnormal decrease in the number of blood platelets). Acidosis is often present and may be life threatening. Methylmalonic acidemia occurs in humans in association with vitamin B_{12} deficiency, since coenzymatically active B_{12} is required for the conversion of methylmalonyl-coenzyme A to succinyl-coenzyme A. At least six different genetially determined biochemical defects (all autosomal recessive) can result in accumulation of methylmalonic acid. Both B_{12}-responsive and B_{12}-unresponsive variants of the disorder have been identified.[44]

The prenatal diagnosis and successful prenatal treatment of a female infant with B_{12}-responsive MMA was first reported in 1975. Maternal excretion of methylmalonate was monitored. Since the mother did not excrete methylmalonate when she was not pregnant, the appearance of this compound in her urine could be used as a biochemical index of fetal status. During the last trimester, large doses of vitamin B_{12} produced a marked decrease in methylmalonate. The infant was shown to have elevated vitamin B_{12} stores at birth as a result of the dose given to the mother. Subsequent follow-up studies showed the infant developing normally on a restricted protein diet alone. This was a marked contrast to an affected, untreated earlier sibling who died of severe acidosis and dehydration at the age of 3 months.

Although in this case treatment certainly improved fetal—and secondarily maternal—biochemistry, it has been questioned whether this therapy was more effective than immediate treatment at birth with large doses of cyanohydroxycobalamin or hydroxycobalamin.[45]

Multiple Carboxylase Deficiency

Biotin responsive multiple carboxylase deficiency is a rare autosomal recessively inherited inborn error of metabolism in which three biotin dependent mitochondrial enzymes (namely, pyruvate carboxylase, proprionyl-CoA carboxylase, and B-methylcrotonyl-CoA carboxylase) show diminished activity. Affected infants show a clinical picture of severe metabolic acidosis, hypertonia, and irritability. If left untreated, they become lethargic, lapse into a coma, and die. If infants with this disorder are given pharmacologic doses of biotin (250 to 1,000 times the usual daily intake of this vitamin), there is rapid normalization of their chemical derangements, accompanied by dramatic clinical improvement.

In one case, a woman presented at 34 weeks' gestation with a twin pregnancy.[46] Earlier, a posthumous diagnosis of multiple carboxylase deficiency had been made in a previous child of this couple, and another sibling had died within three days of birth (undiagnosed but with a similar clinical picture). Prenatal diagnosis was not attempted because of the very late stage of pregnancy. But, because of the previous family history of neonatal onset of this disorder, these investigators believed it imperative to attempt prenatal therapy by oral administration of large doses of biotin to the mother. After the birth of clinically normal nonidentical twins, one unaffected and one later shown to be affected, the investigators concluded the prenatal therapy for the disease was efficacious.

In another case the mother started to receive oral biotin at 23½ weeks' gestation. The full-term female infant exhibited no clinical or chemical aberrations during the first four days of life, before the start of postnatal biotin supplementation. Growth and development were normal at age 1¼ years. The investigators speculated that prenatal treatment can prevent a specific and potential irreversible cerebellar degeneration.[47]

Although these cases demonstrate that prenatal treatment can alter the biochemical abnormalities in affected fetuses, they have not proved that such management provides any greater advantage as compared to that offered by prompt postnatal treatment.[45]

Congenital Adrenal Hyperplasia (21-Hydroxylase Deficiency)

The most common form of congenital adrenal hyperplasia (CAH) is due to a deficiency of the enzyme 21-hydroxylase. The most prominent clinical feature of this autosomal recessive disorder is virilization of the external genitalia in genetic females, which is manifest at birth and results from excessive prenatal secretion of adrenal androgens. Further complications arise at puberty in untreated patients with CAH. The female fails to develop breasts, remains amenorrheic, and develops a male habitus. In the male, the testes generally remain small and fail to develop and function. Without appropriate therapy adults may be expected to be sterile.

In one case, a woman with mild 21-hydroxylase deficiency had a previous female child who had classic CAH with masculinization.[48] The mother was given dexamethasone orally, beginning at the tenth week of gestation and treatment was continued until birth. Fetal adrenal suppression was demonstrated by serial measurements of maternal estriol excretion, and quantitation of various steroid metabolites in midtrimester amniotic fluid. A female was born who had normal clinical findings; she was subsequently shown not to have CAH. The investigators considered it likely that similar suppression could be achieved with classic CAH; however, they acknowledged that determination of whether such suppression would prevent external genital masculinization in CAH awaits definitive testing.

Other Metabolic Disorders

Additional prenatal medical therapies have been speculated upon for the treatment of fetuses at risk for various metabolic diseases. Maternal copper supplementation has been given for *Menkes' kinky-hair syndrome* (an X-linked recessive disorder that causes defective copper absorption and leads to abnormal and depigmented (steely) hair, a characteristic face, and brain degeneration). Maternal dietary galactose restriction has been recommended for *galactosemia* (an autosomal recessive defect of the enzyme galactose-1-phosphate uridyl transferase that can lead to lethargy, hypotonia, cataracts, mental retardation, and death in infants not treated with galactose-free diets). High-dose therapy with vitamin E has been utilized for *glutathione synthetase deficiency* (an autosomal recessive disorder that results in hemolytic anemia, acidosis, and central nervous system dysfunction). High-doses of vitamin E have been given for *abetalipoproteinemia* (an autosomal recessive disorder that is presumed to be due to failure of synthesis of apoprotein B and is characterized by pigmentary retinal degeneration, intestinal malabsorption, abnormal red blood cells, neonatal psychomotor delay slowly progressing to moderate-to-severe ataxia before age 20, and mental retardation in about a third of patients).[45]

B Vitamin/Mineral Supplementation

Periconceptual vitamin/mineral supplementation to prevent neural tube defects (NTDs) is one of the most promising prevention technologies on the horizon today.[49] Studies in the United Kingdom suggest a protective effect in high-risk pregnancies of women who have previously had a child with an NTD (recurrence risk 1:10 to 1:50).[50–52] Despite potential difficulties in recruiting women and ensuring compliance, the Medical Research Council in the United Kingdom has initiated a five-year multicenter clinical trial to determine whether vitamin supplementation prior to and during early pregnancy can prevent the recurrence of NTDs.[53, 54] An anticipated 5,000 participants will be allocated blindly into four treatment groups: (1)

minerals plus vitamins; (2) minerals, vitamins, and folate; (3) minerals and folate; and (4) minerals only. Participation in the study requires the following: (1) each woman is fully aware of the issues; (2) her physician agrees that participation is in the interest of the patient; (3) each local center has approval from its ethics committee; and (4) participants may withdraw from the program at anytime.*

Stem Cell Transplantation

A number of cases have been reported of children with hematologic disorders who have been successfully treated by bone marrow transplantation. The disorders included thalassemia major,[55] sickle cell disease,[56] and chronic granulomatous disease and others.[57-61] Using the same basic concept, it has been proposed that hematopoietic stem cells (i.e., cells whose descendants differentiate into the various types of blood cells) could be transplanted. Such prenatal therapy might obviate the potential complications of postnatal hematopoietic stem cell (HSC) transplantation, particularly the so-called "graft versus host" disease. In this disease, bone marrow cells are from immunocompetent donors, and, if lymphocytes and their committed precursors are present in a graft, a rejection could occur. Moreover, the recipients of HSC transplants often have had time to develop the sequelae of their inherited disease state (including growth retardation, recurrent infections, and sensitization to therapeutic blood transfusions) should an HSC graft be later considered.[62]

In theory, in utero fetal HSC transplantation should be feasible because the fetus is an ideal host due to its ontologic readiness for engraftment, i.e., the bone marrow is normally seeded by hematopoietic cells delivered from the liver at around the 20th week of gestation. In addition, the fetus appears to exhibit some degree of "immunotolerance" to allogeneic grafts from unmatched donors. The fetus may also be regarded as an ideal donor because the richest and most available source of HSC is fetal liver. Current areas of investigation are focusing on the development of methods to minimize the potential for graft versus host disease and the development of models to assess the effectiveness of an in utero HSC transplantation to cure various genetic disorders. Attention is also being directed toward determining the

---

*In the United States the National Institute of Child Health and Human Development (NICHD) is sponsoring a collaborative retrospective case-control study of vitamin supplementation and neural tube defects, which is being conducted at Northwestern University Medical School, Chicago (Joe L. Simpson, principal investigator) and at the California Public Health Foundation, Berkeley (George C. Cunningham, principal investigator) in coordination with James L. Millis and George G. Rhodes from NICHD. Also, the Spina Bifida Association of America, in conjunction with the Center for Disease Control, has initiated a prospective randomized clinical trial evaluating vitamin/mineral supplementation.

optimal technique for introducing HSC into the fetus: (1) intraperitoneally, as is currently done with intrauterine transfusions, or (2) directly into a blood vessel in the placenta or the umbilical cord using fetoscopy or ultrasound guidance.[62]

Gene Therapy

Gene therapy is concerned with treating genetic disease by the replacement or correction of a defective mutant gene.[2, 63] There are four potential levels of application of genetic engineering for the insertion of a gene into a human being:

1. *Somatic cell gene therapy* involves correction of a genetic defect in the somatic (i.e. body) cells of a patient; the genetic changes would *not* be transmitted to future generations.

2. *Germ line gene therapy* entails insertion of the gene into the reproductive cells of the patient in such a way that the disorder in his or her offspring would also be corrected.

3. *Enhancement genetics* involves insertion of a gene to "enhance" a specific characteristic; for example, adding an extra gene that codes for growth hormone into a normal child in an attempt to achieve a tall individual.

4. *Eugenic genetic engineering* includes attempts to alter or "improve" complex human traits that are at least in part genetically determined; for example, intelligence, personality, or athletic ability.[64]

Somatic cell gene therapy is technically the most feasible and ethically the least controversial.

Somatic Cell Gene Therapy

As in the case of stem cell transplantation, somatic cell gene therapy could be undertaken either preconceptually or postconceptually. The rationale for prenatal therapy is that the fetus will benefit from in utero activity of the inserted gene. For example, a metabolic disorder may cause irreversible adverse effects that could have been prevented if gene therapy had been performed during fetal development. However, postnatal therapy might prove equally or even more efficacious as compared to prenatal therapy, at least for some of the genetic disorders in which this technology might be applied.

Gene therapy should be beneficial primarily for the replacement of a defective or missing enzyme or protein that must function inside the cell that makes it, or a deficient circulating protein whose level does not need to be exactly regulated.[64] Opinions differ in the scientific community as to which diseases will be among the first to be treated with gene therapy. Those diseases currently being proposed include combined immune deficiency diseases attributed to deficiencies in adenosine deaminase or in purine nucleoside phosphorylase; metabolic disorders of the urea cycle, including citrullinemia and ornithine transcarbamoylase deficiency; and possibly α_1-antitrypsin deficiency. A great deal of research is also being done on the gene that codes for hypoxanthine-guanine phosphoribosyl transferase, a deficiency that leads to the devastating Lesch-Nyhan syndrome, characterized by mental retardation, self-mutilation, and choreoathetosis.

Current research has been primarily directed at integrating the appropriate gene into the DNA of primordial (stem) cells of an individual's own aspirated bone marrow. These transformed cells would then be reimplanted into the patient where they would multiply to produce colonies of cells that would express the new inserted genes at an appropriate level. Techniques for transferring cloned genes into cells can be grouped into four categories: (1) *viral*, both RNA viruses (or retroviruses) and DNA viruses (for example, simian virus 40, adenovirus, and bovine papilloma); (2) *chemical*, such as calcium phosphate-mediated DNA uptake; (3) *fusion*, that is fusion of DNA-loaded membrane vesicles (such as red blood cell ghosts or protoplasts) to cells; and (4) *physical*, that is microinjection or electroporation.[64] Efficiency is needed because stem cells—the target of gene transfer—are not morphologically distinct and compose a minor proportion of nucleated bone marrow cells. The most promising of these approaches uses retroviruses as vectors for gene transfer.[65]

There are formidable technical problems to be overcome before somatic gene therapy becomes possible. Nevertheless, animal experiments are beginning to yield useful results. General requirements that should be met in animal models before proceeding to human clinical trials: (1) the new gene should be inserted into the correct target cells and will remain there long enough to be effective; (2) the new gene should be expressed in the cells at an appropriate level; and (3) the new gene should not harm the cell or, by extension, the animal.[66]

The following steps must be taken before a rational strategy of somatic cell gene therapy becomes a clinical reality:

- Ascertaining that benefit-risk assessment favors gene therapy;

- Isolating and cloning the normal gene;

- Defining and cloning regulatory sequences necessary for the expression of the cloned gene;

- Integrating the cloned gene and the regulatory sequences into the genome of the recipient cells;

- Propagating the recipient cells in appropriate tissue of the patient and providing them with selective advantage;

- Regulating the production of the gene product by the recipient cells; and

- Continuing evaluation for untoward effects of treatment.[67]

SOCIETAL ISSUES

Fetal surgery is controversial because it raises issues involving potential maternal/fetal conflicts. Genetic therapy is controversial because it seems to point to human manipulation of the "gene pool" and thus of the future of the race. Moreover, the "eugenics movement" has left a bad taste in almost everyone's mouth regarding our abilities to determine what characteristics to "enhance" or selectively breed or engineer. Accordingly, it is very important to distinguish between gene therapy designed to help an individual sick person by treatment of somatic cells and all other types of potential "genetic engineering." Research on the first differs from other medical research only by the target of manipulation (the gene) rather than by the overall goal (to treat diseased individuals). Thus, for example, it is difficult to identify any unique legal or ethical issues in trying to activate, supplement, or replace the gene responsible for the production of the enzyme hypoxanthine-guanine phosphoribosyltransferase (HPRT), the absence of which produces Lesch-Nyhan syndrome in an individual with that disease.

Nonetheless, there are those who argue eloquently that we can make gains in genetic engineering only by giving up our view of "humanness" as unique and reducing our self-image to that of a biotechnologically designed product. Most prominent among these is Jeremy Rifkin, who has argued that the transporter of Captain Kirk's USS Enterprise represents biotechnology's own vision of immortality. In the transporter room, watchers of *Star Trek* will certainly recall, crew members of the starship are "beamed down" to the planet surface by having their bodies transformed into billions of bits of information, which are electronically transported to a preset place and then reassembled in their original form. In Rifkin's words, "the ability to reduce all biological systems to information and then to use that information to overcome time and space limitations is the ultimate dream of biotechnologists."[68]

Our position in this book has been informed by science, rather than by science fiction, but also by a firm commitment to individual rights and human dignity. Thus, while we have strongly argued in favor of attempting to identify and cure genetic diseases, we have consistently urged that this only be done with the informed consent of individual patients, and with informed public discussion of the myriad issues and interests involved. In fetal surgery, for example, we see a potentially very positive development, one that enhances that status of the fetus and gives both mother and child a better opportunity for a happy and healthy life together. Done with informed consent and reasonable, scientific protocols, it can reinforce our central values of autonomy and respect for human dignity. Done forcibly, however, it threatens to turn back the clock to the days pregnant women were considered no more than incubators, only dehumanized means to an end, rather than ends in themselves.

Likewise, human gene therapy is a potential good that can help correct numerous devastating genetic disorders in time. Applied to fetuses, it can also help reduce the number of abortions by giving women with affected fetuses a third alternative to the current choice of either abortion or having a handicapped child. As John Fletcher has noted, "the growing ability to conduct fetal therapy will result in a fresh respect for the moral status of the treatable but unviable fetus, reduce the number of late abortions in desired pregnancies, and ease the psychological injury to parents who face the choice to abort."[69] The possibility of helping the fetus without in any way harming the mother is exciting, can enhance fetal interests without diminishing the mother's interests, and can decrease suffering in specific individuals.

More difficult questions are, of course, presented by gametic gene therapy, which lead some to oppose it completely,[70, 71] and others to propose guidelines for its use. Fletcher, for example, has argued that it is acceptable so long as the therapy (1) will benefit the subjects and their offspring with no demonstrable harm; (2) can be confined to medically necessary goals; and (3) will not threaten the ethical systems most treasured by society.[69]

Others, however, have suggested that this scheme puts too much faith in our ability to define what is "medically necessary." Biologist Clifford Grobstein, for example, believes we need more stringent policy guidelines and has suggested four principles to initiate discussion:

> 1. No genetic intervention shall be attempted on any human being with the intention or reasonable expectation that it will reduce either somatic or germ-line potential (intended to prevent gene transfer from becoming a tool for government tyranny).
>
> 2. Any human genetic modification that is intended or may reasonably be expected to alter germ line cells shall not be attempted without special review and sanction by a body suitably constituted to evaluate not only technical risks

of effects on the human gene pool but political, social, and moral aspects as well (this affirms the special problems raised by germ line modification).

3. Except as demonstrably required under principles 1 and 2, no restriction shall be placed on research intended to increase understanding of human heredity and its expression (a freedom to research principle).

4. Principles regarding human genetic therapy should be incorporated into both national policy and international covenants, since the human gene pool knows no geographical boundaries within the species.[72]

These principles replace "medically necessary" as a requirement for germ cell modification with prior approval of "a body suitably constituted to evaluate not only technical risks of effects on the human gene pool, but political, social and moral aspects as well." This may seem slight progress but it is real. Like many others discussed in this book, the issues involved in human germ cell research are not only, or even primarily, medical. Putting research oversight into a multidisciplinary review body[73] with public representation, recognizes this fact, and that recognition alone is a giant step toward further constructive dialogue and reasonable policy development.

The twin tests for *all* genetic interventions, from chorionic villus sampling (CVS) to amniocentesis, from abortion to adoption, from fetal surgery to gene therapy should be: (1) is there reasonable scientific evidence to believe that it will cure or prevent a disabling disease; and (2) is the intervention done with the informed, voluntary, competent, and understanding consent of the individuals involved? If these two conditions are met, we believe a reasonable balance is likely to be struck between human health and human values that can produce healthier offspring who retain their personhood, human rights, and human dignity.

References

Chapter 1: Principles of Genetics

1. Watson JD, Crick FHC: Molecular structure of nucleic acids: A structure for deoxyribose nucleic acid. *Nature* 1953; 171:737.
2. Jeffreys AJ, Flavell RA: The rabbit β-globin gene contains a large insert in the coding sequence. *Cell* 1977; 12:1097.
3. Paris Conference: Standardization of human cytogenetics. *Birth Defects* 1975; 8 (suppl 1).
4. Clermont Y: Kinetics of spermatogenesis in mammals: Seminiferous epithelium cycle and spermatogonial renewal. *Physiol Rev* 1972; 52:198.
5. Mikkelsen M: Down's syndrome: Current stage of cytogenetic research. *Hum Genet* 1971; 12:1.
6. Elias S, Simpson JL: Evaluation and clinical management of patients at apparent increased risk for spontaneous abortions, in Porder IH, Hook EB (eds): *Human Embryonic and Fetal Death*. New York, Academic Press, 1980, pp 331–353.
7. Boué J, Boué A, Lazar P: Retrospective and prospective epidemiological studies of 1500 karyotyped spontaneous human abortions. *Teratology* 1975; 12:11.
8. Evans HJ: Chromosome anomalies among livebirths. *J Med Genet* 1977; 14:309.
9. Zellweger H, Simpson J: *Chromosomes of Man*. Philadelphia, JB Lippincott Co, 1977.
10. De Grouchy J, Turleau C: *Clinical Atlas of Human Chromosomes*, ed 2. New York, John Wiley & Sons, 1984.
11. Lejune J, Gautier M, Turpin R: Etude des chromosomes somatiques de neul enfants mongolines. *Compt Rend* 1959; 248:1721.

12. Magenis RE, Chamberlin J: Parental origin in nondisjunction, in de la Cruz FF, Gerald PS (eds): *Trisomy 21: Research Perspectives*. Baltimore, University Park Press, 1981, pp 77–93.

13. Stene J, Fisher G, Stene E, et al: Paternal age effect in Down syndrome. *Ann Hum Genet* 1977; 40:299.

14. Matsunga E, Tonomura A, Oishi H, et al: Re-examination of paternal age effect in Down syndrome. *Hum Genet* 1978; 40:259.

15. Stene J, Stene E, Stenge-Rutkowski S, et al: Paternal age and Down's syndrome: Data from prenatal diagnosis (DFG). *Hum Genet* 1981; 55:119.

16. Hook EB, Gross PK: Interpretation of recent data pertinent to genetic counseling for Down syndrome: Maternal-age-specific rates, temporal trends, adjustments for paternal age, recurrence risks after remarriage, in Wiley AM, Carter YP, Kelly S, et al (eds): *Clinical Genetics: Problems in Diagnosis and Counseling*. New York, Academic Press, 1982, pp 119–143.

17. Mikkelsen M: Down syndrome: Current stage of cytogenetic epidemiology, in Bonne-Tamir B, Cohen T, Goodman RM (eds): *Human Genetics: Medical Aspects*. New York, Alan R Liss, 1982, pp 297–309.

18. Hamerton JL: *Human Cytogenetics. Clinical Cytogenetics*. New York, Academic Press, 1971, vol 11, pp 196–275.

19. Edwards JH, Harnden DG, Cameron AH, et al: A new trisomic syndrome. *Lancet* 1960; 1:787.

20. Conen PE, Erkman B: Frequency and occurrence of chromosomal syndromes: II. E-trisomy. *Am J Hum Genet* 1966; 18:387.

21. Smith DW: *Recognizable Patterns of Human Malformation: Genetic, Embryological and Clinical Aspects*, ed 3. Philadelphia, WB Saunders Co, 1982, pp 14–17.

22. Hamerton J, Boué A, Ferguson-Smith M, et al: Workshop in collaborative studies in prenatal diagnosis of chromosome disease, in Bonne-Tamin B, Cohen T, Goodman RM (eds): *Human Genetics: Medical Aspects*. New York, Alan R Liss, 1982, pp 369–373.

23. Patua K, Smith DW, Therman E, et al: Multiple congenital anomaly caused by an extra autosome. *Lancet* 1960; 1:790.

24. Lejune J, Lafourcade J, Berger R, et al: Trois cas de deletion partielle du bras court d'un chromosome 5. *C R Seances Acad Sci* 1963; 257:3098.

25. Gorlin RJ: Classical chromosome disorders, in Yunis JJ (ed): *New Chromosomal Syndromes*. New York, Academic Press, 1977, p 60.

26. Turner HH: A syndrome of infantilism, congenital webbed neck and cubitus valgus. *Endocrinology* 1938; 23:566.

27. Ford CE, Jones KW, Polani PE, et al: A sex-chromosome anomaly in a case of gonadal dysgenesis (Turner's syndrome). *Lancet* 1959; 1:711.

28. Simpson JL: *Disorders of Sexual Differentiation in Etiology and Clinical Delineation*. New York, Academic Press, 1976.

29. Garron DC, Vander Stoep LR: Personality and intelligence in Turner's syndrome. *Arch Gen Psychiatry* 1969; 21:339.

30. King CR, Magenis E, Bennett S: Pregnancy and the Turner syndrome. *Obstet Gynecol* 1978; 52:617.

31. Hamerton JL: *Human Cytogenetics: Clinical Cytogenetics.* New York, Academic Press, 1971, vol 2.

32. Simpson JL; Pregnancies in women with chromosomal abnormalities, in Schulman JD, Simpson JL (eds): *Genetic Diseases in Pregnancy: Maternal Effects and Fetal Outcome.* New York, Academic Press, 1981, pp 440–471.

33. Elias S: Klinefelter syndrome, in Sciarra JJ (ed): *Gynecology and Obstetrics.* Hagerstown, Md, Harper and Row, 1981, vol 5, pp 1–10.

34. Leonard MF, Landy G, Ruddle FH, et al: Early development of children with abnormalities of the sex chromosomes: A prospective study. *Pediatrics* 1974; 54:208.

35. Becker KL: Clinical and therapeutic experiences with Klinefelter's syndrome. *Fertil Steril* 1972; 23:568.

36. Robach J, Sipova I: The mental level in 47 cases of true Klinefelter's syndrome. *Acta Endocrinol (Copenh)* 1961; 36:404.

37. Sandberg AA, Koeph GF, Ishihara R, et al: An XYY human male. *Lancet* 1961; 2:488.

38. Jacobs PA, Brunton M, Melville MM, et al: Aggressive behavior, mental subnormality and the XYY male. *Nature* 1965; 208:1351.

39. Casey MD, Segall LJ, Street DRK, et al: Sex chromosome abnormalities in two state hospitals for patients requiring special security. *Nature* 1966; 209:641.

40. Robinson A, Lubs HA, Nielsen J, et al: Summary of clinical findings: Profiles of children with 47,XXY, 47,XXX and 47,XYY karyotypes. *Birth Defects* 1979; 15:261.

41. Elias S: Males with polysomy Y and females with polysomy X, in Sciarra JJ (ed): *Gynecology and Obstetrics,* Hagerstown, Md, Harper & Row, 1981, vol 5 pp 1–8.

42. Jacobs PA, Price WH, Court-Brown WM, et al: Chromosome studies in man in a maximum security hospital. *Ann Human Genet* 1968; 31:339.

43. Alvesalo L, Kari M: Size of deciduous teeth in 47,XYY males. *Am J Hum Genet* 1977; 29:485.

44. Holt SB: Dermatoglyphics and sex chromosomes, in Rashad MN, Morton MRW (eds): *Genital Anomalies.* Springfield, Ill, Charles C Thomas Publisher, 1969, p 375.

45. Borgoankar DS, Mules E: Comments on patients with sex chromosome aneuploidy, dermatoglyphes, parental ages, Xg^a blood group. *J Med Genet* 1970; 7:345.

46. Price WH: The electrocardiogram in males with extra Y chromosome. *Lancet* 1968; 1:1106.

47. Price WH, Lander IJ, Wilson J: The electrocardiograph and sex chromosomal aneuploidy. *Clin Genet* 1974; 6:1.

48. Volavka J, Mednick SA, Sergeant J, et al: Electroencephalograms of XYY and XXX men. *Br J Psychiatry* 1977; 130:43.

49. Price WH, Strong JA, Whatmore PB, et al: Criminal patients with XYY sex-chromosome complement. *Lancet* 1966; 1:565.

50. Price WH, Whatmore PB: Behavioral disorders and pattern of crime among XYY males identified at a maximum security hospital. *Br Med J* 1967; 1:533.
51. Witken HA, Mednick SA, Schulsinger F, et al: Criminality in XYY and XXY men. *Science* 1976; 193:547.
52. Hook EB: Extra sex chromosomes and human behavior: The nature of the evidence regarding XYY, XXY, XXYY, and XX genotypes, in Vallet HL, Porter IH (eds): *Genetic Aspects of Sexual Differentiation*. New York, Academic Press, 1978.
53. Kessler S, Moos RH: Behavioral aspects of chromosomal disorders. *Ann Rev Med* 1973; 24:89.
54. Jones HW Jr, Scott WH: *Hermaphroditism, Genital Anomalies and Related Endocrine Disorders*, ed 2. Baltimore, Williams & Wilkins Co, 1971.
55. Robinson A, Lubs HA, Bergsma D (eds): Sex chromosome aneuploidy: Prospective studies on children. *Birth Defects* 1979; 15:1.
56. Tennes S, Puck M, Bryant K, et al: A developmental study of girls with trisomy X. *Am J Hum Genet* 1975; 27:71.
57. Smith HC, Seale JP, Posen S: Premature ovarian failure in a triple X female. *J Obstet Gynaecol Br Commonw* 1974; 81:405.
58. Kadotoni T, Ohama K, Makino S: A case of 21-trisomic Down's syndrome from the triplo-X mother. *Proc Jap Acad* 1970; 46:709.
59. Singer J, Sachdeva S, Smith GR, et al: Triple X female with a Down's syndrome offspring. *J Med Genet* 1972; 9:238.
60. McKusick VA: *Mendelian Inheritance in Man*, ed 6. Baltimore, Johns Hopkins Press, 1982.
61. Vogel F, Motulsky AG: *Human Genetics: Problems and Approaches*. New York, Springer-Verlag, 1979, pp 594–596.
62. Edwards JH: Simulation of Mendelism. *Acta Genet Stat Med* 1960; 10:63.

Chapter 2: Genetic Counseling

1. Fraser FC: Heredity counseling: The darker side. *Eugene Quart* 1956; 3:45.
2. Fraser FC: Introduction: The development of genetic counseling, in Capron AM, Lappe M, Burray RF, et al (eds): *Genetic Counseling: Facts, Values, and Norms. Birth Defects* 1979; 15(2):5–15.
3. Nadler HL, Gerbie AB: Role of amniocentesis in the intrauterine detection of genetic disorders. *N Engl J Med* 1970; 282:599.
4. Fraser FC: Genetic counseling. *Am J Hum Genet* 1974; 26:636.
5. Hsia YE, Hirschhorn K: What is genetic counseling? in Hsia YE, Hirschhorn K, Silverberg RL, et al (eds): *Counseling in Genetics*. New York, Alan R Liss, 1979, pp 1–29.
6. Kessler S: The psychological foundations of genetic counseling, in Kessler S (ed): *Genetic Counseling: Psychological Dimensions*. New York, Academic Press Inc, 1979, pp 17–33.
7. Motulsky AG, Hecht F: Genetic prognosis and counseling. *Am J Obstet Gynecol* 1964; 90:1227.

8. Nora JJ, Fraser FC: *Medical Genetics: Principles and Practice*. Philadelphia, Lea & Febiger, 1981.

9. Murray RF Jr: The technique of genetic counseling, in Jackson LG, Schimke RN (eds): *Clinical Genetics: A Source Book for Physicians*. New York: John Wiley & Sons, 1979, pp 597–616.

10. Healey JM: The legal obligations of genetic counselors, in Milunsky A, Annas GJ (eds): *Genetics & the Law II*. New York, Plenum, 1980, pp 69, 73.

11. Rimoin D, American Board of Medical Genetics Inc: *Bulletin of Information, Description of Examinations, Application Form, 1984*. Harbor-UCLA Medical Center, American Board of Medical Genetics Inc, 1984.

12. Simpson JL, Elias S, Gatlin M, et al: Genetic counseling and genetic services in obstetrics and gynecology: Implications for educational goals and clinical practice. *Am J Obstet Gynecol* 1981; 140:70.

13. Hsia YE: Approaches to the appraisal of genetic counseling, in Lubs HA, de la Cruz F (eds): *Genetic Counseling*. New York, Raven Press, 1977, pp 53–79.

14. Skinner R: Genetic counseling, in Emery AH, Rimoin DL (eds): *Principles and Practice of Medical Genetics*. Edinburgh, Churchill Livingstone, 1983, pp 1427–1436.

15. Shaw MW: Review of published studies of genetic counseling: A critique, in Lubs HA, de la Cruz F (eds): *Genetic Counseling*. New York, Raven Press, 1977, pp 35–52.

16. Pearn J: Decision-making and reproductive choice, in Hsia YE, Hirschhorn K, Silverberg RL, et al (eds): *Counseling in Genetics*. New York, Alan R Liss, 1979, pp 223–238.

17. Pearn JH: Patient's subjective interpretation of risks offered in genetic counseling. *J Med Genet* 1973; 10:129.

18. Sorenson JR, Culbert AJ: Genetic counselors and counseling orientations: Unexamined topics in evaluation, in Lubs HA, de la Cruz F (eds): *Genetic Counseling*. New York, Raven Press, 1977, pp 131–154.

19. Fort AT, Morrison JC, Berreras L, et al: Counseling the patient with sickle cell disease about reproduction: Pregnancy outcome does not justify maternal risk! *Am J Obstet Gynecol* 1971; 111:324.

20. Silverberg RL, Godmilow L: The process of genetic counseling, in Hsia YE, Hirschhorn K, Silverberg RL, et al (eds): *Counseling in Genetics*. New York, Alan R Liss, 1979, pp 281–283.

21. Annas GJ: Problems of informed consent and confidentiality in genetic counseling, in Milunsky A, Annas GJ (eds): *Genetics and the Law*. New York, Plenum, 1976, p 111.

22. Harper FV, James F: *The Law of Torts* (1968 supp) sec 171.1, 61.

23. World Health Organization Expert Committee: *Genetic Counseling*. *WHO Tech Rep Ser* 1969; 416:1.

24. Elias S, Simpson JL: Genetic counseling, in Sciarra JJ (ed): *Gynecology and Obstetrics*. Philadelphia, Harper & Row, vol 5, 1984, pp 1–5.

25. McCollum AT, Silverberg RL: Psychosocial advocacy, in Hsia YE, Hirschhorn K, Silverberg RL, et al (eds): *Counseling in Genetics*. New York, Alan R Liss, 1979, pp 239–260.

26. Kessler S: The process of communication, decision making and coping in genetic counseling, in Kessler S (ed): *Genetic Counseling: Psychological Dimensions.* New York, Academic Press, 1979, pp 35–51.
27. Falek A: Sequential aspects of coping and other issues in decision making in genetic counseling, in Emery AEH, Pullen I (eds): *Psychological Aspects of Genetic Counseling.* London, Academic Press Inc, 1984, pp 25–36.
28. Falek A: Use of the coping process to achieve psychological homeostasis in genetic counseling, in Lubs HA, de la Cruz F (eds): *Genetic Counseling.* New York, Raven Press, 1977, pp 179–188.
29. Hollerback PE: Reproductive attitudes and the genetic counselee, in Hsia YE, Hirschhorn K, Silverberg RL, et al (eds): *Counseling in Genetics.* New York, Alan R Liss, 1979, pp 155–187.
30. Pullen I: Physical handicap, in Emery AE, Pullen I (eds): *Psychological Aspects of Genetic Counseling.* London, Academic Press Inc, 1984, pp 107–124.
31. Annas GJ: Law and psychiatry: When must a doctor warn others of the potential dangerousness of his patient's condition? *Medicolegal News* 1975; 3:173.
32. Annas GJ, Glantz LH, Katz BF: *The Rights of Doctors, Nurses and Allied Health Professionals.* Cambridge, Mass, Ballinger, 1981, chap 9.
33. Tarasoff v. Regents of U. of California, 131 Cal. Rptr. 14, 551 P. 2d 334 (1976).
34. Evers-Kiebooms G, van den Berghe H: Impact of genetic counseling: A review of published follow-up studies. *Clin Genet* 1979; 15:465.
35. Sorenson JR, Swazey JP, Scotch NA: *Reproductive Pasts Reproductive Futures: Genetic Counseling and Its Effectiveness.* New York, Alan R Liss, 1981.
36. Emery AEH: Introduction: The principles of genetic counseling, in Emery AEH, Pullen IM (eds): *Psychological Aspects of Genetic Counseling.* New York, Academic Press, 1984, pp 1–9.
37. Emery AEH, Raeburn JA, Skinner R, et al: Prospective study of genetic counseling. *Br Med J* 1979; 1253.
38. Wertz DC, Sorenson JR, Heeren TC: Genetic counseling and reproductive uncertainty. *Am J Med Genet* 1984; 18:79.
39. Sorenson JR: Personal communication, July 1986. (A list of the 39 studies reviewed is available from the author.)

Chapter 3: Genetic Screening

1. Reilly P: *Genetics, Law and Social Policy.* Cambridge, Mass, Harvard University Press, 1977.
2. Andrews LB: *State Laws and Regulations Governing Newborn Screening.* Chicago, American Bar Association, 1985.
3. National Academy of Sciences: *Genetic Screening: Programs, Principles and Research.* Washington, DC, National Academy of Sciences, 1975.
4. Holtzman NA: Newborn screening for heredity metabolic disorders: Desirable characteristics, experience, and issues, in Kaback MM (ed): *Genetic Issues in Pediatric and Obstetric Practice.* Chicago, Year Book Medical Publishers Inc, 1981, pp 455–470.

5. Holtzman NA: *Newborn Screening for Genetic-Metabolic Diseases: Progress, Principles and Recommendations.* US Dept of Health, Education and Welfare, Publication No (HSA) 78-5207, 1977.
6. Nora JJ, Fraser FC: *Medical Genetics: Principles and Practice,* ed 2. Philadelphia, Lea & Febiger, 1981.
7. Levy HL: *Genetic Screening for Inborn Errors of Metabolism.* US Dept of Health, Education and Welfare, Publication No (HSA) 78-5124, 1978.
8. Veale AMO: Screening for phenylketonuria, in Bicknell H, Guthrie R, Hammersen G (eds): *Neonatal Screening for Inborn Errors of Metabolism.* Berlin, Springer-Verlag, 1980, pp 7–18.
9. Partington MW: The early symptoms of phenylketonuria. *Pediatrics* 1961; 27:464.
10. Koch R, Blaskavics M, Wenz E, et al: Phenylalanemia and phenylketonuria, in Nyhan WL (ed): *Heritable Disorders of Amino Acid Metabolism.* New York, John Wiley & Sons, 1974, pp 109–140.
11. Tourain A, Sidbury JB: Phenylketonuria and hyperphenylalaninemia, in Stanbury JB, Wyngaarden JB, Fredrickson DS, et al (eds): *The Metabolic Basis of Inherited Disease,* ed 5. New York, McGraw-Hill Book Co, 1983, pp 270–286.
12. Jarvis GA: Studies on phenylpyruvic oligophrenia: The position of the metabolic error. *J Biol Chem* 1947; 169:651.
13. Bicket H, Gerrard J, Hickmans EM: The influence of phenylalamine intake on the chemistry and behavior of a phenylketonuria child. *Acta Paediatr* 1954; 43:64.
14. Armstrong MD, Tyler FH: Studies on phenylalamine intake in phenylketonuria. *J Clin Invest* 1955; 34:565.
15. Holtzmank NA, Welcher DW, Mellitis ED: Termination of restricted diet on children with phenylketonuria: A randomized controlled study. *N Engl J Med* 1975; 293:1121.
16. Koff E, Kammerer B, Boyle P, et al: Intelligence and phenylketonuria: Effects of diet termination. *J Pediatr* 1979; 94:534.
17. Cabalaka B, Duczynska N, Borymowska J, et al: Termination of dietary treatment on phenylketonuria. *Eur J Pediatr* 1977; 126:253.
18. Smith I, Lobascher ME, Stevenson JE, et al: Effect of stopping low phenylalamine diet on intellectual progress of children with phenylketonuria. *Br Med J* 1978; 2:723.
19. Williamson M, Koch R, Berlow S: Diet discontinuation in phenylketonuria, letter. *Pediatrics* 1979; 63:823.
20. Scriver CR, Clow CL: Phenylketonuria: I. Epitome of human biochemical genetics. *N Engl J Med* 1980; 303:1336.
21. Scriver CR, Clow CL: Phenylketonuria: II. Epitome of human biochemical genetics. *N Engl J Med* 1980; 303:1394.
22. Guthrie R, Susi A: A simple phenylalamine method for detecting phenylketonuria in large populations of newborn infants. *Pediatrics* 1963; 32:338.
23. McCaman M, Robins E: Fluorometric method for the determination of phenylalamine in serum. *J Lab Clin Med* 1962; 59:885.

24. American College of Obstetricians and Gynecologists: *Neonatal Metabolic Disease.* Tech Bull No. 60, Jan. 1981.
25. Bush JW, Chen MM, Patrick DL: Health status index in cost-effectiveness: Analysis of PKU program, in Berg RL (ed): *Health Status Indexes.* Chicago, Hospital Research and Educational Trust, 1973, pp 172–209.
26. MacCready RA: Admissions of phenylketonuric patients to residential institutions before and after screening programs of neonates. *J Pediatr* 1974; 85:383.
27. Massachusetts Department of Public Health: Cost-benefit analysis of new-born screening for metabolic disorders. *N Engl J Med* 1974; 291:1414.
28. Raine DN: Inherited metabolic disease. *Lancet* 1974; 2:996.
29. Dent CE: Discussion of M.D. Armstrong, Relation of biochemical abnormality to development of mental defect in phenylketonuria, in Ross Laboratories: *Etiologic Factors in Mental Retardation: Report of Twenty-third Ross Pediatric Research Conference.* Nov 8–9, 1956. Ross Laboratories, Columbus, Ohio, 1957, pp 32–33.
30. Lenke RR, Levy HL: Maternal phenylketonuria and hyperphenylalinemia. *N Engl J Med* 1980; 303:1202.
31. Lamon JM, Lenke RR, Levy HL, et al: Selected metabolic diseases, in Schulman JD, Simpson JL (eds): *Genetic Disease in Pregnancy.* New York, Academic Press Inc, 1981, pp 1–55.
32. Segal S: Disorders of galactose metabolism, in Stanbury JB, Wyngaarden JB, Fredrickson DS, et al (eds): *The Metabolic Basis of Inherited Disease,* ed 5. New York, McGraw-Hill Book Co, 1983, pp 167–191.
33. Levy HL: Genetic screening. *Adv Hum Genet* 1973; 4:1–104.
34. Donnell GN, Lann SH: Galactosemia: Report of four cases. *Pediatrics* 1951, 7:503.
35. Gitzelman R: Newborn screening for inherited disorders of galactose metabolism, in Bicknel H, Guthrie R, Hammersen G (eds): *Neonatal Screening for Inborn Errors of Metabolism.* New York, Springer-Verlag, 1980, pp 67–79.
36. Donnell GN, Collado M, Koch R: Growth and development of children with galactosemia. *J Pediatr* 1961; 58:836.
37. Hsia DY-Y, Walker FA: Variability in the clinical manifestations of galactosemia. *J Pediatr* 1961; 59:872.
38. Koch R, Acosta P, Donnell GN, et al: Nutritional therapy of galactosemia. *Clin Pediatr (Phila)* 1965; 4:571.
39. Donnell GN, Koch R, Bergren WR: Observations on results of management of galactosemia patients, in Hsia DY-Y (ed): *Galactosemia.* Springfield, Ill, Charles C Thomas Publisher, 1969, pp 247–275.
40. Nadler HL, Inouge T, Hsia DY-Y: Classical galactosemia: A study of fifty-five cases, in Hsia DY-Y (ed): *Galactosemia.* Springfield, Ill, Charles C Thomas Publisher, 1969, pp 127–139.
41. Anderson EP, Kalckar HM, Kurashi K, et al: A specific enzymatic essay for the diagnosis of congenital galactosemia. *J Lab Clin Med* 1957; 50:569.
42. Levy HL, Hammersen G: Newborn screening for galactosemia and other galactose metabolic defects. *J Pediatr* 1978; 92:871.

43. Menkes JH, Hurst PL, Craig JM: A new syndrome: Progressive familial infantile cerebral dysfunction associated with an unusual urinary substance. *Pediatrics* 1954; 14:462.
44. Naylor EW: Newborn screening for maple syrup urine disease (branched-chain ketoaciduria), in Bicknel J, Guthrie G, Hammersen G (eds): *Errors of Metabolism*. Berlin, Springer-Verlag, 1980, pp 19–28.
45. Tanaka K, Rosenberg LE: Disorders of branched-chain amino acid and organic acid metabolism, in Stanbury JB, Wyngaarden JB, Fredrickson DS (eds): *The Metabolic Basis of Inherited Disease*, ed 5. New York, McGraw-Hill Book Co, 1983, pp 440–473.
46. Synderman SE, Norton PM, Roitman E, et al: Maple syrup urine disease with particular reference to dietotherapy. *Pediatrics* 1964; 34:454.
47. Fisher DA, Burrow GN, Dussault JH, et al: Recommendations for screening programs for congenital hypothyroidism. *J Pediatr* 1976; 89:692.
48. Dussault JH, Parlow A, Letarte J, et al: TSH measurement from blood spots on filter paper: A confirmatory screening test for neonatal hypothyroidism. *J Pediatr* 1976; 89:550.
49. Dussault JH, Morisette J, Letarte J, et al: Modification of a screening program for neonatal hypothyroidism. *J Pediatr* 1978; 92:274.
50. Neel JV, Carr EA, Beierwaltes WH, et al: Genetic studies on the congenitally hypothyroid. *Pediatrics* 1967; 27:269.
51. Mitchell ML, Larsen PR, Levy HL, et al: Screening for congenital hypothyroidism. *JAMA* 1973; 239:2348.
52. Raiti S, Newns GH: Cretinism: Early diagnosis and its relation to mental retardation prognosis. *Arch Dis Child* 1971; 46:692.
53. DeJonge GA: Congenital hypothyroidism in the Netherlands. *Lancet* 1976; 2:143.
54. Dussault JH, Letarte J, Guyda H: Neonatal screening for congenital hypothyroidism: 4 years experience, in Bicknel H, Guthrie R, Hammersen G (eds): *Neonatal Screening for Inborn Errors of Metabolism*. Berlin, Springer-Verlag, 1980, pp 167–178.
55. Klein A, Meltzer S, Kenny M: Improved prognosis in congenital hypothyroidism. *J Pediatr* 1972; 81:912.
56. Levy HL, Mitchell ML: Regional newborn screening for hypothyroidism. *Pediatrics* 1979; 63:340.
57. Fisher DA, Dussault JH, Foley TP Jr, et al: Screening for congenital hypothyroidism: Results of screening one million North American infants. *J Pediatr* 1979; 94:700.
58. New England Congenital Hypothyroid Collaborative: Effects of neonatal screening for hypothyroidism: Prevention of mental retardation by treatment before clinical manifestations. *Lancet* 1981; 2:1095.
59. Rowley PT: Genetic screening: Marvel or menace? *Science* 1984; 255:138.
60. Lappé M: Genetic screening, in Hsia, YE, Hirschhorn K, Silverberg RL, et al (eds): *Counseling in Genetics*. New York, Alan R Liss Inc, 1979, pp 295–309.

61. Kabach MM: Heterozygote screening, in Emery AEH, Rimoin DL (eds): *Principles and Practice of Medical Genetics.* New York, Churchill Livingstone Inc, 1983, pp 1451–1457.

62. Aronson SM, Volk BW: Genetic and demographic considerations concerning Tay-Sachs disease, in Aronson SM, Volk BW (eds): *Cerebral Sphingolipidoses.* New York, Academic Press, 1962, pp 375–394.

63. Kabach MM, Nathan TJ, Greenwald S: Tay-Sachs disease: Heterozygote screening and prenatal diagnosis: US experience and world perspective, in Kabach MM (ed): *Tay-Sachs Disease: Screening and Prevention.* New York, Alan R Liss Inc, 1977, pp 13–36.

64. O'Brien JS: The gangliosidoses, in Stanbury JB, Wyngaarden JB, Fredrickson DS, et al (eds): *The Metabolic Basis of Inherited Disease,* ed 5. New York, McGraw-Hill Book Co, 1983, pp 945–969.

65. O'Brien JS, Okada S, Fillerup DL, et al: Tay-Sachs disease: Prenatal diagnosis. *Science* 1971; 172:61.

66. Kabach MM: Heterozygote screening and prenatal diagnosis in Tay-Sachs disease: A worldwide update, in Callahan JW, Lowden A (eds): *Lysosomes and Lysosomal Storage Diseases.* New York, Raven Press, 1981, pp 331–343.

67. O'Brien JS: Tay-Sachs disease: From enzyme to prevention. *Fed Proc* 1973; 32:191.

68. Nelson WB, Swint JM, Caskey CT: An economic evaluation of a genetic screening program for Tay-Sachs disease. *Am J Hum Genet* 1978; 30:160.

69. Powers DR: Natural history of sickle cell disease: The first ten years. *Semin Hematol* 1975; 12:267.

70. Brain P: Sickle cell anemia in Africa. *Br Med J* 1952; 2:880.

71. Lehman H, Huntsman RG: *Man's Haemoglobins,* ed 2. Philadelphia, JB Lippincott, 1974.

72. Bunn HF, Forget BG, Ranney HM: *Human Hemoglobins.* Philadelphia, WB Saunders Co, 1977.

73. Weatherall DG, Clegg JB: Recent developments in the molecular genetics of human hemoglobin. *Cell* 1979; 16:467.

74. Kan YW: The thalassemias, in Stanbury JB, Wyngaarden JB, Fredrickson DS, et al (eds): *The Metabolic Basis of Inherited Disease,* ed 5. New York, McGraw-Hill Book Co, 1983, pp 1711–1725.

75. Sansone G, Sciarratta GV, Agosti-Vallerino S, et al: Geographic distribution and heterogeneity of thalassemias in the Italian population. *Birth Defects* 1982; 18:189.

76. Russo G: Types of thalassemia in Sicily. *Birth Defects* 1982; 18:185.

77. Carcassi U, Cacace E, Mela Q, et al: Thalassemia phenotypes in Sardinia. *Birth Defects* 1982; 18:165.

78. Weatherall DJ: The thalassemias, in Williams WJ, Beutler E, Erslev AJ, et al (eds): *Hematology,* ed 3. New York, McGraw-Hill Book Co, 1983, pp 493–521.

79. Kattamis C, Efremov G, Pootrakul S: Effectiveness of one tube osmotic fragility screening in detecting β-thalassemia. *J Med Genet* 1981; 18:266.

80. Screening for β-thalassemia, editorial. *Lancet* 1981; 2:566.
81. Cao A, Pintus L, Lecca U, et al: Control of homozygous β-thalassemia by carrier screening and antenatal diagnosis in Sardinians. *Clin Genet* 1984; 26:12.
82. WHO Working Group: Hereditary anemias: Genetic basis, clinical features, diagnosis and treatment. *Bull WHO* 1982; 60:643.
83. Consensus Conference: The use of diagnostic ultrasound imagery during pregnancy. *JAMA* 1984; 252:669.
84. De Grouchy J, Trebuchet C: Transfusion foeto-maternelle de lymphocytes sanguins et detection du sexe de foetus. *Ann Genet* 1971; 14:133.
85. Walknowska J, Conte FA, Grumbach MM: Practical and theoretical implications of fetal-maternal lymphocyte transfer. *Lancet* 1969; 1:1119.
86. Schindler AM, Martin-du-Pan R: Prenatal diagnosis of fetal lymphocytes in the maternal blood. *Obstet Gynecol* 1972; 40:340.
87. Parks DR, Herzenberg LA: Fetal cells from maternal blood: Their selection and prospects for use in prenatal diagnosis, in Latt SA, Darlington GI (eds): *Methods in Cell Biology: Prenatal Diagnosis: Cell Biological Approaches*. New York, Academic Press, 1982, vol 26, pp 277–295.
88. Covone AE, Mutton D, Johnson PM, et al: Trophoblast cells in peripheral blood from pregnant women. *Lancet* 1984; 2:841.
89. Schulman D: Anencephaly, in Bergsma D (ed): *Birth Defects Atlas and Compendium*. Baltimore, Williams & Wilkins Co, 1974, p 161.
90. Holmes LB: The health problem: Neural tube defects, in Gastel B, Haddow JE, Fletcher JC, et al (eds): *Maternal Serum α-Fetoprotein: Issues in the Prenatal Screening and Diagnosis of Neural Tube Defects*. US Government Printing Office, 1981.
91. Weiss RR, Macri JN, Elligers KW: Origin of amniotic fluid α-fetoprotein in normal and defective pregnancies. *Obstet Gynecol* 1976; 47:697.
92. Brock DJH, Bolton AE, Monaghan JM: Prenatal diagnosis of anencephaly through maternal serum α-fetoprotein measurement. *Lancet* 1973; 2:923.
93. UK Collaborative Study on α-Fetoprotein in Relationship to Neural Tube Defects: Maternal serum α-fetoprotein measurement in antenatal screening for anencephaly and spina bifida in early pregnancy. *Lancet* 1977; 1:1323.
94. Macri JN, Haddow JE, Weiss RR: Screening for neural tube defects in the United States. *Am J Obstet Gynecol* 1979; 133:119.
95. Burton BK, Sowers SG, Nelson LH: Maternal serum α-fetoprotein screening in North Carolina: Experience with more than twelve thousand pregnancies. *Am J Obstet Gynecol* 1983; 146:439.
96. Milunsky A, Alpert J: Results and benefits of a maternal serum α-fetoprotein screening program. *JAMA* 1984; 252:1438.
97. *Federal Register* 27780-27782, June 17, 1983.
98. American College of Obstetricians and Gynecologists: *Prenatal Detection of Neural Tube Defects*. Technical Bulletin No. 67, Oct 1982.
99. Macri JN, Weiss RR; Prenatal serum α-fetoprotein screening for neural tube defects. *Obstet Gynecol* 1982; 59:633.

100. Leonard CO: Serum AFP screening for neural tube defects. *Clin Obstet Gynecol* 1981; 24:1121.
101. Crandall BF, Robertson RD, Lebherz TB, et al: Maternal serum α-fetoprotein screening for neural tube defects: Report of a pilot program. *West J Med* 1983; 138:524.
102. Hamilton MPR, Abdalla MI, Whitfield CR: Significance of raised maternal serum α-fetoprotein in singleton pregnancies with normally formed fetuses. *Obstet Gynecol* 1985; 65:465.
103. Davenport DM, Macri JN: The clinical significance of low maternal serum α-fetoprotein. *Am J Obstet Gynecol* 1983; 146:657.
104. Merkatz IR, Nitowsky HM, Macri JN, et al: An association between low maternal serum α-fetoprotein and fetal chromosomal abnormalities. *Am J Obstet Gynecol* 1984; 148:886.
105. Cuckle HC, Wald NJ, Lindenbaum RH: Maternal serum α-fetoprotein measurement: A screening test for Down syndrome. *Lancet* 1984; 1:926.
106. Cuckle HS, Wald NJ, Lindenbaum RH, et al: Amniotic fluid AFP levels and Down syndrome. *Lancet* 1985; 1:290.
107. Guibaud S, Bonnet-Capela M, Germain D, et al: Prenatal screening for Down syndrome. *Lancet* 1984; 1:1359.
108. Fuermann W, Wendt P, Wetzel HK: Maternal serum-AFP as screening test for Down syndrome. *Lancet* 1984; 2:413.
109. Tabor A, Norgaard-Pedersen B, Jacobsen JC: Low maternal serum AFP and Down syndrome. *Lancet* 1984; 2:161.
110. Hagard S, Carter F, Milne RG: Screening for spina bifida cystica: A cost-benefit analysis. *Br J Prev Soc Med* 1976; 30:40.
111. Layde PM, von Allen S, Milne RG: Maternal serum α-fetoprotein screening: A cost-benefit analysis. *Am J Public Health* 1979; 69:566.
112. Cowchock S, Jackson L: Use of α-fetoprotein for diagnosis of neural tube and other anomalies. *Clin Obstet Gynecol* 1980; 7:83.
113. Sadovnick A, Baird PC: A cost-benefit analysis of a population screening program for neural tube defects. *Prenat Diagn* 1983; 3:117.
114. Nadler HL, Simpson JL: Maternal serum AFP screening promise not yet fulfilled. *Obstet Gynecol* 1979; 54:333.
115. Milunsky A, Haddow JE: Cautions about maternal serum α-fetoprotein screening, letter to the editor. *N Engl J Med* 1985; 313:694.
116. Turner RH, Bowden C: More on maternal serum α-fetoprotein: Problems with a test kit, letter to the editor. *N Engl J Med* 1986; 315:194.
117. Annas GJ, Elias S: Maternal serum AFP: Educating physicians and the public, editorial. *Am J Public Health* 1985; 75:1374.
118. Helling v. Carey, 519 P.2d 981 (Wash. 1974).
119. T.J. Hooper, 60 F.2d. 737,740 (2d Cir. 1932).
120. American College of Obstetricians and Gynecologists: *ACOG Newsletter.* Sept, 1985, p 3.
121. Swazey J: Phenylketonuria: A case study in biomedical legislations. 48 *J Urban L* 883 (1971).

122. Naccarato v. Grob, 180 N.W. 2d 788 (Mich. 1970).
123. Annas GJ, Coyne B: "Fitness" for birth and reproduction: Legal implications of genetic screening, 9 *Family Law Q* 463, 482 (1975).
124. Curran WJ: The questionable virtues of genetic screening laws. *Am J Pub Health* 1974; 64:1003.
125. Shah S: *Report on the XYY Chromosomal Abnormality.* US Government Printing Office, 1970.
126. Faden R, Chwalow AJ, Horn SD, et al: A survey to evaluate parental consent as public policy for neonatal screening. *Am J Public Health* 1982; 72:1347–1352.
127. Faden R, Holtzman NA, Chwalow AJ: Parental rights, child welfare and public health: The case of PKU screening. *Am J Public Health* 1982; 72:1396–1400.
128. Callahan D: Genetic disease and human health. *Hastings Center Rep* 4(4):7–10, Aug, 1974.
129. Annas GJ: Mandatory PKU screening: The other side of the looking glass. *Am J Public Health* 1982; 72:1401–1403.
130. President's Commission for the Study of Ethical Problems in Medicine and Biomedical and Behavioral Research: *Screening and Counseling for Genetic Conditions.* US Government Printing Office, 1983.

Chapter 4: Prenatal Diagnosis: Indications

1. Hook EB, Chambers GC: Estimated rates in Down syndrome in livebirths by one year maternal age intervals for mothers aged 20–49, in New York State study: Implication of the risk figures for genetic counseling and cost benefit analysis of prenatal diagnosis programs. *Birth Defects* 1977; 13:123.
2. Hook EB, Cross PK, Lamson SH, et al: Paternal age and Down syndrome in British Columbia. *Am J Hum Genet* 1981; 33:123.
3. Hook EB, Cross PK, Schreinemachers DM: Chromosomal abnormality rates at amniocentesis and live-born infants. *JAMA* 1983; 249:2034.
4. Ferguson-Smith MA: Advanced maternal age, in Murken J-D, Stengel-Rutkowski S, Schwinger E (eds): *Prenatal Diagnosis. Proceedings 3rd European Conference on Prenatal Diagnosis of Genetic Disorders.* Stuttgart, Germany, Ferdinand Enke Publishers, 1979 pp 1–14.
5. Stene J, Stene E, Mikkelsen M: Risk for chromosome abnormality at amniocentesis following a child with a non-inherited chromosome aberration: A European collaborative study on prenatal diagnosis, 1981. *Prenat Diagn* 1984; 4:81.
6. Elias S, Verp MS: Prenatal diagnosis of genetic disorders. *Obstet Gynecol Annu* 1983; 12:79.
7. Wright SW, Day RW, Muller H, et al: Frequency of trisomy and translocation in Down's syndrome. *J Pediatr* 1967; 70:420.
8. Boué A, Gallano P: A collaborative study of the segregation of inherited chro-

mosome structural rearrangements in 1256 prenatal diagnoses. *Prenat Diagn* 1984; 4:45.

9. Lubs HA: A marker X chromosome. *Am J Hum Genet* 1969; 21:231.
10. Blomquist HK, Gustavson KH, Holmgren G, et al: Fragile site X chromosomes and X-linked mental retardation in severely retarded boys in a northern Swedish county-prevalence study. *Clin Genet* 1982; 21:209.
11. Carpenter NJ, Leichtman LG, Say B: Fragile X-linked mental retardation. *Am J Dis Child* 1982; 136:392.
12. Jenkins E, Brown T, Duncan C, et al: Fragile X chromosome prenatal diagnosis. *Am J Hum Genet* 1982; 34:130A.
13. Shapiro LR, Wilmot PL, Brenholz P, et al: Prenatal diagnosis of fragile X chromosome. *Lancet* 1982; 1:99.
14. Simpson JL: Pregnancies in women with chromosomal abnormalities, in Schulman JD, Simpson JL (eds): *Genetic Diseases in Pregnancy.* New York, Academic Press, 1981, pp 440–471.
15. Verp MS, Simpson JL: Amniocentesis for cytogenetic studies, in Filkins K, Russo JF (eds): *Human Prenatal Diagnosis.* New York, Marcel Dekker Inc, 1985, pp 13–48.
16. Miles JH, Kaback MM: Prenatal diagnosis of hereditary disorders. *Pediatr Clin North Am* 1978; 25:593.
17. Souther EM: Detection of specific sequences among DNA fragments separated by gel electrophoresis. *J Mol Biol* 1975; 98:503.
18. Emery AEH: *An Introduction to Recombinant DNA.* New York, John Wiley & Sons, 1984.
19. Watson JD, Tooze J, Kurtz DT: *Recombinant DNA.* New York, WH Freeman, 1983.
20. Kan YW, Golbus MS, Dozy AM: Prenatal diagnosis of α-thalassemia: Clinical application of molecular hybridization. *N Engl J Med* 1976; 295:1165.
21. Botstein D, White RL, Skolnick M, et al: Construction of a genetic linkage map using restriction fragment length polymorphism. *Am J Hum Gen* 1980; 32:314.
22. Tsui LC, Guchwald M, Barker D, et al: Cystic fibrosis locus defined by a genetically linked polymorphic DNA marker. *Science* 1985; 230:1054.
23. Knowlton RG, Cohen-Haguenauer O, Van Cong N, et al: A polymorphic DNA marker linked to cystic fibrosis is located on chromosome 7. *Nature* 1985; 318:380.
24. White R, Woodward S, Leppert M, et al: A closely linked genetic marker for cystic fibrosis. *Nature* 1985; 318:382.
25. Wainwright BJ, Scambler PJ, Schmidtke J, et al: Localization of cystic fibrosis locus to human chromosome 7cen-q22. *Nature* 1985; 318:384.
26. Dean M, Park M, LeBeau MM, et al: The human met-oncogene is related to the tyrosine kinase oncogenes. *Nature* 1985; 318:385.
27. Carter CO, David PA, Laurence KM: A family study of major central nervous system malformations in South Wales. *J Med Genet* 1968; 5:81.
28. Elwood HH: Anencephalus in Belfast. *Br J Prev Soc Med* 1970; 34:78.

29. Fedrick J: Anencephalus in Scotland 1961–1972. *Br J Prev Soc Med* 1973; 30:383.
30. Nakano KK: Anencephaly: A review. *Dev Med Child Neurol* 1973; 15:383.
31. Milunsky A: Prenatal diagnosis of neural tube defects, in Milunsky A (ed): *Genetic Disorders and the Fetus.* New York, Plenum Press, 1979, p 379.
32. Janerich DT, Piper J: Shifting genetic patterns in anencephaly and spina bifida. *J Med Genet* 1978; 15:101–105.
33. Main DM, Mennuti MT: Neural tube defects: Issues in prenatal diagnosis and counseling. *Obstet Gynecol* 1986; 67:1.
34. Brock DJH: *Early Diagnosis of Fetal Defects.* Edinburgh, Churchill Livingstone Inc, 1982, pp 67–95.
35. Brock DJH, Sutcliffe RG: α-Fetoprotein in the antenatal diagnosis of anencephaly and spina bifida. *Lancet* 1972; 2:197.
36. Weiss RR, Macre JN, Ellegers KW: Origin of amniotic fluid α-fetoprotein in normal and defective pregnancies. *Obstet Gynecol* 1976; 47:697.
37. Second Report of the UK Collaborative Study on α-Fetoprotein in Relation to Neural Tube Defects. *Lancet* 1979; 2:651.
38. Crandall BF, Matsumoto M: Routine amniotic fluid α-fetoprotein measurement in 34,000 pregnancies. *Am J Obstet Gynecol* 1984; 149:744.
39. Milunsky A: Prenatal detection of neural tube defects: VI. Experience with 20,000 pregnancies. *JAMA* 1980; 244:2731.
40. Report of the Collaborative Acetylcholinesterase Study: Amniotic fluid acetylcholinesterase electrophoresis as a secondary test in the diagnosis of anencephaly and open spina bifida in early pregnancy. *Lancet* 1981; 2:321.
41. Smith AD, Wald NJ, Cuckle HS, et al: Amniotic fluid acetylcholinesterase as a possible diagnostic test for neural tube defects in early pregnancy. *Lancet* 1979; 1:685.
42. Milunsky A, Sapirstein VS: Prenatal diagnosis of open neural tube defects using amniotic fluid acetylcholinesterase assay. *Obstet Gynecol* 1982; 59:1.
43. Brock DJH, Hayward C: Gel electrophoresis of amniotic fluid acetylcholinesterase as an aid to the prenatal diagnosis of fetal defects. *Clin Chim Acta* 1980; 108:135.
44. Brock DJH, Barron L, Van Heyninger V: Prenatal diagnosis to neural tube defects with a monoclonal antibody specific for acetylcholinesterase. *Lancet* 1985; 1:5.
45. Rogers TD: Wrongful life and wrongful birth: Medical malpractice in genetic counseling and prenatal testing. 33 *SC L Rev* 713 (1982).
46. Troppi v. Scarf, 187 N.W.2d 511 (Mich. App. 1971).
47. Sherlock v. Stillwater Clinic, 260 N.W.2d 169 (Minn. 1977).
48. Lambert T: Tort liability for inadequate genetic counseling. 26 *ATLA L Rep* 106 (April, 1983).
49. Turpin v. Sortini, 182 Cal. Rptr. 337, 340 (1982).
50. Gleitman v. Cosgrove, 49 N.J. 22, 227 A.2d 689 (1967).
51. Annas GJ: Medical paternity and 'wrongful life.' *Hastings Center Rep* 9:15, June, 1979.
52. Berman v. Allan, 80 N.J. 421, 404 A.2d 8 (1979).

53. Jacobs v. Theimer, 519 S.W.2d 846, 849 (Tex. 1975).
54. Annas GJ, Coyne B: 'Fitness' for birth and reproduction: Legal implications of genetic screening. 9 *Family L Q* 463 (1975).
55. Phillips v. U.S., 508 F. Supp. 544 (S.C. 1981).
56. Phillips v. U.S., 575 F. Supp. 1309 (S.C. 1983).
57. Becker v. Schwartz, and Park v. Chessin, 46 N.Y.2d 401, 413 N.Y.S.2d 895 (1978).
58. Capron AM: The wrong of 'wrongful life,' in Milunsky A, Annas GJ (eds): *Genetics and the Law II*. New York, Plenum Press, 1980, pp 81–93.
59. Capron AM: Tort liability in genetic counseling. 79 *Columbia L Rev* 618 (1979).
60. Curlender v. Bio-Science Laboratories, 165 Cal. Rptr. 477 (Ct. App. 2d Dist. Div. 1, 1980).
61. Steinbock B: The logical case of 'wrongful life.' *Hastings Center Rep* 16:15–20, April, 1986.
62. Feinberg J: *Harm to Others*. New York, Oxford University Press, 1984, pp 97–104.
63. Shaw M: Preconception and prenatal torts, in Milunsky A, Annas GJ (eds): *Genetics and the Law II*. New York, Plenum Press, 1980, pp 225–232.

Chapter 5: Prenatal Diagnosis: Techniques

1. Gerbie AB, Elias S: Technique for midtrimester amniocentesis for prenatal diagnosis. *Semin Perinatol* 1980; 4:159.
2. Simpson JL: Genetic counseling and prenatal diagnosis, in Gabbe SG, Niebyl JF, Simpson JL (eds): *Obstetrics: Normal and Abnormal Pregnancies*. New York, Churchill-Livingstone Inc, 1986, pp 211–244.
3. Elias S, Simpson JL: Amniocentesis, in Milunsky A (ed): *Genetic Disorders of the Fetus*, ed 2. New York, Plenum Press, 1986.
4. Emery AEH: Antenatal diagnosis of genetic disease. *Mod Trends Hum Genet* 1970; 1:267.
5. Wagner G, Fuchs F: The volume of amniotic fluid in the first half of pregnancy. *J Obstet Gynaecol Br Commonw* 1962; 69:131.
6. Nelson MM: Amniotic fluid volumes in early pregnancy. *J Obstet Gynaecol Br Commonw* 1972; 79:50.
7. Elias S, Simpson JL: Ultrasound and amniocentesis, in Sabbagha RE (ed): *Diagnaostic Ultrasound Applied to Obstetrics and Gynecology*. Hagerstown, Md, Harper & Row, 1980, pp 165–177.
8. Elias S: Prenatal diagnosis of genetic disorders, in Givens JR (ed): *Endocrinology of Pregnancy*. Chicago, Year Book Medical Publishers Inc, 1980, pp 327–354.
9. Elias S, Martin AO, Patel V, et al: Amniotic fluid crystallization in second trimester amniocentesis. *Am J Obstet Gynecol* 1979; 133:401.
10. Crane JP, Roland B, Larson D: Rh immune globulin after genetic amniocentesis: Impact on pregnancy outcome. *Am J Med Genet* 1984; 19:763.

11. Golbus MS, Stephens JD, Cann HM, et al: Rh-isoimmunization following genetic amniocentesis. *Prenat Diagn* 1982; 2:149.

12. Miles JH, Kaback MD: Rh immune globulin after genetic amniocentesis. *Clin Genet Res* 1979; 27:103A.

13. Elias S, Gerbie AB, Simpson JL, et al: Genetic amniocentesis in twin gestations. *Am J Obstet Gynecol* 1980; 138:169.

14. Goldstein AI, Stills SM: Midtrimester amniocentesis in twin pregnancies. *Am J Obstet Gynecol* 1983; 62:659.

15. Rodeck CH, Mibashan J, Abramowicz J, et al: Selective feticide of the affected twin by fetoscopic air embolism. *Prenat Diagn* 1982; 2:189.

16. Aberg A, Mitelman F, Cantz M, et al: Cardiac puncture of fetus with Hurler's disease avoiding abortion of unaffected co-twin. *Lancet* 1978; 2:990.

17. Petres RE, Redwine F: Selective birth in twin pregnancy. *N Engl J Med* 1981; 305:1218.

18. Kerenyi T, Chitkara U: Selective birth in twin pregnancy with discordancy for Down's syndrome. *N Engl J Med* 1981; 304:1525.

19. Antsaklis A, Politis J, Karagiannopoulos C, et al: Selective survival of only the healthy fetus following prenatal diagnosis of thalassemia major in binovular twin gestation. *Prenat Diagn* 1984; 4:289.

20. Rodeck CH, Wass D: Sampling pure fetal blood in twin pregnancy by fetoscopy using a single uterine puncture. *Prenat Diagn* 1981; 1:43.

21. Robertson J: The right to procreate and in utero fetal therapy. 3 *J Legal Med* 333 (1982).

22. Annas GJ, Glantz LH, Katz BF: *Informed Consent to Human Experimentation: The Subject's Dilemma.* Cambridge, Mass, Ballinger Publishing Co, 1977.

23. Singer P: *Animal Liberation.* New York, New York Review, 1975.

24. Murken JA, Stengel-Rutkowski S, Schwinger E: Prenatal diagnosis, in *Proceedings, 3rd European Conference on Prenatal Diagnosis of Genetic Disorders.* Stuttgart, Germany, Ferdinand Enke Publishers, 1979.

25. Turnbull AC, MacKenzie IZ: Second-trimester amniocentesis and termination of pregnancy. *Br Med Bull* 1983; 39:315.

26. NICHD National Registry for Amniocentesis Study Group: Midtrimester amniocentesis for prenatal diagnosis: Safety and accuracy. *JAMA* 1976; 236:1471.

27. Lamb MP: Gangrene of a fetal limb due to amniocentesis. *Br J Obstet Gynaecol* 1975; 82:829.

28. Karp LE, Hayden PW: Fetal puncture during midtrimester amniocentesis. *Obstet Gynecol* 1977; 49:115.

29. Rickwood AMK: A case of ileal atresia and ileocutaneous fistula caused by amniocentesis. *J Pediatr* 1977; 91:312.

30. Eply SL, Hanson JW, Cruikshank DP: Fetal injury with mid-trimester diagnostic amniocentesis. *Obstet Gynecol* 1979; 53:77.

31. Youroukos S, Papadelis F, Matsaniotis N: Porencephalic cysts after amniocentesis. *Arch Dis Child* 1980; 55:814.

32. Merin S, Byth Y: Uniocular congenital blindness as a complication of midtrimester amniocentesis. *Am J Ophthamol* 1980; 80:299.

33. Simpson NE, Dallaire L, Miller JR, et al: Prenatal diagnosis of genetic disease in Canada: Report of a collaborative study. *Can Med Assoc J* 1976; 115:739.
34. Working Party on Amniocentesis: An assessment of the hazards of amniocentesis. *Br Jr Obstet Cynaecol* 1978; 85 (suppl 2):1.
35. Tabor A, Philip J, Madsen M, et al: Randomized controlled trial of genetic amniocentesis in 4606 low risk women. *Lancet* 1986; 1:1288.
36. Kullander S, Sandahl B: Fetal chromosome analysis after transcervical placental biopsies in early pregnancy. *Acta Obstet Cynaecol Scand* 1973; 52:355.
37. Department of Obstetrics and Gynecology, Tietung Hospital of Ansham Iron and Steel Company, Ansham, China: Fetal sex prediction by sex chromatin of chorionic villi cells during early pregnancy. *Chin Med J* 1975; 1:117.
38. Old JM, Ward RHT, Karagozlu F, et al: First trimester fetal diagnosis for haemoglobinopathies: Three cases. *Lancet* 1982; 2:1413.
39. Simoni G, Brambati B, Danesino C, et al: Diagnostic application of first trimester trophoblast sampling in 100 pregnancies. *Hum Genet* 1984; 66:252.
40. Fletcher JC: Ethical aspects of a controlled clinical trial of chorion biopsy approaches to prenatal diagnosis, in Berg N (ed): *Genetics: Past, Present and Future*. New York, Alan R Liss, 1985, pp 213–248.
41. Fletcher JC: *Coping with Genetic Disorders*. New York, Harper & Row, 1982, pp 127–128.
42. Elias S, Simpson JL, Martin AO, et al: Chorionic villus sampling for first-trimester prenatal diagnosis: Northwestern University program. *Am J Obstet Gynecol* 1985; 152:204.
43. Maxwell D, Lilford R, Czepulkowski B, et al: Transabdominal chorionic villus sampling. *Lancet* 1986; 1:123.
44. Martin AO, Simpson JL, Martin AO, et al: Chorionic villus sampling in continuing pregnancies: II. Cytogenetic reliability. *Am J Obstet Gynecol* 1986; 154:1353.
45. Chorionic Villus Sampling Newsletter, Dec 1, 1986. Philadelphia, Division of Medical Genetics, Jefferson Medical College.
46. Elias S, Simpson JL, Martin AO, et al: Chorionic villus sampling in continuing pregnancies: I. Low fetal loss rates in initial 109 cases. *Am J Obstet Gynecol* 1986; 154:1349.
47. Elias S: Fetoscopy in prenatal diagnosis. *Semin Perinatol* 1980; 4:199.
48. Elias S: Fetoscopy in prenatal diagnosis. *Clin Perinatol* 1983; 10:357.
49. Daffos F, Capella-Pavlovshy M, Forester F: Fetal blood sampling during pregnancy with use of a needle guided by ultrasound: A study of 606 consecutive cases. *Am J Obstet Gynecol* 1985; 153:655.
50. Grannum PA, Copel JA, Plaxe SC, et al: In utero exchange transfusion by direct intravascular injection in severe erythroblastosis fetalis. *N Engl J Med* 1986; 314:1431.
51. Chang JC, Kan YW: A sensitive new prenatal test for sickle cell anemia. *N Engl J Med* 1982; 307:30.
52. Elias S, Esterly NB: Prenatal diagnosis of hereditary skin disorders. *Clin Obstet Gynecol* 1981; 24:1069.

53. Esterly NB, Elias S: Antenatal diagnosis of genodermatoses. *J Am Acad Dermatol* 1983; 8:655.
54. Elias S: Use of fetoscopy for the prenatal diagnosis of hereditary skin disorders, in Gedde-Dahl T, Wuepper KD (eds): *Proceedings of the 35th Annual Symposium on the Biology of the Skin: Antenatal Diagnosis of Heritable Dermatoses*. Basel, Switzerland, Karger, 1986.
55. Nicolaides KH, Rodeck CH, Gosden CM: Rapid karyotyping in non-lethal fetal malformations. *Lancet* 1986; 1:283.
56. International Fetoscopy Group: Special Report: The status of fetoscopy of fetal tissue sampling. *Prenatal Diagn* 1984; 4:79.
57. Working Party on Amniocentesis of the Medical Research Council: An assessment of hazards of amniocentesis. *Br J Obstet Gynaecol* 1978; 85 (suppl 2).
58. Hobbins JC: Doing fetoscopy. *Contemp Ob/Gyn* 1985; 25:31.
59. Eady RAJ, Rodeck CH: Prenatal diagnosis of the skin, in Rodeck CH, Nicolaides KH (eds): *Prenatal Diagnosis. Proceedings of the Eleventh Study Group of the Royal College of Obstetricians and Gynaecologists*. Chichester, England, John Wiley & Sons, 1984, pp 147–158.
60. Anton-Lamprecht I: Prenatal diagnosis of the skin by means of electron microscopy. *Hum Genet* 1981; 59:392.
61. Mass. Gen. Laws, c. 112, sec. 12J.
62. Sabbagha RE: Ultrasonic evaluation of fetal congenital anomalies. *Clin Obstet Gynaecol* 1980; 7:103.
63. Sabbagha RE, Sheikh Z, Tamwia RK, et al: Predictive value, sensitivity, and specificity of ultrasonic targeted imaging for fetal anomalies in gravid women at high risk for birth defects. *Am J Obstet Gynecol* 1985; 152:822.
64. Rutledge JC, Weinberg AG, Friedman JM, et al: Anatomic correlates of ultrasonographic prenatal diagnosis. *Prenat Diag* 1986; 6:51.

Chapter 6: Reproductive Liberty

1. Eisenstadt v. Baird, 405 U.S. 438 (1972).
2. Griswold v. Connecticut, 381 U.S. 479 (1965).
3. Woodward B, Armstrong S: *The Brethren: The Inside Story of the Supreme Court*. New York, Simon & Schuster, 1979.
4. Roe v. Wade, 410 U.S. 113 (1973).
5. Callahan D: *Abortion: Law, Choice and Morality*. New York, Macmillan Publishing Co, 1970.
6. Lamanna MA: Social science and ethical issues: The policy implications of poll data on abortion, in Callahan S, Callahan D (eds): *Abortion: Understanding Differences*. New York, Plenum Press, 1984.
7. Bayles MD: *Reproductive Ethics*. Englewood Cliffs, NJ, Prentice-Hall, 1984, pp 66–68.
8. Ely J: The wages of crying wolf: A commentary on *Roe v. Wade*. 82 *Yale L J* 920, 924 (1973).
9. Beal v. Doe, 432 U.S. 438 (1977).

10. Maher v. Roe, 432 U.S. 464 (1977).
11. Poelker v. Doe, 432 U.S. 519 (1977).
12. Tribe LH: *American Constitutional Law*. Mineola, NY, Foundation Press, 1978.
13. Harris v. McRae, 448 U.S. 297 (1980).
14. Annas GJ: The irrelevance of medical judgment. *Hastings Center Rep* 10:23–24, Oct, 1980.
15. Danforth v. Planned Parenthood of Missouri, 428 U.S. 52 (1976).
16. Annas GJ: Abortion: Round II. *Hastings Center Rep,* 6:15–16, Oct, 1976.
17. Bellotti v. Baird, 423 U.S. 982 (1975).
18. Bellotti v. Baird, 443 U.S. 622 (1979).
19. Glantz LH: Abortion: A decade of decisions, in Milunsky A, Annas GJ (eds): *Genetics and the Law III*. New York, Plenum Press, 1985.
20. Akron v. Center for Reproductive Health, 462 U.S. 416 (1983).
21. Thornburgh v. American College of Obstetricians and Gynecologists, 90 L. Ed.2d 776 (1986).
22. Planned Parenthood Association of Kansas City, Missouri v. Ashcroft, 462 U.S. 476 (1983).
23. Annas GJ: *Roe v. Wade* reaffirmed. *Hastings Center Rep* 13:21–22, Aug, 1983.
24. Skinner v. Oklahoma, 316 U.S. 535 (1942).
25. Buck v. Bell, 274 U.S. 200 (1927).
26. Lombardo PA: Three generations, no imbeciles: New light on *Buck v. Bell*. 60 *NYU Law Rev* 20 (1985).
27. Lederberg S: State channeling of gene flow by regulation of marriage and procreation, in Milunsky A, Annas GJ (eds): *Genetics and the Law*. New York, Plenum, 1976.
28. Baron CH: Voluntary sterilization of the mentally retarded, in Milunsky A, Annas GJ (eds): *Genetics and the Law*. New York, Plenum, 1976.
29. Kindregan C: Sixty years of compulsory eugenic sterilization: 'Three generations of imbeciles' and the constitution of the United States. 43 *Chicago-Kent L Rev* 123 (1966).
30. Sherlock RK, Sherlock RD: Sterilizing the retarded: Constitutional, statutory and policy alternatives, 60 *No Carolina L Rev* 943 (1982).
31. Note, Protection of the mentally retarded individual's right to choose sterilization: The effect of the clear and convincing evidence standard. 12 *Capital U L Rev* 413 (1983).
32. Note, Exclusive juvenile jurisdiction to authorize sterilization of incompetent minors. 16 *Indiana L Rev* 835 (1983).
33. Note, Procreation: A choice for the mentally retarded. 23 *Washburn L J* 359 (1984).
34. Wing KR: *The Law and the Public's Health*, ed 2. Ann Arbor, Mich, Health Administration Press, 1985, p 29.
35. In the Matter of Lee Ann Grady, 85 N.J. 235, 426 A.2d 467 (1981).
36. Annas GJ, Glantz LH, Katz BF: *Informed Consent to Human Experimentation: The Subject's Dilemma*. Cambridge, Mass, Ballinger, 1977, pp 80–87.

Chapter 7: Treatment of Handicapped Newborns

1. Singer P: Sanctity of life or quality of life. *Pediatrics* 1983; 72:128–129.
2. Kushe H, Singer P: *Should the Baby Live?* New York, Oxford University Press, 1985.
3. Robertson J: Involuntary euthanasia of defective newborns: A legal analysis, 27 *Standford L Rev* 213–269 (1975).
4. Robertson J: Dilemma at Danville. *Hastings Center Rep* 11:5–8, Nov, 1981.
5. Lyon J: *Playing God in the Nursery.* New York, WW Norton, 1985, pp 190–192.
6. Duff RS, Campbell AGM: Moral and ethical dilemmas in the special care nursery. *N Engl J Med* 1973; 289:890–894.
7. Gross RH, Cox A, Tatyrek R, et al: Early management and decision making for the treatment of myelomeningocele. *Pediatrics* 1983; 72:450–458.
8. Hentoff N: The awful privacy of Baby Doe. *Atlantic Monthly* Jan 1985, 54–62.
9. Fost N: Putting hospitals on notice. *Hastings Center Rep* 12:5–8, Aug, 1982.
10. 48 *Federal Register* 9630–9632 (March 7, 1983).
11. American Academy of Pediatrics v. Heckler, 561 F.Supp. 395 (D.D.C. 1983).
12. Annas GJ: Disconnecting the Baby Doe hotline. *Hastings Center Rep* 13:14–16, June, 1983.
13. 48 *Federal Register* 30846–30852 (July 5, 1983).
14. Annas GJ: Baby Doe redux: Doctors as child abusers. *Hastings Center Rep* 13:26–27, Oct, 1983.
15. 49 *Federal Register* 1622–1654 (Jan 12, 1984).
16. Annas GJ: The Baby Doe regulations: Governmental intervention in neonatal rescue medicine. *Am J Public Health* 1984; 74:618–620.
17. Steinbock B: Baby Jane Doe in the courts. *Hastings Center Rep* 14:13–19, Feb, 1984.
18. Weber v. Stony Brook Hospital, 467 N.Y.S. 2d 685 (AD 2 Dept. 1983).
19. Burt R: Authorizing death for anomalous newborns: Ten years later, in Milunsky A, Annas GJ (eds): *Genetics and the Law III.* New York, Plenum Press, 1985, pp 259–282.
20. Weber v. Stony Brook Hospital, 456 N.E. 2d 1186, 469 N.Y.S. 2d 63 (1983).
21. United States v. University Hospital, State U. of New York at Stony Brook, 575 F. Supp. 607 (E.D.N.Y. 1983).
22. United States v. University Hospital, State U. of New York at Stony Brook, 729 F.2d 144 (2d Cir. 1984).
23. Child Abuse and Neglect Prevention and Treatment Program: Final Rule, 50 *Federal Register* 14877–14892, April 15, 1985.
24. Bowen v. American Hospital Association, 90 L.Ed. 2d 584 (1986).
25. Shaw A, Randolph R, Manard M: Ethical issues in pediatric surgery: A national survey of pediatricians and pediatric surgeons. *Pediatrics* 1977; 60:588.
26. Arras J: Toward an ethic of ambiguity. *Hastings Center Rep* 14:25–33, April, 1984.

27. American Academy of Pediatrics. Joint Policy Statement: Principles of treatment of disabled infants. *Pediatrics* 1984; 73:559.
28. Burt R: The ideal of community in the work of the President's Commission. 6 *Cardozo L Rev* 267 (1984).
29. Brahans D: Severely handicapped babies and the law. *Lancet* 1986; 1:984–985.
30. In the Matter of Earle Spring, 380 Mass. 629 (1980).
31. Johnson AR, Garland MJ: A moral policy of life/death decisions in the intensive care nursery, in Jonsen AR, Garland MJ (eds): *Ethics of Intensive Care.* San Francisco, Health Policy Program, University of California, 1976, pp 150–151.
32. Burt R: Authorizing death for anomalous newborns, in Milunsky A, Annas GJ (eds): *Genetics and the Law.* New York, Plenum Press, 1976.
33. Stinson P, Stinson R: *The Long Dying of Baby Andrew.* Boston, Little, Brown & Co, 1983.
34. President's Commission for the Study of Ethical Problems in Medicine and Biomedical and Behavioral Research: *Deciding to Forego Life-Sustaining Treatment.* US Government Printing Office, 1983.
35. Roe v. Wade, 410 U.S. 113 (1973).
36. Doe v. Bolton, 410 U.S. 179 (1973).
37. 45 CFR 46, Protection of Human Subjects, 1983.
38. Annas GJ: Informed consent and review committees, in Valenstein ES (ed): *The Psychosurgery Debate.* San Francisco, Freeman, 1980, pp 494–498.
39. Annas GJ: The lion and the crocodiles: Consent to the artificial heart. *Hastings Center Rep* 13:20–22, April, 1983.
40. Fox R, Swazey J: *The Courage to Fail.* Chicago, University of Chicago Press, 1978.
41. In re Quinlan, 70 N.J. 10, 355 A.2d 647 (1976).
42. Annas GJ: Reconciling *Quinlan* and *Saikewicz:* Decision making for the terminally ill incompetent. 4 *Am J Law & Med* 367 (1979).
43. In re Claire Conroy, 486 A.2d 1209 (N.J. 1985).
44. President's Commission for the Study of Ethical Problems in Medicine and Biomedical and Behavioral Research: *Defining Death.* US Government Printing Office, 1981.
45. Cramton RC: A comment on trial-type hearings in nuclear power plant siting. 58 *Va L Rev* 585 (1972).
46. Calabresi G, Bobbitt P: *Tragic Choices.* New York, WW Norton, 1978.
47. Sewall RB: The tragic form, in Michel L, Sewall RB (eds): Tragedy: Modern Essays in Criticism. Englewood Cliffs, NJ, Prentice-Hall, 1963, p 120.

Chapter 8: Teratology

1. Nora JJ, Fraser FC: *Medical Genetics: Principles and Practice,* ed 2. Philadelphia, Lea & Febiger, 1981.

2. Golbus MS: Teratology for the obstetrician: Current status. *Obstet Gynecol* 1980; 55:269.
3. Lee DHK: Foreword, in Wilson JG (ed): *Environment and Birth Defects*. New York, Academic Press, 1973, pp xi–xii.
4. Warkany J, Nelson RC: Appearance of skeletal abnormalities in the offspring of rats reared on a deficient diet. *Science* 1940; 92:383.
5. Warkany J, Schraffenberger E: Congenital malformations induced in rats by roentgen rays. *Am J Roentgenol Radium Ther* 1947; 57:455.
6. Gregg N: Congenital cataract following German measles in the mother. *Trans Ophthalmol Soc Aust* 1941; 3:35.
7. London Times: *Suffer the Children: The Story of Thalidomide*. New York, Viking Press, 1979.
8. Heinonen OP, Slone D, Shapiro S: *Birth Defects and Drugs in Pregnancy*. Littleton, Mass, Publishing Science Group Inc, 1977.
9. Briggs, GG, Bodendorter TW, Freeman RK, et al: *Drugs in Pregnancy and Lactation: A Reference Guide to Fetal and Neonatal Risk*. Baltimore, Williams & Wilkins Co, 1983.
10. Wilson JG, Fraser FC (eds): *Handbook of Teratology: General Principles and Etiology*. New York, Plenum Press, 1977, vol 1.
11. Nishimura H, Tanimua T: *Clinical Aspects of the Teratogenicity of Drugs*. New York, Elsevier, 1976.
12. Wilson JG: *Environment and Birth Defects*. New York, Academic Press, 1973.
13. Brent RL: The production of congenital malformations using tissue antisera IV: Evaluation of the mechanisms of teratogenesis by varying the time of administration of anti-rat-kidney-antiserum. *Am J Anat* 1966; 119:555.
14. Dyban AP, Akimova IM: Features of the pathogenic action of chloridin at various stages of embryonic development. *Akush I Genek* 1966; 6:21.
15. Krauer B: Introduction, in Krauer B, Krauer F, Hytten FE, et al (eds): *Drugs and Pregnancy*. New York, Academic Press, 1984, p 105.
16. Wilson JG: Current status of teratology: General principles and mechanisms derived from animal studies, in Wilson JG, Fraser FC (eds): *Handbook of Teratology: General Principles and Etiology*. New York, Plenum Press, 1977, vol 1, pp 47–74.
17. Vesell ES: Pharmacokinetics and pharmacodynamics as techniques in environmental pathology, in Hill RB, Terzian JA (eds): *Environmental Pathology: An Evolving Field*. New York, Alan R Liss, 1982, pp 243–285.
18. Propping P: Pharmacogenetics. *Rev Physiol Biochem Pharmacol* 1978; 83:124.
19. Fraser FC: The use of teratogens in the analysis of abnormal developmental mechanisms, in *First International Conference on Congenital Malformations*. Philadelphia, JB Lippincott, 1961, p 179.
20. Jacobson BD: Hazards of norethindrone therapy during pregnancy. *Am J Obstet Gynecol* 1962; 84:962.
21. Hahn EW, Feingold SM: Abscopal delay of embryonic development after prefertilization X-irradiation. *Radiat Res* 1973; 53:267–272.
22. Jauchau MR, Faustman-Watts E: Pharmacokinetic considerations in the maternal-placental-fetal unit. *Clin Obstet Gynecol* 1983; 26:379.

23. MacMahon B, Pugh TF: *Epidemiology: Principles and Methods*. Boston, Little, Brown & Co, 1970.
24. Schlesselman JJ: *Case-Control Studies: Design, Conduct, Analysis*. New York, Oxford University Press, 1982.
25. Simpson JL, Golbus MS, Martin AO, et al: *Genetics in Obstetrics and Gynecology*. New York, Grune & Stratton, 1982.
26. Perrin EVDK: Teratology, "dysmorphology," and related subjects, in Hill RB, Tarzian JA (eds): *Environmental Pathology: An Evolving Field*. New York, Alan R Liss, 1982, pp 129–153.
27. Shepard TH: *Catalog of Teratogenic Agents*, ed 4. Baltimore, Johns Hopkins University Press, 1983.
28. Legator MS, Rosenberg M, Zenick H (eds): *Environmental Influences on Fertility, Pregnancy, and Development: Strategies for Measurement and Evaluation*. New York, Alan R Liss, 1984.
29. Zielhuis RL, Stijkel A, Verberk MM, van de Poel-Bot M: *Health Risks to Female Workers in Occupational Exposure to Chemical Agents*. New York, Springer-Verlag, 1984.
30. Lemoine P, Harouseau H, Borteyru JP, et al: Les infants de parents alcoholiques: Anomalies obse'erves. *Quest Med* 1968; 25:476.
31. Jones K, Smith DW, Ulleland CN, et al: Patterns of malformation in offspring of chronic alcoholic mothers. *Lancet* 1973; 1:267.
32. Rosett HL: A clinical perspective of the fetal alcohol syndrome. *Alcoholism Clin Exp Res* 1980; 4:119.
33. Deheaene P, Samaille-Villette C, Samaille PP, et al: Le Syndrome d'alcolisme foetal dans le Nord de la France (Fetal alcohol syndrome in the North of France). *Rev l'Alcolisme* 1977; 23:145.
34. Hanson JW, Streissguth AP, Smith DW: The effects of moderate alcohol consumption during pregnancy on fetal growth and morphogenesis. *J Pediatr* 1978; 92:457.
35. Olegord R, Sabel KG, Aronsson M, et al: Effects on the child of alcohol abuse during pregnancy: Retrospective and prospective studies. *Acta Paediatr Scand* 1979; 275(suppl):112.
36. Aase JM: The fetal alcohol syndrome in American Indians: A high risk group. *Neurobehav Toxicol Teratol* 1981; 3:153.
37. May PA, Hymbaugh KJ: A pilot project on fetal alcohol syndrome among American Indians. *Alcohol Health Res World* 1982; 7:3.
38. *Testimony of EN Brandt: Alcohol Consumption During Pregnancy: Hearings Before the Subcommittee on Alcoholism and Drug Abuse of the Committee on Labor and Human Resources*. US Senate, Sept 21, 1982. US Government Printing Office, 1983, pp 9–23.
39. King JC, Fabro S: Alcohol consumption and cigarette smoking: Effect on pregnancy. *Clin Obstet Gynecol* 1983; 26:437.
40. Little RE, Asker RL, Sampson PD, et al: Fetal growth and moderate drinking in early pregnancy. *Am J Epidemiol* 1986; 123:270.
41. Rosett HL: A clinical perspective of the fetal alcohol syndrome. *Alcoholism Clin Exp Res* 1980; 4:119.

42. Sulik KK, Johnston MC, Webb MA: Fetal alcohol syndrome: Embryogenesis in a mouse model. *Science* 1981; 214:936.

43. Fabro S: Alcohol beverage consumption and outcome of pregnancy, in *The Fetal Alcohol Syndrome-Public Awareness Campaign, Progress Report Concerning the Advance Notice of Proposed Rulemaking on Warning Labels on Containers of Alcoholic Beverages and Addendum.* The Department of the Treasury and the Bureau of Alcohol, Tobacco and Firearms, Feb 1979, pp 37–199.

44. American Council on Science and Health: *Alcohol Use During Pregnancy.* Summit, NJ, ACSH, 1981.

45. American Medical Association, Council on Scientific Affairs: Fetal effects of maternal alcohol use. *JAMA* 1983; 249:2517.

46. Pritchard JA, MacDonald PD, Gant NF: *Williams Obstetrics,* ed 17. Norwalk, Conn, Appleton-Century-Crofts, 1985, pp 258–259.

47. Meyer MB: Smoking and pregnancy, in Niebyl JR (ed): *Drug Use in Pregnancy.* Philadelphia, Lea & Febiger, 1982, pp 133–153.

48. Kullander S, Kaellen B: A prospective study of smoking and pregnancy. *Acta Obstet Gynecol Scand* 1971; 50:83.

49. Kline J, Stein YA, Susser M, et al: Smoking: A risk factor for spontaneous abortion: *N Engl J Med* 1977; 297:793.

50. Boué J, Boué A, Lazar P: Retrospective and prospective epidemiological studies of 1500 karyotyped spontaneous human abortions. *Teratology* 1975; 12:11.

51. Meyer MB, Torascia JA, Buck C: The interrelationship of maternal smoking and increased perinatal mortality and other risk factors: Further analysis of the Ontario Mortality Study 1960–61. *Am J Epidemiology* 1975; 199:443.

52. Naeye RL: Relationship of cigarette smoking to congenital anomalies and perinatal death. *Am J Pathol* 1978; 90:289.

53. Underwood PB, Kessler KF, O'Lane JM, et al: Parental smoking empirically related to pregnancy outcome. *Obstet Gynecol* 1967; 29:1.

54. Simpson WJ: Preliminary report on cigarette smoking and the incidence of prematurity. *Am J Obstet Gynecol* 1957; 73:808.

55. Stein ZA, Susser M: Intrauterine growth retardation: Epidemiological issues and public health significance. *Semin Perinatol* 1984; 8:5.

56. Naeye RL, Peters EC: Mental development of children whose mothers smoked during pregnancy. *Obstet Gynecol* 1984; 64:601.

57. Hinds MW, Kolonel LN: Maternal smoking and cancer risk to offspring. *Lancet* 1980; 2:703.

58. Steele R, Longworth JT: The relationship of antenatal and postnatal factors to sudden unexpected death in infancy. *Can Med Assoc J* 1966; 94:1165.

59. *The Health Consequence of Smoking for Women: A Report of the Surgeon General.* Pub no. 410-899/1284, Department of Health and Human Services, 1983, pp 191–249.

60. Neiberg P, Marks JS, McLaren NM, et al: The fetal tobacco syndrome. *JAMA* 1986; 253:2998.

61. American College of Obstetricians and Gynecologists (ACOG): *Cigarette Smoking and Pregnancy.* Technical Bulletin No. 53., Sept, 1979.

62. Christoffel T, Stein S: Using the law to protect health: The frustrating case of smoking. *7 Medicolegal News* 5, Winter, 1979.
63. Cobey C: The resurgence and validity of anti-smoking legislation. *7 UC Davis L Rev* 167 (1974).
64. Matthews D: Where there's smoke, there's ire. *7 Medicolegal News* 4, Winter, 1979.
65. Cohen CI, Cohen EJ: Health education: Panacea, pernicious or pointless? *N Engl J Med* 1978; 299:718.
66. Carlo GL: Systematic account and critical appraisal of current epidemiological approaches for monitoring reproductive outcome in industry, in Lockey JE, Lemasters GK, Keye WR Jr (eds): *Reproduction: The New Frontier in Occupational and Environmental Health Research.* New York, Alan R Liss, 1984, pp 139–145.
67. John JA, Wroblewski DJ, Schwetz BA: Teratogenicity of experimental and occupational exposure to industrial chemicals, in Kalter H (ed): *Issues and Reviews in Teratology.* New York, Plenum Press, 1984, pp 267–324.
68. American College of Obstetricians and Gynecologists (ACOG): *Pregnancy, Work, and Disability.* Technical Bulletin No. 58., May, 1980.
69. Council on Scientific Affairs: Effects of toxic chemicals on the reproductive system. *JAMA* 1985; 253:3431.
70. Barlow SM, Sullivan FM (eds): *Reproductive Hazards of Industrial Chemicals.* New York, Academic Press, 1982.
71. Kurzel RB, Certulo CL: Chemical teratogenesis and reproductive failure. *Obstet Gynecol Surv* 1985; 40:397.
72. Murphy DP: Outcome of 625 pregnancies in women subjected to pelvic radium or roentgen irradiation. *Am J Obstet Gynecol* 1929; 18:179.
73. Yamazaki JN: A review of the literature on the radiation dose required to cause manifest central nervous system disturbances from in utero and post-natal exposure. *Pediatrics* 1966; 27:877.
74. Plummer G: Anomalies occuring in children exposed in utero to atomic bombs in Hiroshima. *Pediatrics* 1952; 10:687.
75. Griem ML, Meier P, Dobben GD: Analysis of the morbidity and mortality of children irradiated in fetal life. *Radiology* 1976; 88:347.
76. Dekaban AS: Abnormalities in children exposed to X-radiation during various stages of gestation: I. Tentative timetable of radiation injury to the human fetus. *J Nucl Med* 1968; 9:471.
77. Brent RL: The effects of embryonic and fetal exposure to X-ray, microwaves, and ultrasound. *Clin Obstet Gynecol* 1983; 26:484.
78. Americal College of Obstetricians and Gynecologists: *Guides for diagnostic X-ray examination of fertile women.* Chicago, ACOG, 1977.
79. Jones KL: Teratogens: What we know and don't know about them, in Kabak MM (ed): *Genetic Issues in Pediatric and Obstetric Practice.* Chicago, Year Book Medical Publishers Inc, 1981, pp 109–130.
80. Center for Disease Control: Valproic acid and spina bifida: A preliminary report—France. *Morbidity Mortality Weekly Rep* 1982; 31:565.

81. Fuchs VR: Sex differences in economic well-being. *Science* 1986; 232:459.
82. Office of Technology Assessment: *Reproductive Health Hazards in the Work-place.* Washington, DC, US Congress, 1985.
83. Hayes v. Shelby Memorial Hospital, 726 F.2d 2095 (11th Cir. 1984) [Firing a pregnant X-ray technician who worked in a hospital radiation department because she announced she was pregnant was a violation of Title VII].
84. Zuniga v. Klenberg County Hospital, 692 F.2d 986 (5th Cir. 1982) [Firing a pregnant X-ray technician upon her announcement that she was pregnant is a violation of Title VII, because a less discriminatory alternative would have been to grant leave of absence].
85. Wright v. Olin Corp., 697 F.2d 1172 (4th Cir. 1982) [Suit involved a challenge to Olin's fetal protection policy].
86. Brodeur P: *Outrageous Misconduct.* New York, Pantheon Books, 1986.

Chapter 9: Noncoital Reproduction

1. Bustillo M, Buster JE, Cohen SW: Nonsurgical ovum transfer as a treatment in infertile women: Preliminary experience. *JAMA* 1984; 251:1171–1173.
2. Dept. of Health and Social Security: *Report of the Committee of Inquiry into Human Fertilization and Embryology.* London, 1984.
3. Committee to Consider the Social, Ethical and Legal Issues Arising from In Vitro Fertilization: *Report on the Disposition of Embryos Produced by In Vitro Fertilization,* Melbourne, 1984.
4. Ontario Law Reform Commission: *Report on Human Artifical Reproduction and Related Matters.* Toronto, Ministry of the Attorney General, 1985.
5. *Hearings on the Extracorporeal Embryo Before the Investigations and Oversight Subcommittee of the Science and Technology Committee.* US House of Representatives August 8–9, 1984, US Government Printing Office, 1984.
6. *People,* March 5, 1984, p 73.
7. Grobstein C, Flower M, Mendeloff J: External human fertilization: An evaluation of policy. *Science* 1983; 222:127–133.
8. Robertson JA: Procreative liberty and the control of conception, pregnancy, and childbirth. 69 *Virginia Law Rev* 405–464 (1983).
9. Andrews L: *New Conceptions.* New York, St Martins Press, 1984.
10. Rohleder H: *Test Tube Babies: A History of the Artificial Impregnation of Human Beings.* New York, Panurge Press, 1934.
11. Rothman BK: Choice in reproductive technology, in Arditti R, Klein RD, Minden S (eds): *Test-Tube Women: What Future for Motherhood?* London, Pandora Press, 1984.
12. President's Commission for the Study of Ethical Problems in Medicine and Biomedical and Behavioral Research: *Summing Up.* US Government Printing Office, 1983, p 85.
13. Annas GJ, Elias S: In vitro fertilization and embryo transfer: Medicolegal aspects of a new technique to create a family. 17 *Family Law Q* 199–223 (1983).

14. Ethics Advisory Board: *Report and Conclusions: HEW Support of Research Involving Human In Vitro Fertilization and Embryo Transfer.* US Government Printing Office, 1979.
15. Annas GJ: Fathers anonymous: Beyond the best interests of the sperm donor. 14 *Family Law Q* 1–13 (1980).
16. Kass LR: *Toward A More Natural Science.* New York, The Free Press, 1985.
17. Mascola, Guinan: Screening to reduce transmission of sexually transmitted diseases in semen used for artificial insemination. *N Eng J Med* 1986; 314:1354.
18. Annas GJ: The baby broker boom. *Hastings Center Rep* 16:30–31, June, 1986.
19. The Ethics Committee of the American Fertility Society: Ethical considerations of the new reproductive technologies. *Fertil Steril* 1986; 46:1S.
20. Blumberg GG: Legal issues in nonsurgical human ovum transfer. *JAMA* 1984; 251:1178–1181.
21. Rowland R: in Singer P, Wells D (eds): *The Reproductive Revolution.* New York, Oxford University Press, 1984.
22. *American Medical News,* March 14, 1986, p 46.
23. Grobstein C, Flower M, Mendeloff J: Frozen embryos: Policy issues. *N Engl J Med* 1985; 312:1584–1588.
24. Annas GJ, Glantz LH, Katz BF: *Informed Consent to Human Experimentation: The Subject's Dilemma.* Cambridge, Mass, Ballinger, 1977, pp 195–213.
25. President's Commission for the Study of Ethical Problems in Medicine and Biomedical and Behavioral Research: *Screening and Counseling for Genetic Conditions.* US Government Printing Office, 1983.
26. Culliton BJ: Gene therapy: Research in public. *Science* 1985; 227:493–496.
27. Annas GJ: Making babies without sex: The law and the profits. *Am J Pub Health* 1984; 74:1415–1417.
28. Tittmus RM: *The Gift Relationship: From Human Blood to Social Policy.* London, Alan R Liss, 1970.
29. US House of Representatives: *Hearings on the Sale of Organs before the Investigations and Oversight Subcommittee of the Science and Technology Committee.* US House of Representatives. Nov 7–9, 1983, US Government Printing Office, 1984.
30. Annas GJ: Life, liberty and pursuit of organ sales. *Hastings Center Rep* 14:22–23, Feb, 1984.
31. Kennedy I: Let the law take on test tube. *London Times,* May 26, 1984.
32. Annas GJ: Surrogate embryo transfer: The perils of patenting. *Hastings Center Rep* 14:25–26, Oct, 1984.
33. American Fertility Society: Ethical statement on in vitro fertilization. *Fertil Steril* 1984; 41:12.
34. Royal College of Obstetricians and Gynecologists: *Report of the RCOG Ethics Committee on In Vitro Fertilization and Embryo Replacement or Transfer.* London, RCOG, 1983.
35. Brahams D: In-vitro fertilisation and related research: Why Parliament must legislate. *Lancet* 1983; 2:726–729.

36. Wadlington W: Artificial conception: The challenge for family law. 69 *Virginia Law Rev* 465–514 (1983).
37. Working Party of Council for Science and Society: *Human Procreation: Ethical Aspects of New Techniques*. Oxford, England, Oxford University Press, 1984.
38. Capron AM: The new reproductive possibilities: Seeking a moral basis for concerted action in a pluralistic society. *Law Med Health Care* 1984; 12:192–198.
39. *Contra;* Hollinger JH: From coitus to commerce: Legal and social consequence of noncoital reproduction. 18 *J Law Reform* 865–932 (1985).
40. Fraser FC, Forse RA: On genetic screening of donors for artificial insemination. *Am J Genetics* 1981; 10:399–405.
41. Huxley A: *Brave New World Revisited*. New York, Harper & Row, 1958, pp 24–25.

Chapter 10: Fetal and Gene Therapy

1. Elias S, Annas GJ: Perspectives on fetal surgery. *Am J Obstet Gynecol* 1983; 145:807.
2. Office of Technology Assessment: *Human Gene Therapy*. OTA-BP-BA-32. US Government Printing Office, 1984.
3. Harrison MR, Golbus MS, Berlowitz RS, et al: Fetal treatment 1982, occasional notes. *N Engl J Med* 1982; 307:1651–1652.
4. Council on Scientific Affairs Report: In utero fetal surgery: Resolution 73(I-81). *JAMA* 1983; 250:1443–1444.
5. Liley AW: Intrauterine transfusions of fetus in haemolytic disease. *Br Med J* 1963; 2:1107.
6. Grannum PA, Copel JA, Plaxe SC, et al: In utero exchange transfusion by direct intravascular injection in severe erythroblastosis fetalis. *N Engl J Med* 1986; 314:1431.
7. Campbell S: Early prenatal diagnosis of neural tube defects by ultrasound. *Clin Obstet Gynecol* 1977; 20:351.
8. Chervenak FA, Berkowitz RL, Romero R, et al: The diagnosis of fetal hydrocephalus. *Am J Obstet Gynecol* 1983; 147:703.
9. Clewell WH, Johnson ML, Meier PR, et al: Placement of ventriculoamniotic shunt for hydrocephalus in a fetus. *N Engl J Med* 1981; 305:944.
10. Manning FA, Harrison MR, Rodeck C, and Members of the International Fetal Medicine and Surgery Society: Catheter shunts for fetal hydronephrosis and hydrocephalus. Report of the International Fetal Surgery Registry. *N Engl J Med* 1986; 315:336.
11. Depp R, Sabbagha RE, Brown JT, et al: Fetal surgery for hydrocephalus: Successful in utero ventriculoamniotic shunt for Dandy-Walker syndrome. *Obstet Gynecol* 1983; 61:710.
12. Harrison MR, Golbus MS, Filly RA: *The Unborn Patient: Prenatal Diagnosis and Treatment*. Orlando, Fla, Grune & Stratton, 1984.
13. Hobbins HC, Grannum PAT, Berkowitz RL, et al: Ultrasound in the diagnosis of congenital anomalies. *Am J Obstet Gynecol* 1979; 134:331.

14. Harrison MR, Golbus MS, Filly RA, et al: Fetal surgery for congenital hydronephrosis. *N Engl J Med* 1982; 305:591.
15. Golbus MS, Harrison MR, Filly RA, et al: In utero treatment of urinary tract obstruction. *Am J Obstet Gynecol* 1982; 142:383.
16. Harrison MR, Golbus MS, Filly RA, et al: Management of the fetus with congenital hydronephrosis. *J Pediatr Surg* 1982; 17:728.
17. Golbus MS, Filly RA, Callen PW, et al: Fetal urinary tract obstruction: Management and selection for treatment. *Semin Perinatol* 1985; 9:91.
18. Harrison MR, Ross NA, de Lorimier AA: Correction of congenital diaphragmatic hernia in utero: III. Development of a successful surgical technique using abdominoplasty to avoid compromise of umbilical blood flow. *J Pediatr Surg* 1981; 16:934.
19. Hodgen GK: Antenatal diagnosis and treatment of fetal skeletal malformations with emphasis on in utero surgery for neural tube defects and limb bud regeneration. *JAMA* 1981; 246:1079.
20. Haller JA Jr, Kehrer BH, Shaker IJ, et al: Studies of the pathophysiology of gastroschisis in fetal sheep. *J Pediatr Surg* 1974; 9:627.
21. Oshio AT, Komi N: An experimental study of gastroschisis using fetal surgery. *J Pediatr Surg* 1980; 15:252.
22. Michejda M, Bacher J, Kuwabara T, et al: In utero allogeneic bone transplantation in primates: Roentgenographic and histologic observations. *Transplantation* 1981; 32:96.
23. Hodgen GD: Antenatal diagnosis and treatment of fetal skeletal malformations with emphasis on in utero surgery for neural tube defects and limb bud generation. *JAMA* 1981; 246:1079.
24. Roe v. Wade, 410 U.S. 113 (1973).
25. Jonsen A: Fetal surgery, in Milunsky A, Annas GJ (eds): *Genetics and the Law III*. New York, Plenum, 1985.
26. Annas GJ, Glantz LH, Katz BF: *Informed Consent to Human Experimentation: The Subject's Dilemma*. Cambridge, Mass, Ballinger, 1977.
27. Fox R, Swazey J: *The Courage to Fail*. Chicago, University of Chicago Press, 1974.
28. Annas GJ, Glantz LH, Katz BF: *The Rights of Doctors, Nurses, and Allied Health Professionals*. Cambridge, Mass, Ballinger, 1981.
29. Karp v. Cooley, 349 F. Supp. 827 (S.D. Tex. 1972), aff'd, 493 F.2d 408 (5th Cir. 1974).
30. Annas GJ, Densberger JE: Competence to refuse medical treatment: Autonomy vs. paternalism. 15 *Toledo L Rev* 561 (1984).
31. Danforth v. Planned Parenthood, 428 U.S. 52 (1976).
32. Fletcher JC: The fetus as patient: Ethical issues. *JAMA* 1981; 246:772.
33. Robertson J: Procreative liberty, and the control of conception, pregnancy, and childbirth. 69 *Virginia Law Rev* 405, 441–7 (1983).
34. Leiberman JR, Mazor M, Chaim W: The fetal right to live. *Obstet Gynecol* 1979; 53:515.
35. Jefferson v. Griffin Spalding Co. Hospital Authority, 247 Ga. 86, 274 S.E.2d 457 (1981).

36. Raleigh Fitkin-Paul Morgan Memorial Hospital v. Anderson, 201 A.2d 537, 538 (N.J. 1964).
37. *American Medical News,* Feb 19, 1982, p 11.
38. Goldman EB: Fetal versus maternal rights: Who is the patient? *Mich Hospitals* April 1983, pp 23–25.
39. Gallager J: The fetus and the law—whose life is it anyway? *Ms Magazine* 1984; 62:134–135.
40. Bowes WA, Salgestad B: Fetal v. maternal rights: Medical and legal perspectives. *Am J Obstet Gynecol* 1981; 58:209.
41. Application of the President and Directors of Georgetown College, 331 F.2d 1000 (1964).
42. Ruddick W, Wicox W: Operating on the fetus. *Hastings Center Rep* 12:10–14, Oct, 1982.
43. Johnson DE: The creation of fetal rights: Conflicts with women's constitutional rights to liberty, privacy and equal protection. 95 *Yale Law Review* 599 (1986).
44. Matsui SM, Mahoney JM, Rosenberg LE: The natural history of inherited methylmalonic acidemias. *N Engl J Med* 1983; 308:857.
45. Schulman JD: Prenatal treatment of biochemical disorders. *Semin Perinatol* 1985; 9:75.
46. Roth KS, Yang W, Allan L, et al: Prenatal administration of biotin in biotin responsive multiple carboxylase deficiency. *Pediatr Res* 1982; 16:126.
47. Packman S, Cowan MJ, Golbus MS, et al: Prenatal treatment of biotin responsive multiple carboxylase deficiency. *Lancet* 1982; 1:1435.
48. New MI, Dupont B, Grumbach K, et al: Congenital adrenal hyperplasia and related conditions, in Stanbury JB, Wyngaarden JB, Fredrickson DS, et al (eds): *The Metabolic Basis of Inherited Disease,* ed 5. New York, McGraw-Hill Book Co, 1983, pp 973–1000.
49. Edwards JH: Vitamin supplementation and neural tube defects. *Lancet* 1982; 1:275.
50. Laurence KM, James N, Miller MH, et al: Double blind randomised controlled trial of folate treatment before conception to prevent recurrence of neural tube defects. *Br Med J* 1981; 282:1509.
51. Smithells RW, Sheppard S, Schorah CJ, et al: Apparent prevention of neural tube defects by periconceptual vitamin supplementation. *Arch Dis Child* 1981; 56:911.
52. Seller MJ: Preconceptual vitamin supplementation to prevent recurrence of neural tube defects. *Lancet* 1985; 1:1392.
53. MRC: Trial of multivitamin prophylaxis in pregnancies at risk of neural tube defects. *Lancet* 1982; 2:1412.
54. Vitamins to prevent neural tube defects. *Lancet* 1982; 2:1255.
55. Thomas ED, Buckner C, Sanders JE: Marrow transplantation for thalassemia. *Lancet* 1982; 2:227.
56. Johnson F, Look AT, Gockerman J: Bone-marrow transplantation in a patient with sickle-cell anemia. *N Engl J Med* 1984; 311:780.

57. Rappeport JM: Allogenic bone marrow transplantation for chronic granulomatous disease. *J Pediatr* 1982; 101:952.

58. Westminster Hospitals BMT Team: Bone-marrow transplant from an unrelated donor for chronic granulomatous disease. *Lancet* 1977; 1:210.

59. Coccia PF, Krivit W, Cervenka J: Successful bone marrow transplantation for infantile malignant osteopetrosis. *N Engl J Med* 1980; 302:701.

60. Virelizier JL, Lagrue A, Duranoy A: Reversal of natural killer defect in a patient with Chediak-Higashi syndrome after bone-marrow transplantation. *N Engl J Med* 1982; 306:1055.

61. Krivit W, Piepont ME, Ayaz K: Bone-marrow transplantation in the Maroteaux-Lamy syndrome (mucopolysaccharidosis VI). *N Engl J Med* 1984; 311:1606.

62. Simpson TJ, Golbus MS: In utero fetal hematopoietic stem cell transplantation. *Semin Perinatol* 1985; 9:68.

63. Emery AEH: *An Introduction to Recombinant DNA.* Chichester, England, John Wiley & Sons, 1984.

64. Anderson WF: Human gene therapy: Scientific and ethical considerations. *Recombinant DNA Tech Bull* 1985; 8:55.

65. Mann R, Mulligan RC, Baltimore D: Construction of a retrovirus packaging mutant and its use to produce helper-free defective retrovirus. *Cell* 1983; 33:153.

66. Anderson WF, Fletcher JC: Gene therapy in human beings: When is it ethical to begin? *N Engl J Med* 1980; 303:1293.

67. Rosenberg LE: Can we cure genetic disorders?, in Milunsky A, Annas GJ (eds): *Genetics and the Law III.* New York, Plenum, 1985, pp 5–13.

68. Rifkin J: *Algeny.* New York, Penguin Books, 1984.

69. Fletcher JC: Moral problems and ethical issues in prospective human gene therapy. 69 *Virginia Law Rev* 515–546 (1983).

70. Kass L: *Toward a More Natural Science.* New York, Free Press, 1985.

71. Ramsey J: *Fabricated Man: The Ethics of Genetic Control.* New Haven, Yale University Press, 1970.

72. Grobstein C, Flower M: Gene therapy: Proceed with caution. *Hastings Center Rep* 14:13–17, April, 1984.

73. Culliton BJ: Gene therapy: Research in public. *Science* 1985; 227:493–496.

Index